The ECG in Clinical Decision-Making

The ECG in Clinical Decision-Making

Patrick Davey

Consultant Cardiologist, Northampton General Hospital;
Honorary Consultant Cardiologist, John Radcliffe Hospital, Oxford;
Honorary Senior Lecturer, Oxford University

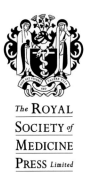

The ROYAL
SOCIETY *of*
MEDICINE
PRESS *Limited*

Published by the Royal Society of Medicine Press Ltd
1 Wimpole Street, London W1G 0AE, UK
Tel: +44 (0)20 7290 2921
Fax: +44 (0) 20 7290 2929
E-mail: publishing@rsm.ac.uk
Website: www.rsmpress.co.uk

British Library Cataloguing in Publication Data
A catalogue record for this book is available from the British Library

ISBN 1-85315-535-7

Distribution in Europe and Rest of World:
Marston Book Services Ltd
PO Box 269
Abingdon
Oxon OX14 4YN, UK
Tel: +44 (0)1235 465500
Fax: +44 (0)1235 465555

Distribution in the USA and Canada:
Royal Society of Medicine Press Ltd
c/o Jamco Distribution Inc
1401 Lakeway Drive
Lewisville, TX 75057, USA
Tel: +1 800 538 1287
Fax: +1 972 353 1303
E-mail: jamco@majors.com

Distribution in Australia and New Zealand:
Elsevier Australia
30-52 Smidmore Street
Marrickville NSW 2204
Australia
Tel: + 61 2 9517 8999
Fax: + 61 2 9517 2249

Phototypeset by Phoenix Photosetting, Chatham, Kent
Printed and bound by Krips b.v., Meppel, The Netherlands

iv

Preface

The ECG is a wonderful test – what other investigation can decide so quickly, easily and cheaply whether the heart is undergoing necrosis, where the pathology is located, indicate whether the lining of the heart is inflamed, whether the patient has a background of long-standing high blood pressure, an underactive thyroid, or an important genetic disease, whether the patient is going to blackout, why they have blacked out, how fit they are, when they go to bed, when they get up?

The ECG is one of the most powerful of clinical investigations. However, there is a down-side – the ECG doesn't always tell the truth. It is liable to misinterpretation and can fool the unwary. It may suggest critical coronary disease, when in fact the coronary arteries are normal; it can appear to indicate a myocardial infarct, when the heart muscle is actually perfectly healthy. It can also suggest that the heart is completely normal, when in fact the coronary arteries are critically diseased. It can imply that the pumping function of the heart is normal, when it is substantially impaired. It can suggest that there is no serious cause for an arrhythmia, when in fact the heart is prone to stopping for prolonged periods of time.

So, used correctly the ECG allows great insights into the functioning of the heart, but used incorrectly it can lead the unwary clinician into all sorts of errors. The aim of this book is to provide the information that will turn the reader into a 'savvy' ECG reader, one who can handle the ECG calmly, confidently and accurately. He/she will not be led astray, and will understand when the ECG tells the truth and when it does not.

Understanding the basic mechanisms that underline the generation of the ECG signals is crucial to such an understanding – this book enables this, using a multitude of diagrams. However, mere mechanics are not sufficient for a full understanding – one needs to know how clinical factors interact with the ECG. The reader of this book will have the information needed to correctly interpret the clinical ECG in a plethora of clinical contexts. Indeed, the fundamental philosophy of this book is that the ECG will only be useful when it is combined with data on the clinical situation – furthermore, that the ECG cannot be understood without this clinical data. This is the key message of the book.

I hope this book leaves you with a full understanding of the ECG, a confident sense of its uses and limitations, and a thirst to learn even more about this fascinating test.

Patrick Davey

Acknowledgements

Many people have made this book possible, to all of whom my thanks go. I thank my colleagues, who were generous in their provision of ECGs, especially Andrew Beswick from the Coronary Care Unit in Northampton, along with John Birkhead and David Sprigings, my colleague cardiologists. A number of textbooks have been helpful: *Arrhythmia Diagnosis and Management: A Clinical Electrocardiographic Guide*. St Gallen: Fachmed, by Erik Sandøe and Bjarne Sigurd, *Marriot's Practical Electrocardiography*, 10th edition, by S Wagner, *Chou's Electrocardiography in Clinical Practice*, 5th edition, by Borys Surawicz and Timothy Knilans, *Making Sense of the ECG*, by Andrew Houghton and David Grey, *Cardiology*, by Michael Crawford and John DiMarco, and *Mayo Clinic Cardiology Review*, 2nd edition, by Joseph Murphy. The *New England Journal of Medicine*, The *Lancet*, *Circulation* and the *Journal of the American Medical Association* all rendered helpful data. However, towering above all else, this book would not have been possible without the many patients with cardiac and other disease I have seen, some of whose ECGs are shown here. My indispensable thanks must go especially to them.

About the author

Patrick Davey is both an interventional and a general cardiologist, as well as a busy general physician working in two large hospitals. This broad range of professional activities has given him a unique exposure to the ECGs of many varied patients and a detailed understanding of how these correlate with subsequent investigative findings. He is also the editor of a best-selling textbook of medicine.

List of abbreviations

ACE	Angiotensin-converting enzyme
ACS	Acute coronary syndrome
AF	Atrial fibrillation
ASD	Atrial septal defect
AT	Atrial tachycardia
AV	Atrioventricular
AVNRT	Atrioventricular nodal reentrant tachycardia
AVRT	Atrioventricular reentrant tachycardia
BMI	Body mass index (kg/m^2)
CAD	Coronary artery disease
CHB	Complete heart block
CHF	Chronic heart failure
COPD	Chronic obstructive pulmonary disease
CVA	Cerebrovascular accident
DCM	Dilated cardiomyopathy
EPS	Electrophysiological study
ESR	Erythrocyte sedimentation rate
HF	High-frequency
HOCM	Hypertrophic obstructive cardiomyopathy
HRV	Heart rate variability
ICD	Implantable cardioverter defibrillator
IHD	Ischaemic heart disease
IRA	Infarct-related artery
JVP	Jugular venous pressure
LAD	Left anterior descending coronary artery
LBBB	Left bundle branch block
LF	Low-frequency
LV	Left ventricle/ventricular
LVF	Left ventricular failure
LVOT	Left ventricular outflow tract
LVH	Left ventricular hypertrophy

MI	Myocardial infarction
MR	Mitral regurgitation
MRI	Magnetic resonance imaging
NIDDM	Non-insulin-dependent diabetes mellitus
NSVT	Nonsustained ventricular tachycardia
OSA	Obstructive sleep apnoea
PAN	Polyarteritis nodosum
PAP	Pulmonary arterial pressure
PE	Pulmonary embolus
RBBB	Right bundle branch block
RCA	Right coronary artery
RV	Right ventricle/ventricular
RVH	Right ventricular hypertrophy
SBP	Systolic blood pressure
SLE	Systemic lupus erythematosus
SCD	Sudden cardiac death
SN	Sinus node
SVC	Superior vena cava
SVT	Supraventricular tachycardia
STEMI	ST elevation myocardial infarction
TIMI	Thrombolysis In Myocardial Infarction Study Group
TOE	Transoesophageal echocardiography
TTE	Transthoracic echocardiography
VLF	Very low-frequency
VF	Ventricular fibrillation
VPC	Ventricular premature contraction
$\dot{V}/\dot{Q}$	Ventilation–perfusion
VSD	Ventricular septal defect
VT	Ventricular tachycardia
WPW	Wolff–Parkinson–White (syndrome)

Contents

Chapter 1
Introduction to the ECG

The ECG allows a simple and reproducible assessment of aspects of cardiac function. Used correctly, the 12-lead ECG is a very powerful clinical tool for:

- diagnosis
- monitoring disease progression and response to treatment.

Equally, the unwary may by misled by an ECG into incorrect diagnosis and treatment. As a generalization, the ECG should be used to confirm a diagnosis already made on standard clinical grounds rather than to make a completely unexpected diagnosis. (Like any rule, this one should on occasion be broken.)

One important principle is that what is true for history-taking and physical examination is equally true for ECG interpretation: one interpretation (a single 'cast-iron' diagnosis) is often not possible. Rather a range of interpretations is necessary (a 'differential diagnosis'). In interpreting the ECG a differential diagnosis ordered by probability should always be drawn up in conjunction with other clinical features. If the student ignores this approach, and gambles all on a single diagnosis, he/she will not infrequently be caught out. This may be embarrassing; more importantly, the patient may suffer, sometimes permanently. Thus the student must learn when it is reasonable to rely on an ECG and when it is more useful to reject the diagnosis suggested by the ECG and instead rely on other clinical clues to understand what is going on with a patient. This book aims to put the ECG into the overall context of clinical decision-making.

Importance of the clinical situation in ECG diagnosis

Clinical features are crucial to ordering the list of potential diagnoses correctly. Why is this? In essence, because any ECG abnormality can have several causes and conversely any single disease process can often cause several different ECG abnormalities. Thus, to determine the correct diagnosis, or at least to draw up a list of possible diagnoses in order of probability, it is vital to have data on the clinical situation.

ECGs are useful if pretest probability of disease is medium (not high or low)

If there is a medium pretest probability of disease, an ECG can be used to significantly increase or decrease this probability. When the pretest probability of disease is very low, an abnormal ECG often adds little to the diagnosis. This is particularly true of ST segment changes, although it is also true for many QRS changes (eg amplitude) or T wave abnormalities. For example, an ECG showing planar ST depression can indicate critical multivessel coronary disease in an elderly diabetic male smoker with classic angina, but may occur with entirely normal epicardial coronary arteries in a young nonsmoking woman with atypical chest pain.

The ECG therefore often cannot be interpreted reliably in the absence of clinical data, including patient demographics.

Diagnostic ECG patterns

There are of course exceptions to the above rules and, like other clinical investigations, ECG abnormalities can occasionally be diagnostic. For example, classic Wolff–Parkinson–White syndrome can often be diagnosed unambiguously from the ECG regardless of whether or not symptoms (usually sudden-onset rapid palpitations terminated by vagotonic manoeuvres) are present. Likewise, even in the presence of very atypical symptoms it is often possible to diagnose correctly ST segment elevation myocardial infarct. However, in numerical terms, most unexpected ECG findings are unlikely to reflect diagnostic gold and often should be ignored.

'Unexpected' ECG findings

Usually, unexpected ECG findings are relatively mild (eg mild T wave changes, conducting tissue disease, etc) and often either reflect remote non-relevant pathology (eg a previous episode of pericarditis) or minor but still non-relevant pathology (eg T wave changes in an asymptomatic elderly patient are of very little diagnostic use). Thus the ECG should be used, like all other tests, to confirm the clinical diagnosis already made.

The normal ECG

Underlying electrical processes

The fundamental basis of the ECG relies on the fact that the heart uses electricity for its basic functions and that disease processes interfere with the generation and transmission of this electricity.

Myocyte action potential

In order to understand the ECG, one needs to have some understanding of the cardiac action potential. The key points of the myocyte action potential (Figure 1.1a), as follows, must be appreciated.

The resting membrane potential, around −80 to −90 mV, is largely determined by the relative differences in potassium concentration on either side of the myocyte membrane, as the resting membrane is poorly permeable to ions other than potassium. The internal K^+ concentration is around 140 mmol/l and the external level around 4–5 mmol/l. When the cell is resting, as the membrane is only permeable to K^+ ions, a small number of K^+ ions leave the cell, rendering the inside negatively charged with respect to the outside. This internal negative charge and external positive charge prevents further positively charged K^+ ions from leaving the cell; this occurs usually when the internal membrane voltage is about 80–90 mV negative to the external voltage. The resting membrane potential can be calculated from a knowledge of the permeability of the membrane to the different ions and the concentration of these ions either side of the membrane, using the Henderson–Hasselbach equation.

Depolarization is due to the rapid entry of sodium ions into the cell, ie the cell membrane transiently becomes very permeable to Na^+, allowing these ions to flow down their concentration gradient (the external level is approximately 140 mmol/l and the internal level approximately 4 mmol/l).

Myocytes, unlike neural tissue, remains depolarized for a very long time period following initial depolarization, often several 100 ms. This long depolarization period is due to a long 'plateau' phase of the action potential, which in part relates to sodium–calcium exchange, though many other currents are contributory. The contribution of these currents varies in different parts of the heart, accounting for the variation in action potential shape (Figure 1.1b).

(a)

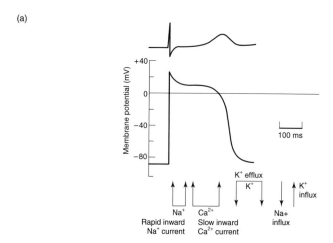

(b)

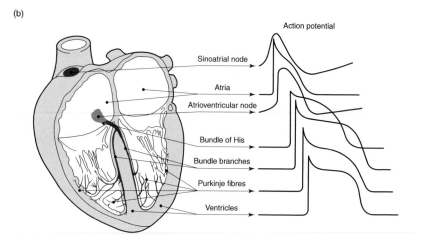

Figure 1.1
(a) Myocyte action potential measured using an intracellular electrode. The three phases are
shown – depolarization, plateau phase and repolarization. The surface ECG consequence of this is
shown above. (b) Shape of the action potential in different parts of the heart. The duration of the
action potential gets progressively longer from the sinus node to the Purkinje fibres. Reprinted
with permission from Sandøe E, Sigurd B. *Arrhythmia Diagnosis and Management: A Clinical
Electrocardiographic Guide*. St Gallen: Fachmed.

The plateau phase ends when repolarization occurs and the membrane
returns to the resting potential. Repolarization mainly involves the opening
of potassium channels, which allows positively charged K+ ions to flow out
of the cell, thus restoring the negative resting potential of the cell.

Whole-heart consequences of depolarization and repolarization

During the cardiac cycle a wave of electricity spreads over the heart, as cells in some parts of the heart are depolarized (ie have a positive intracellular voltage of about +30 mV) whereas cells in other parts of the heart continue with normal resting transmembrane potentials (ie are 'polarized', with intracellular voltages of about –90 mV relative to the extracellular space). When cells depolarize, small amounts of positive charge (K^+ ions) move into them. Thus the area immediately adjacent to the cell becomes depleted of positive charge relative to other extracellular areas of the heart adjacent to cells that have yet to depolarize.

This has two consequences (Figure 1.2). First, electrical current, as negatively charged electrons, will flow from these negatively charged areas adjacent to depolarized cells to the areas adjacent to cells yet to depolarize. Second, there will be a different charge density (ie in electrical terms a different potential difference) in different parts of the heart. These potential differences within the heart are reflected as potential differences between different areas of the chest wall, and can be measured using a sensitive voltage detector (ie one capable of measuring millivolt potential differences accurately), an 'ECG machine' connected to electrodes placed on the body surface. Potential differences between different parts of the chest are only seen when the heart is partially depolarized or partially repolarized; if the heart is fully depolarized or fully repolarized, there are no potential differences and thus no ECG signal. The ECG machine is designed so that a wave of depolarization moving towards an electrode generates a positive deflection (ie one above the isoelectric line) and a wave of depolarization moving away from the electrode produces a negative deflection (ie one below the isoelectric line). The reverse is true for repolarization waves.

An ECG machine is therefore in essence no more than a sensitive voltmeter, although modern machines often have additional features such as electronic filters designed to remove extraneous 'electrical noise' (eg, a 50-Hz filter that removes any nearby mains current AC 'hum', or a high-frequency filter to remove skeletal muscle artefact noise). The signal from an ECG machine is conventionally recorded on paper, although electronic storage means are increasingly being used. It is usual for the paper speed to be set at 25 mm/s and the deflection sensitivity to be set at 10 mm/mV.

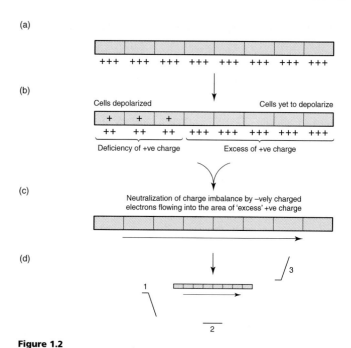

Figure 1.2

How cell depolarization causes current flow in and around the heart. (a) Imagine a row of cells resting quietly. There is an excess of negative charge inside the cell and a relative excess of positive charge outside. All the cells are in a similar state and there is no current flow between the different cells. (b) When cells at one end of the strip depolarize, they allow positive charge to flow in. This reduces the positive charge outside these cells and causes a charge imbalance between the two ends of the row. (c) To neutralize this charge imbalance, electrons flow from the less positively charged end to the more positively charged end. (d) According to physical principles, 'lines' of current flow outside the row of cells. 'Isopotential' lines run at right angles to these lines of current. An observer at 1 will see current flow away from them, ie the ECG will show a negative deflection; an observer at 2 (at right angles to the current flow) will see no current, ie the ECG will show a flat line; and an observer at 3 will observe current flowing towards them, ie the ECG will show a positive deflection.

Summary of electrical changes during the cardiac cycle

When the heart is fully repolarized or depolarized, no current flows and the ECG shows no deflection.

When an area of the heart depolarizes, the positively charged ions flow into the cell, rendering the immediately adjacent external environment negatively charged. Areas more distant to this, adjacent to cells yet to depolarize, are (relatively) positively charged. Electrons (ie current) will flow from these 'depolarized' areas to those areas 'yet to depolarize'.

When an area of the heart repolarizes, the positively charged ions flow out of the cell, rendering the immediately adjacent external environment positively charged. Areas more distant to this, adjacent to cells that have yet to repolarize, are (relatively) negatively charged. Electrons (ie current) will flow from these 'yet-to-repolarize' areas to those areas that have repolarized.

Standard lead positions

A variety of body attachments were used in the very early days of ECG recording. However, for decades now a standard set of ECG attachments have been used, which 'look' at the heart from a variety of different directions (Figures 1.3 and 1.4). It is, however, important to realize that, despite what is suggested by this comment, each ECG lead does not 'look' purely at one anatomical area of the heart. Rather the signal obtained from one lead looks predominantly at one area but is also influenced by neighbouring areas of the heart. These neighbouring signals can sometimes be useful. For example, one may be uncertain whether ST segment elevation genuinely reflects myocardial infarction (MI) or not; if neighbouring ECG leads do not show this abnormality then it is less likely that infarction is present. Conversely, if ST elevation is present in the neighbouring leads then it is more likely that infarction is present.

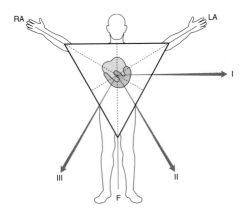

Figure 1.3
For the standard leads four electrodes are attached to the right and left shoulder and right and left leg. These leads allow six views of the heart. The standard leads 'look' at the heart according to their position in Einthoven's triangle. RA, right arm; LA, left arm; F, foot. Reproduced with permission from Timmis AD, Nathan AW. *Essentials of Cardiology*, 2nd edn. Oxford: Blackwell Science.

(a)

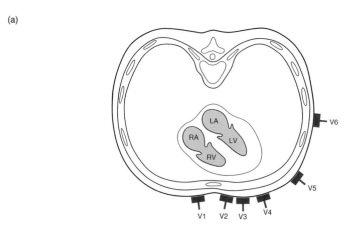

(b)

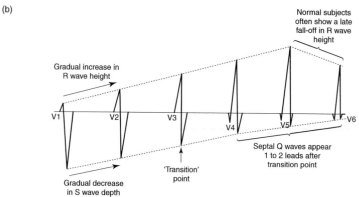

Figure 1.4
How the chest leads 'look' at the heart. (a) As the position of the septum within the chest varies between individuals, so the lead directly in line with the septum will vary. The lead in front of the septum in this example is lead V4. (b) The 'transition point' occurs when the size of the positive deflection equals the size of the negative one, here in lead V3. The transition point reflects the position of the septum. Displacement towards leads V1/2 is termed 'clockwise' rotation of the heart; displacement towards leads V5/6 is termed 'anticlockwise' rotation (eg due to obesity).

Sequence of electrical events

Nomenclature

The different components of the ECG signal are given the letters P, Q, R, S and T (U). The J point occurs when the QRS complex finishes and the ST segment starts (Figure 1.5). The P wave and QRS complex reflect respectively atrial and ventricular depolarization and the T (U) wave reflects ventricular

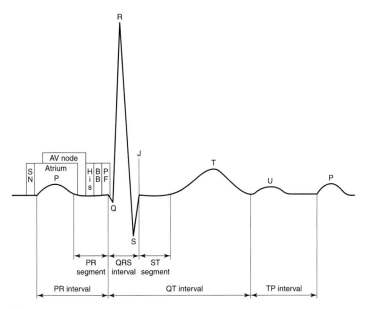

Figure 1.5
Nomenclature and components of the PQRSTU complex. SN, sinoatrial node; AVN, atrioventricular node; His, bundle of His; BB, bundle branch; PF, Purkinje fibres. Adapted with permission from Damato AN, Lau SH. Clinical value of the electrocardiogram of the conduction system. *Prog Cardiovasc Dis* 1970; **13**: 119.

repolarization. Atrial repolarization is not seen on the surface ECG as the currents and voltages involved are too small.

Atrial depolarization and the P wave

The normal ECG complex starts off with a P wave, which reflects atrial depolarization. The duration of the P wave reflects how long it takes for full atrial depolarization to occur, whereas the amplitude of the P wave reflects the muscle mass of the atria. The vector of atrial depolarization will determine the shape of the P wave. The normal shape is shown in Figures 2.1 and 2.2. This in turn relates to where depolarization first started, ie whether the pacemaker is in the sinoatrial node (SN) or elsewhere. After the P wave, the ECG signal returns to the isoelectric line until the QRS complex occurs.

Atrioventicular conduction

The time taken for the cardiac electrical impulse to start at the SN and be conducted down to the ventricle to initiate ventricular depolarization (Figure 1.6) is reflected in the time from the onset of the P wave to the onset of the QRS complex, known as the PR interval.

There are two major components to this time (Figure 1.6). The first is the time taken for the impulse to be propagated through the atria to the atrioventricular node (AVN), then to traverse the AVN and reach the bundle of His. This time is known as the AH interval. As the current generated within the AVN is too small to reach the surface of the body, during its passage through the node the ECG is isoelectric with the baseline (this time can only be accurately measured invasively; Figure 9.4).

The second component is the time taken for the impulse to travel from the bundle of His to the ventricle: the HV interval. The HV interval can only be accurately measured invasively. Together, the AH and HV intervals make up the PR interval.

Thus diseases of the AVN that prolong the time taken for the electrical impulse to propagate through the AVN cause a lengthening of the PR interval, mainly due to a lengthening of the AH interval, which is seen on the

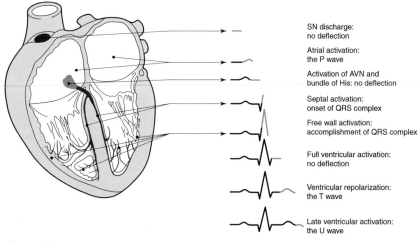

Figure 1.6
Atrioventricular conduction, ventricular depolarization and the QRS complex. SN, sinoatrial node; AVN, atrioventricular node.

surface ECG as PR interval prolongation. Likewise, disease of the bundle of His also leads to PR interval prolongation, this time due to HV interval prolongation.

Ventricular depolarization and the QRS complex

Ventricular depolarization commences once the electrical signal has reached the ventricle and is seen as the first deflection of the QRS complex. The depolarizing current is spread throughout the ventricles very quickly via the specialized conducting tissue, resulting in a systematic spread of depolarization throughout the ventricle (Figure 1.7). The time taken for full ventricular depolarization is reflected in the duration of the QRS complex and so quick ventricular depolarization results in a narrow QRS complex in health (Figure 1.6), usually less than 120 ms. As the specialized conducting cells run just under the endocardium and from there into the more general myocardial tissue, depolarization spreads first into the endocardium and then proceeds outwards towards the epicardium. This has implications for whether or not Q waves are found in health, and for the polarity of the T wave.

The terminology of the QRS complex depends on whether the initial deflection is upwards or downwards.

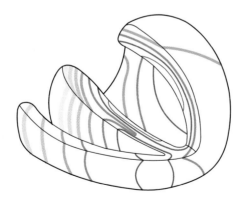

Figure 1.7
Sequence of ventricular depolarization from pale shaded areas to darker shaded areas. Reprinted with permission from Durrer D. Electrical aspects of human cardiac activity: a clinical–physiological approach to excitation and stimulation. *Cardiovasc Res* 1968; **2**: 1.

If the first deflection is upwards, the deflection is termed an R wave. Subsequent downward deflections below the isoelectric line are called S waves. If there is a further subsequent deflection upwards above the isoelectric line following an S wave, it is termed an R' (R prime) wave.

If the first deflection is downwards, the deflection is termed a Q wave. The following upward deflection is termed an R wave provided it rises above the isoelectric line. Deflections downward below the isoelectric line following an R wave are termed S waves. By definition, a Q wave cannot occur in a QRS complex that starts with an R wave.

Why do some leads in health start with R waves and others with small Q waves?

As the specialized conducting tissue runs along the endocardial surface of the heart, depolarization of the main body of the ventricle proceeds from the endocardium to the epicardium. Thus current flows in the direction of most leads at the start of ventricular depolarization. As many ECG leads look at the main body of the heart, in health many normal ECG leads start with an R wave. However, leads looking at the left side of the normal heart usually show an initial, small Q wave. The reason for this is that early on in ventricular repolarization such leads look at the interventricular septum, which in health depolarizes from left to right (Figure1.8). Thus the current

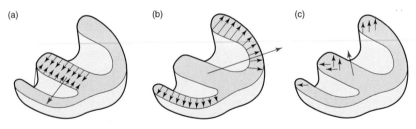

Figure 1.8
Septal depolarization causes small Q waves in the left-facing leads. (a) As depolarization initially occurs mainly in the septum, from left to right, leads facing the right side start with a positive deflection, whereas leads facing the left side start with a small Q wave. (b) Later depolarization of the bulk of the left ventricle dominates the QRS complex. (c) At the end of depolarization there is a small, superiorly directed vector. Red arrows indicate the overall vector of depolarization. Reproduced with permission from Sandøe E, Sigurd B. *Arrhythmia Diagnosis and Management: A Clinical Electrocardiographic Guide*. St Gallen: Fachmed.

will initially flow away from left-sided chest leads, and consequently any such leads looking at the septum from the left side initially will show a Q wave. However, this Q wave will be small as the muscle mass of the septum is small. After this short-duration Q wave, the left-sided chest leads will be dominated by the large mass of left ventricular myocardium as it depolarizes. This depolarizes from inside (ie the endocardial surface) to outside (ie the epicardial surface), thus generating a current that flows towards the ECG electrode. Thus, after an initial small Q wave, a large R wave develops in left-sided leads.

Large Q waves

QRS complexes starting with a Q wave imply that initial ventricular depolarization occurs in a direction away from the electrode. The endocardial-to-epicardial sequence of activation in health means that most leads have current flowing towards them at the start of depolarization. Pathological (ie large) Q waves can only occur when there is an electrical 'window' (ie electrically neutral view) on the ventricle, such that that part of the ventricle closest to the electrode does not generate any electrical activity. Rather, the window allows the electrical current from the ventricular wall opposite the electrode to 'pass through'. Thus the electrode that abuts an electrical window looks at the opposite wall of the heart to the one facing it 'from the inside'. As the current passes from the inside of the heart to the outside, the initial deflection is away from the electrode, so a Q wave is produced (Figure 1.9). There are two principle causes of an electrical window onto the heart: first, the electrode is situated facing the AV valve, which is electrically neutral (the only electrode that does this is lead aVR); and second, part of the heart has died, resulting in electrically inert scar tissue (eg following MI or myocarditis).

Interpretation of changes in QRS amplitude and duration

The amplitude of the QRS complex reflects ventricular muscle mass (Figure 1.10), overwhelmingly left ventricular mass, as in health the LV muscle constitutes ≥90% of ventricular muscle mass, whereas QRS duration reflects the time taken for depolarization to spread throughout the normal ventricle. Thus increases or decreases in amplitude often reflect changes in LV mass or a change in the amount of electrical insulation between the heart and the detecting electrode (ie chest wall obesity), whereas increases in QRS

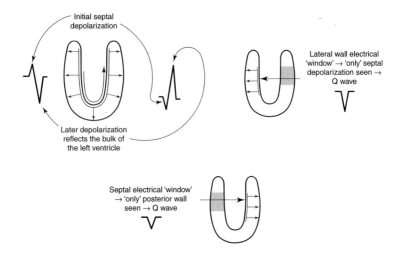

Figure 1.9
Q waves are due to electrical 'windows' on the heart. An electrical window means that any lead looking into the heart through this window only sees the normal inner-to-outer flow of current, resulting in a Q wave.

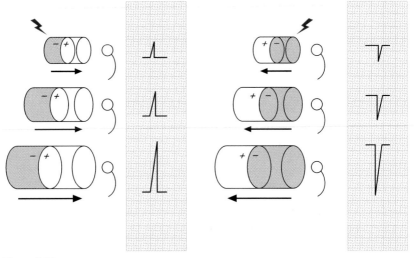

Figure 1.10
The larger the mass of muscle, the greater the size of the deflection detected by an observing electrode, whether the current is flowing towards or away from it. Reprinted with permission from Sandøe E, Sigurd B. *Arrhythmia Diagnosis and Management: A Clinical Electrocardiographic Guide.* St Gallen: Fachmed

duration reflect a prolongation in the time taken for the left ventricle to depolarize. Such an increase in duration can be due to disease of the specialized conducting tissue of the heart.

For any individual lead, the amplitude of the QRS complex will depend not only on how much heart muscle there is but also on the direction from which the lead looks at the depolarizing wave front. The more directly the lead looks at the depolarizing wave the more electricity is detected; conversely, the less directly the lead looks at the depolarizing front the less electricity will be detected – if the lead is at 90° to the wave front, no electricity will be detected.

Axis of ventricular depolarization. During ventricular depolarization a wave of depolarization travels across the heart. The instantaneous direction of this wave can be plotted using an appropriately programmed ECG machine in a process known as 'vectorcardiography', a process rarely used nowadays as (at least until recently) the equipment was heavy, expensive and cumbersome and required a nonstandard set of orthogonal electrodes (X, Y and Z, each at right angles to one another and measuring current flow anteroposteriorly, inferiorly–superiorly and left–right). Furthermore, this difficult recording often added little to the diagnosis.

However, the overall direction of depolarization (ie the sum of the individual instantaneous vectors) can be easily determined from examination of the ECG. The R wave is projected onto a diagram of the standard and augmented limb leads (Figure 1.11) representing a stylized Einthoven's triangle, and the overall axis derived. Another way to determine the axis is to identify which of the standard limb leads is 'isoelectric', ie in which lead the sizes of the upward and downward deflections are equal. The overall axis is at right angles to this isoelectric lead. To determine which of the two possible directions is the right one, inspect a lead at (or close to) right angles to the isoelectric lead. If the QRS complex is positive, then this is the direction of the axis.

Simplified approach to determining the QRS axis. In practice a simple (and usually correct) way to determine the overall axis is to examine the polarity of the R wave in leads I and II: if both are positive, the axis is normal, whereas if either is negative, the axis is either left-shifted (positive R wave in lead I, negative in lead III) or right-shifted (negative R wave in lead I, positive in lead III). The same approach can be used to work out the vector of repolarization (ie the vector of the T wave).

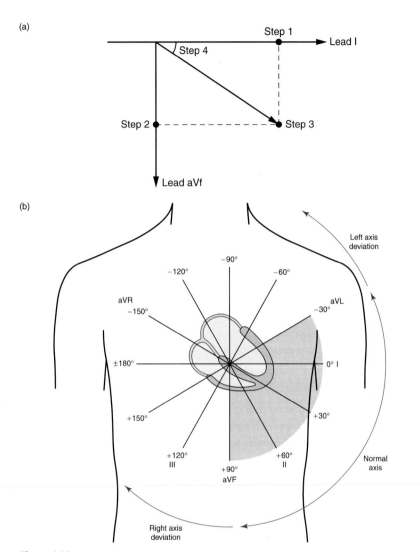

Figure 1.11
(a) Determining the overall QRS axis using leads I, II and III. (b) Interpretation of the overall QRS axis using the standard limb leads. When the mean frontal QRS axis is directed towards lead I it is arbitrarily defined as 0°; the dominant positive deflection is in lead I and the equiphasic deflection is in lead aVF. Axis shifts are given a negative sign if directed leftwards (towards aVL) and a positive sign if directed rightwards (towards aVF). Axes between –30° and +90° are normal (shaded area). Axes less than –30° (left axis deviation) or greater than +90° (right axis deviation) are abnormal. If the ECG complexes are not large enough in either lead I or lead aVF then other leads may be used. Reproduced with permission from Timmis AD, Nathan AW. *Essentials of Cardiology*, 2nd edn. Oxford: Blackwell Science.

Ventricular repolarization

The wave following the QRS complex is termed the T wave and reflects myocardial repolarization. The heart repolarizes in a systematic fashion, from the epicardium to the endocardium. As repolarization proceeds in the reverse direction to depolarization, one might expect that the T wave would be in the reverse direction to the QRS (depolarization) complex. However, as the repolarizing current is the electrical opposite of the depolarizing current (see above), the two 'negatives' cancel each other out, and so the direction of current flow is the same as for depolarization. The important practical implication of this is that the vector of the T wave is very similar to the vector of the QRS complex. Thus, in health those leads that have well-developed R waves usually also have upright T waves.

Duration of electrical systole

Electrical systole reflects the duration of the action potentials of myocytes within the ventricle of the heart. It is reflected in the ECG as the QT interval and is measured from the beginning of the Q wave to the end of the T wave. Influences that prolong or shorten myocyte action potential duration (usually) also prolong or shorten the QT interval.

There are many influences on the QT interval in health, of which heart rate is by far the most powerful influence. The QT interval not only varies with heart rate (increasing heart rate leads to a shorter QT interval, Figure 1.12) but also demonstrates hysteresis; ie a sudden step change in heart rate leads to a slower change in QT interval. Most of the QT adaptation to altered heart rate occurs within 90 seconds. When comparing QT intervals from subjects with different heart rates, some form of correction is thus necessary. There has been considerable debate as to how this should be done. The older Bazett heart rate correction formula has gained widespread acceptance even though it over-corrects (ie artificially prolongs the QT interval) at high heart rates. In its modern form, this formula states:

$$QTc = (QT \text{ interval}) / (RR \text{ interval})^{1/2}$$

where QTc is the rate-corrected QT interval and the RR interval is measured in seconds. In effect, QTc is the QT interval at a heart rate of 60 bpm. Fridericia's formula is preferable:

$$QTc = (QT \text{ interval}) / (RR \text{ interval})^{1/3}$$

this formula does not overcorrect at high heart rates.

17

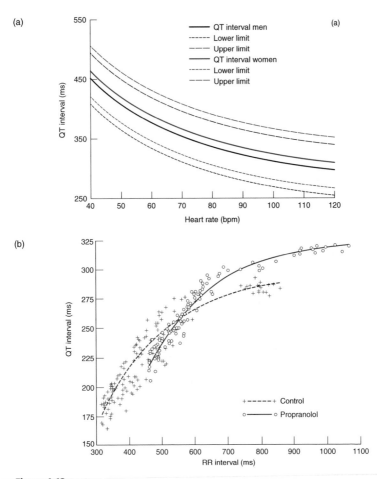

Figure 1.12
The relationship between QT interval and heart rate. (a) Data relating to subjects at rest, from the
Framingham Heart Study. QT intervals outside these limits are regarded as abnormal. (b) The QT
interval varies with exercise, and intervention (in this case a β-blocker) alters the QT–heart rate
relationship. It can be seen that β-blockers prolong the QT interval at low heart rates but shorten it at
high heart rates. This illustrates how a formulaic approach to QT–heart rate correction cannot work.
Part (b) reproduced with permission from Sarma JS, Venkataraman K, Samant DR, Gadgill UG. *Br
Heart J* 1988; **60**: 434–9.

The autonomic nervous system influences the QT interval in two important
situations. First, the autonomic changes associated with exercise (increased
adrenergic tone and withdrawal of vagal tone) shorten the QT interval
regardless of any effects of the autonomic nervous system on heart rate.
Indeed, about one-third of exercise-induced QT interval shortening is due to

these exercise-induced autonomic changes, and about two-thirds is due to the effects of increasing heart rate. Second, the QT interval is also affected by the circadian rhythm, being prolonged at night (probably as the vagal tone is higher and sympathetic tone withdrawn). This can lengthen the nocturnal QT interval (at the same heart rate) by up to 30 ms.

Physical fitness has an impact on the QT interval, probably via its effect on the autonomic nervous system. Gender also has a definite but minor impact on QT interval: women have longer QT intervals than men between puberty and the age of 50 years. Genetic influences are probably important too, but are as yet little understood.

It is important to routinely measure the QT interval as it can be significantly prolonged by some diseases, so predisposing to ventricular arrhythmias. In the modern era this is usually relatively straightforward as most ECG machines have the necessary computer algorithms.

Summary of normal ECG appearance

A normal ECG (Figure 1.13) has:

- normal P wave shape and vector
- normal PR interval, neither too long (suggesting high vagal tone or conducting tissue disease) nor too short (suggesting Wolff–Parkinson–White syndrome)
- normal duration and axis of ventricular depolarization (QRS complex) without pathological Q waves
- normal T wave axis, usually much the same as the normal QRS axis
- normal QT interval.

There are many variations to normal; the best way for the student to learn these is by experience.

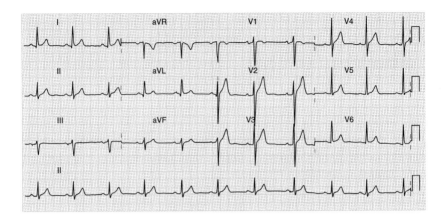

Figure 1.13
Normal 12-lead ECG. Note the normal P wave shape [upright in lead II, biphasic (although predominantly upright) in lead V1], normal PR interval (120–200 ms), absence of pathological Q waves (physiological Q wave in lead aVR), normal QRS axis, normal QRS duration (<120 ms although normally nearer to 100 ms), steady progression of the R wave in the anterior chest leads, small left-sided Q waves in the left chest leads, and normal T wave axis.

Chapter 2
Abnormalities of the P wave

The P wave is normal if atrial depolarization is normal, ie if the vector (direction and velocity) of atrial depolarization and the atrial dimensions are both normal (Figure 2.1a). Normality means:

- P wave amplitude ≤0.25 mV
- P wave duration ≤110 ms
- normal P wave shape (Figure 2.1b), which reflects a normal P wave axis (Figure 2.1a), ie a normal origin and spread of the P wave throughout the atria.

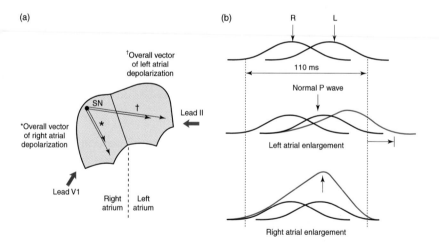

(a)   (b)

Figure 2.1
Atrial depolarization and the P wave. (a) The sinoatrial node (SN) lies in the right atrium and activates it first, so (b) right atrial depolarization occupies the first two-thirds of the P wave and left atrial depolarization the last two-thirds. Right atrial enlargement results in an increased early vector towards leads II and V1; left atrial enlargement results in an increased late vector away from lead V1 and towards lead II. Part (b) reprinted from Murray JG. *Mayo Clinic Cardiology Review*. 2nd edn. Philadelphia: Lippincott, Williams and Wilkins, by permission of Mayo Foundation.

21

The principal abnormalities of the P wave are caused by:

- right atrial enlargement
- left atrial enlargement
- wandering or ectopic pacemaker
- prolonged interatrial conduction time
- rhythm abnormalities.

Right atrial enlargement

Right atrial enlargement prolongs the time taken for right atrial depolarization. Thus the vector of atrial depolarization is dominated by right atrial depolarization and the surface effects of left atrial depolarization are minimized (Figure 2.2). This has two effects. First, in lead V1 the small late negative deflection disappears and the P wave amplitude may also increase. Second, in lead II the P wave vector increases, thus increasing the amplitude of the P wave.

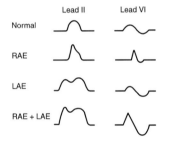

Figure 2.2
Typical findings in right atrial enlargement (RAE) and left atrial enlargement (LAE). The vector of right atrial depolarization is towards leads V1 and almost isoelectric to lead II, whereas the vector of left atrial depolarization is towards lead II and away from lead V1, accounting for the different morphologies of right, left and biatrial enlargement.

As a generalization, the greater the amplitude of the P wave in lead II, the greater the enlargement of the right atrium. Beware, however – substantial right atrial enlargement can occur without any ECG changes.

Causes of right atrial enlargement

There are numerous causes of electrocardiographic right atrial enlargement, some of which can be deduced from spotting concomitant ECG abnormalities.

Right atrial enlargement may be due to pulmonary hypertension of any cause, including: left heart failure [a very common cause; the ECG may also show left ventricular hypertrophy (LVH) or Q waves, especially anteriorly];

chronic lung disease [eg severe chronic obstructive pulmonary disease; this can cause right ventricular hypertrophy (RVH; see below), but ECG changes are often absent]; pulmonary thromboembolic lung disease (rarer); and primary pulmonary hypertension (very rare; there may be ECG signs of RVH, particularly when the pulmonary artery pressure is very high).

Diseases globally affecting the heart, such as dilated cardiomyopathy, may cause right atrial enlargement. The ECG is often globally but rather nonspecifically abnormal, or shows left bundle branch block.

Right atrial enlargement may also be due to disease selectively affecting the right heart, such as right ventricular cardiomyopathy (rarely) and Ebstein's anomaly (congenital displacement of the tricuspid valve upwards into the right ventricular cavity, sometimes with severe tricuspid regurgitation; Figure 2.3).

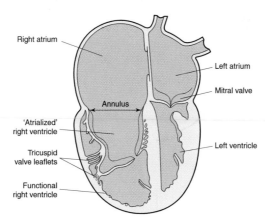

Figure 2.3
Anatomy of Ebstein's anomaly. Reproduced with permission from Crawford MH, DiMarco JP. *Cardiology*. London: Mosby.

Left atrial enlargement

Left atrial enlargement results in the vector of the P wave becoming dominated by left atrial depolarization (Figure 2.2). There are two consequences of this.

First, as the direction of left atrial depolarization is away from V1, left atrial enlargement results in a predominantly negative P wave in lead V1 late on. This is a reasonably sensitive and specific marker for left atrial enlargement.

Second, as left atrial depolarization is normally a late event in atrial depolarization, increasing the dimension of the left atrium delays full atrial depolarization and thus prolongs the duration of the P wave. This is best seen in lead II, where it results in a widened, often bifid, P wave.

Causes of left atrial enlargement

Any disease of the left ventricle that interferes with its pumping performance can cause left atrial enlargement, eg old myocardial infarction (look for Q waves), LVH (eg due to hypertension) or cardiomyopathy (causing a diffusely abnormal ECG or a left bundle branch block pattern).

Disease of the aortic or mitral valves may also result in left atrial enlargement. Aortic valve disease sufficient to enlarge the left atrium usually causes ECG signs of LVH, whereas such ECG signs are less likely with severe mitral regurgitation. Mitral stenosis (very rare in developed countries) has no impact on the left ventricle; often the only early ECG abnormality in pure mitral stenosis is isolated left atrial enlargement (Figure 2.4); atrial fibrillation may occur later.

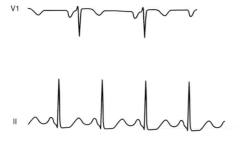

Figure 2.4
Left atrial enlargement. This patient with critical mitral stenosis presented with life-threatening puerperal pulmonary oedema. The P wave in lead II is fairly unremarkable whereas the P wave in lead V1 shows a dramatic late negative deflection. Changes in lead V1 are more sensitive for left atrial enlargement than are changes in lead II.

Wandering (ectopic) pacemaker

The normal cardiac pacemaker is the sinoatrial node (SN). However, on occasions other areas within the atria can develop increased automaticity and 'take over' from the pacemaker function from the SN. As such pacemakers are by definition situated in areas of the atria away from the SN, the vector of depolarization that spreads out from these pacemakers differs from normal (Figure 2.5). This results in an abnormally shaped P wave (best seen in leads II and V1). An ectopic pacemaker may stay in the one spot or may 'wander' around the atria (ie a 'wandering pacemaker'). Although sometimes a normal variant, an ectopic pacemaker may be associated with disease processes such as sinus node disease, 'sinus venosus' atrial septal defect (usually associated with partial or complete right bundle branch block) and digoxin toxicity.

Prolongation of interatrial conduction time

The time taken for the atria to depolarize depends on the velocity of electrical impulse propagation and the size and shape of the atria. Atrial depolarization time can be prolonged if there is disease of the conducting tissue of the atria and/or disease of the atria themselves resulting in slower cell-to-cell depolarization. This increases the breadth of the P wave. The amplitude of the P wave is often diminished also, as most diseases that slow atrial depolarization do so by diminishing the mass of electrically active atrial myocytes

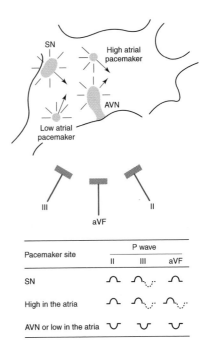

Pacemaker site	P wave		
	II	III	aVF
SN	⌒	⌒	⌒
High in the atria	⌒	⌒	⌒
AVN or low in the atria	⋎	⋎	⋎

Figure 2.5
Ectopic atrial pacemaker. When the dominant atrial pacemaker moves position the morphology of the P wave changes. SN, sinoatrial node; AVN, atrioventricular node. Reproduced with permission from Sandøe E, Sigurd B. *Arrhythmia Diagnosis and Management: A Clinical Electrocardiographic Guide*. St Gallen: Fachmed.

(replacing them with scar tissue, with slower cell-to-cell depolarization). Diseases prolonging atrial depolarization time include cardiomyopathy (especially cardiac amyloidosis) and ischaemic heart disease.

These diseases can end up producing electrically and mechanically inert atria, a powerful substrate for systemic thromboemboli, especially if there is associated heart failure.

Atrial rhythm abnormalities

These include atrial fibrillation, atrial flutter and atrial tachycardia (Figure 2.6).

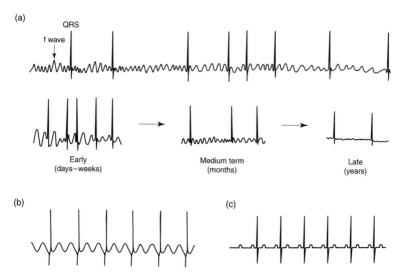

Figure 2.6
(a) Atrial fibrillation (AF). The irregular, completely disorganized baseline shows fibrillatory (f) waves and an irregular QRS response. In early AF the f waves are high-voltage and there is a high QRS rate (>120–140 bpm). In medium-term AF both the f wave voltage and the QRS rate decline. In late AF f waves are very fine and the baseline may appear almost flat. (b) Atrial flutter. The irregular 'saw-tooth' baseline is best seen in the inferior leads (II, III, aVF) and the heart rate is often a ratio of 300 (ie 150, 100 or 75 bpm). (c) Atrial tachycardia. Independent P waves are seen, separated by an isoelectric baseline, often in a two-to-one ratio with QRS complexes. The P wave shape is unusual as the focus is distant from the sinoatrial node.

Atrial fibrillation

Atrial fibrillation is the commonest serious arrhythmia. Instead of coordinated atrial electrical and mechanical activity, the atria are continually electrically active, with six or seven depolarization wavefronts. The absence of coordinated electrical activity prevents coordinated mechanical activity and so the atrial contribution to cardiac output is removed. The ECG shows a random baseline with QRS complexes occurring at irregular intervals.

Atrial flutter

Atrial flutter is due to a reentrant circuit in the right atrium. The ECG shows continual atrial activity and a 'saw-tooth' pattern in the inferior leads. The rate of atrial contractions is usually almost exactly 300 bpm, although a degree of atrioventricular (AV) block means that the rate of QRS complexes is usually in a two- or three-to-one ratio to this, often 150, 100 or 75 bpm.

Atrial tachycardia

Atrial tachycardia is the least common atrial arrhythmia. An automatic focus repeatedly fires within the atria, often at a rate of 140–280 bpm. At the higher heart rates some physiological AV block occurs, often in a two- or three-to-one ratio. The P waves have an unusual axis as the automatic atrial focus is sited ectopically, distant to the normal SA node.

Chapter 3
Abnormalities of the QRS complex

The QRS complex is normal when the speed and direction (ie the vector) of depolarization are normal (Figure 3.1) and the voltage generated in myocardial depolarization is also normal (see Figure 1.10). There are a number of characteristic abnormalities of the QRS complex, including:

- increased or decreased QRS amplitude
- pathological Q waves
- broadened QRS complex (with conducting tissue disease or a delta wave.

In analysing abnormalities of the QRS complex to reach a diagnosis, it is important to determine the distribution of ECG changes, ie which leads are normal and which are not. Characteristic patterns of abnormalities and their common clinical associations are as follows.

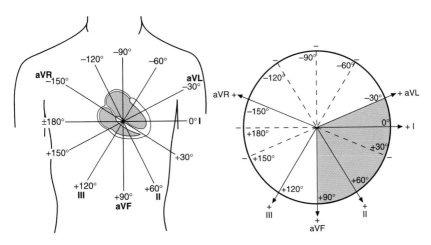

Figure 3.1
A QRS vector directed towards lead I is arbitrarily defined as 0°. Positive axes are directed towards aVL and aVF, and negative axes are directed leftwards towards aVL. Abnormal axes fall outside the −30° (left axis deviation) to +90° (right axis deviation) range.

General increases in QRS voltages:

- thin chest wall
- normal in youth (ie ≤30–40 years)
- left ventricular hypertrophy (LVH)
- Wolff–Parkinson–White syndrome (see p. 201).

Local increases in QRS voltages:

- increased R wave voltages in lead V1: right ventricular hypertrophy (RVH) or right bundle branch block
- increased R wave voltage in leads V5 or V6: LVH.

General loss of QRS amplitude:

- old age
- obesity
- cardiomyopathy, especially ischaemic [previous multiterritory myocardial infarctions (MIs)] or idiopathic dilated cardiomyopathy; rarely, amyloid heart disease
- pericardial effusion
- hypothyroidism.

Local decreases in QRS voltages:

- old MI (very common cause of local loss of R wave height).
- Q waves usually reflect an old MI [the distribution of Q waves usually (but not always) reflects which coronary arteries have been occluded (see below)].

Left ventricular hypertrophy

The impact of LVH on the ECG varies according to aetiology, severity, age and body mass index. However, there is a basic pattern on which additional features are superimposed (Figure 3.2), as follows.

First, there is an increase in the QRS voltage of leads looking at the left ventricle. This is seen as an increase in the R wave amplitude in leads II, aVL, V5 and V6 and an increase in the S wave amplitude in leads V2 and V3. This is by far the most important ECG feature of LVH.

Second, the QRS vector deviates towards the left ventricle ('left axis deviation'). In other words, the QRS vector is directed towards the mass of muscle being depolarized. Most cases of LVH that have left axis deviation

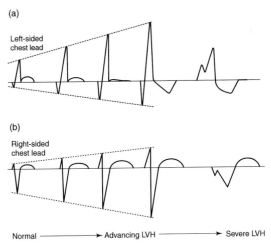

(a)

Left-sided chest lead

(b)

Right-sided chest lead

Normal ⟶ Advancing LVH ⟶ Severe LVH

Figure 3.2
ECG consequences of left ventricular hypertrophy (LVH). (a) Left-sided chest leads: as LVH advances the voltages of the left-sided leads increase, T waves flatten then invert, and left-sided septal Q waves deepen. In severe LVH the ECG often 'converts' to left bundle branch block. (b) Right-sided chest leads: as LVH advances initial R waves slightly increase and S waves deepen, but there is no effect on T waves.

also meet the voltage criteria for LVH. Left axis deviation with normal LV voltages is more likely to be due to conducting tissue disease (see p. 176) than to LVH, although it is occasionally due to LVH (particularly with obesity, which diminishes the size of the QRS complex in the chest leads).

Third, many (but not all) cases of LVH also have left atrial enlargement (see p. 23), and looking for the P wave changes of this condition can be a useful confirmation of significant LVH.

With increasingly severe LVH, several additional features generally develop (Figure 3.2):

- QRS voltages increase further (sometimes dramatically)
- left axis deviation becomes more prominent
- the QRS complex broadens (initially due to a delay in the 'intrinsicoid' deflection; full left bundle branch block or other conducting tissue disease may develop later)
- T wave in the anterolateral leads may decrease in amplitude (early LVH), flatten (later LVH) or invert (severe LVH).

T wave changes tend to be restricted to leads I, II, aVL, V5 and V6 [if ST changes are more extensive then alternative (or additional) diagnoses should be considered]. These changes were previously termed 'strain' but are now referred to as 'repolarization abnormalities'. In hypertension the development of these repolarization changes is ominous (see p. 68 and Figure 3.3).

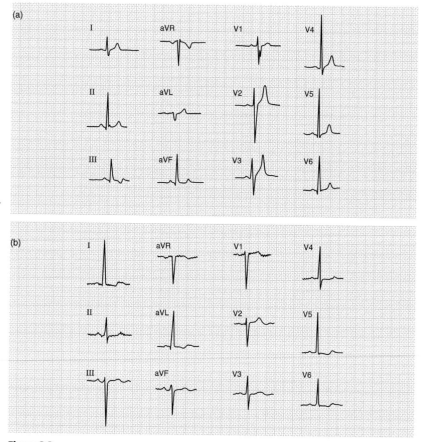

Figure 3.3

(a) Left ventricular hypertrophy (LVH) determined by voltage criteria. S in V2 = R in V5 = 47 mm (normal ≤45 mm), and R in lead II = 21 mm. The patient had asymptomatic aortic stenosis. There was moderate LVH on cardiac ultrasound scanning. (b) Marked LVH due to aortic regurgitation. There is a substantial increase in the amplitude of aVL, to 27 mm (normal ≤12 mm) and an increase in precordial lead voltage [S in V1 + R in V5 is 53 mm, normal ≤45 mm (young) or 35 mm (older)]. Surprisingly, given these substantial voltage increases, with repolarization changes, there is no axis deviation and the left-sided 'physiological' septal Q waves are unremarkable.

Problems with ECG diagnosis of LVH

QRS axis deviation is easy to diagnose (see p. 16). However, it can be quite difficult to state definitively that left-sided voltages in the ECG are pathologically increased, as the magnitude of the QRS complex is affected in an inconsistent manner by body mass and age.

The higher the body mass index (BMI), the smaller will be the QRS complex. Thus thin patients can have substantial QRS complexes without having LVH, and conversely those with unusually high BMIs can have normal-sized QRS complexes and yet still have significant LVH.

With increasing age, normal left ventricular voltages decline. Thus the very elderly may have substantial pathological LVH with very little change in the surface ECG.

Criteria for ECG diagnosis of LVH

To get past these problems, various criteria for the detection of LVH have been proposed (Box 3.1), of which the most widely used are the Lyon and the Sokolov criteria. Unfortunately these criteria and others are so complex that most practising cardiologists stick to one of the following fairly simple voltage changes to diagnose electrical LVH:

- aVL >12 mm
- S in V1 or V2 + R in V5 or V6 >45 mm (under 40 years of age) or >35 mm (over 40 years of age).

Causes of LVH

Aortic stenosis (more rarely, aortic regurgitation). Classical LVH due to aortic stenosis (Figure 3.4a) is associated with a narrow QRS complex, whereas in aortic regurgitation (Figure 3.4b) delayed intrinsicoid deflection is reportedly more common. ST and T wave changes in the lateral leads only are common with both conditions. The diagnosis of aortic valve disease is clinical, confirmed by cardiac ultrasound.

Hypertension. The more severe the LVH and the greater the lateral lead T wave changes, the worse the outlook.

Hypertrophic cardiomyopathy. This is often associated with widespread ST and T wave changes across all the anterior chest leads. There may also be

---

Box 3.1 ECG criteria for diagnosing left ventricular hypertrophy

---

- Romhilt–Estes criteria

1 Voltage criterion: R or S in any limb lead ≥0.20 mV or S in lead V1 or V2 or R in lead V5 or V6 ≥0.30 mV	3 points
2 Left ventricular strain: ST segment and T wave in opposite direction to QRS complex	
– without digitalis	3 points
– with digitalis	1 point
3 Left atrial enlargement: terminal negativity of the P wave in lead V1 ≥0.10 mV in depth and 0.04 s in duration	3 points
4 Axis shift: left axis deviation of ≥–30°	2 points
5 QRS duration: ≥0.09 s	1 point
6 Intrinsicoid deflection in lead V5 or V6 ≥0.05 s	1 point
Total possible score	*13 points*

Probable LVH = 4 points; definite LVH = 5 points

- Sokolow–Lyon criteria

S wave in lead V1 + R wave in lead V5 or V6 >3.50 mV or R wave in lead V5 or V6 >2.60 mV

- Cornell sex-specific voltage criteria
  - women: R wave in lead aVL + S wave in lead V3 >2.00 mV
  - men: R wave in lead aVL + S wave in lead V3 >2.80 mV

- Cornell voltage–QRS duration product criteria

- Gubner–Ungerleider criteria
  - R wave in lead I plus S wave in lead III >2.5 mV

- Minnesota Code 3-1
  - R wave in lead V5–V6 >2.6 mV, or
  - R wave in leads II, III, aVF >2.0 mV, or
  - R wave in lead aVL >1.2 mV

Adapted with permission from Romhilt DW, Estes EH. *Am Heart J* 1968; **75**: 752–8; Sokolow M, Lyon P. *Am Heart J* 1949; **37**: 161–86; Casale PN, Devereux RB, Alonso DR *et al. Circulation* 1987; **75**: 565–72.

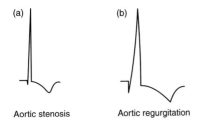

(a)   (b)

Aortic stenosis   Aortic regurgitation

Figure 3.4
Left ventricular hypertrophy in (a) aortic stenosis (small Q wave, narrow QRS complex) compared with (b) aortic regurgitation (deeper Q wave, broader QRS complex). Be aware that these differences between aortic stenosis and regurgitation are perhaps more theoretical than real, and either ECG can be found in either condition.

extraordinarily deep Q waves anteriorly or inferiorly. As these Q waves are due to the hypertrophic process, not to an old MI, they are known as 'pseudo-infarction' Q waves. Some patients with hypertrophic cardiomyopathy have an associated accessory pathway (see p. 201).

Other forms of cardiomyopathy – especially postviral myocarditis (usually associated with widespread ST and T wave changes).

Other causes, including mitral regurgitation. However, many patients with substantial mitral regurgitation do not have clear ECG evidence of LVH.

For most of the above diagnoses the clinical examination can often be suggestive but the cardiac ultrasound will be diagnostic.

Limitations to ECG diagnosis of LVH

Given the above, it is clear that the ECG is a relatively insensitive method for detection of LVH (Table 3.1); cardiac ultrasound is more useful. For example, in hypertension a normal ECG occurs in about half of those with significant LVH (although the severity of LVH tends to be milder if the ECG is normal). Accordingly, if the presence of LVH will significantly alter the patient's management then cardiac ultrasound should be used as the definitive diagnostic tool, regardless of whether or not the ECG suggests this diagnosis. Furthermore, thin and/or young subjects may have prominent (sometimes dramatic) left ventricular voltages without having any LVH. For this reason, 'best practice' is to confirm all ECG diagnoses of LVH via cardiac ultrasound.

Table 3.1 Accuracy of various criteria for the diagnosis of left ventricular hypertrophy

Criterion	Sensitivity (%)	False-positive diagnoses (%)
R + S >45 mm	45	7
SV1 + RV5 or RV6 >35 mm	43	5
OID V5 or V6 = 0.05–0.07 s	29	1
RV5 or RV6 >26 mm	25	2
RaVL >11 mm	11	0
$R_1 + S_3$ >25 mm	11	0
SaVR >14 mm	7	0
RaVF >20 mm	1	1

OID; onset of intrinsicoid deflection. Adapted with permission from Romhilt DW, Bove KE, Norris RJ *et al*. A critical appraisal of the ECG criteria for the diagnosis of left ventricular hypertrophy. *Circulation* 1969; **40**: 185.

Right ventricular hypertrophy

RVH increases the voltages in leads looking at the right side of the heart. Initially (Figures 3.5 and 3.6), the size of the S wave in V1 diminishes; subsequently there may be a rightward shift of the QRS vector. In substantial RVH a 'dominant' R wave appears in V1 [ie in contrast to the usual V1 pattern in health of a very small R wave and a much larger subsequent S wave (Figure 3.5a)]. In substantial RVH the R wave now becomes much larger than the subsequent S wave. Several diseases other than RVH may cause a large R wave in V1 (see below) and sometimes it is not possible to reach a firm diagnosis on ECG grounds alone (see Figure 3.7).

Causes of a dominant R wave in V1

Right ventricular hypertrophy (Figure 3.6 and Box 3.2). The QRS complex is narrow, and there may be right axis deviation of the QRS complex and right atrial enlargement (see p. 22).

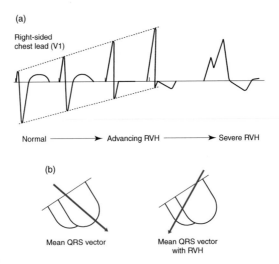

Figure 3.5
ECG consequences of right ventricular hypertrophy (RVH). (a) As RVH increases, the right-sided lead voltages increase, S wave depth decreases and T wave inversion occurs. Advanced RVH may show a right bundle branch block pattern. (b) With increasing RVH the QRS vector shifts to the right.

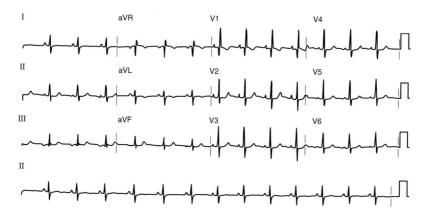

Figure 3.6
This ECG shows RV hypertrophy occurring in Eisenmenger syndrome. There is right axis deviation, and a dominant R wave in lead V1. Unusually, there is also a prominent Q wave in lead V1 – most cases of RV hypertrophy do not show this.

Box 3.2 Criteria for the ECG diagnosis of right ventricular hypertrophy (RVH)

- Butler–Leggett formula*

Directions	Anterior (A)	Rightward (R)	Posterior–leftward (PL)
Amplitude	Tallest R or R′ in lead V1 or V2	Deepest S in lead V1 or V6	S in lead V1

RVH formula: A + R – PL ≥0.70 mV

- Sokolow–Lyon criteria†

– RVH = R wave in lead V1 + S wave in lead V5 or V6 ≥1.10 mV

Adapted with permission from *Butler PM, Leggett SI, Howe CM et al. Identification of electrocardiographic criteria for diagnosis of right ventricular hypertrophy due to mitral stenosis. *Am J Cardiol* 1986; **57**: 639–43: and from †Sokolow M, Lyon TP. The ventricular complex in right ventricular hypertrophy as obtained by unipolar precordial and limb leads. *Am Heart J* 1949; **38**: 273–94.

Right bundle branch block (Figure 3.7) (see p. 173). The QRS complex is broadened >120 ms. The appearances are usually (although not always) highly characteristic: there is a broad 'M' appearance with the second upstroke much larger than the first.

Old posterior wall 'Q wave' myocardial infarction (Figures 3.8 and 3.9). There are often associated Q waves in the inferior leads.

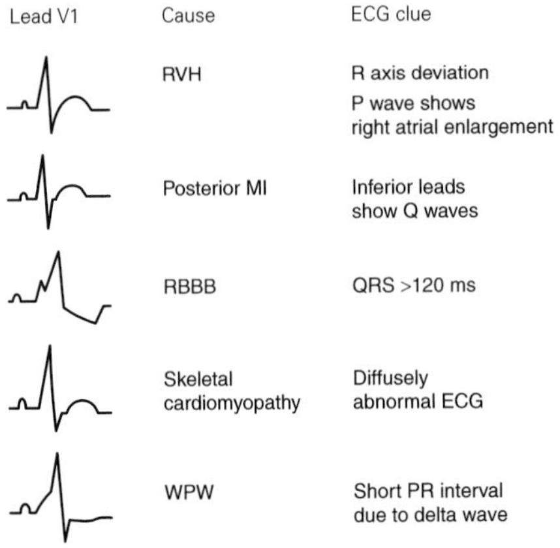

Lead V1	Cause	ECG clue
	RVH	R axis deviation P wave shows right atrial enlargement
	Posterior MI	Inferior leads show Q waves
	RBBB	QRS >120 ms
	Skeletal cardiomyopathy	Diffusely abnormal ECG
	WPW	Short PR interval due to delta wave

Figure 3.7
Different causes of a dominant R wave in lead V1, and ECG patterns. RVH, right ventricular hypertrophy; MI, myocardial infarction; RBBB, right bundle branch block; WPW, Wolff–Parkinson–White syndrome.

Some forms of Wolff–Parkinson–White syndrome (Figure 3.7). A delta wave is seen (see p. 201). Usually this is not a difficult diagnosis to make; adenosine testing may be useful if there is any doubt.

Some cardiomyopathies. These include especially (reputedly) the cardiomyopathies associated with Duchenne muscular dystrophy (Figures 3.7 and 3.10) and Freidrich's ataxia. These diagnoses are established by a physical examination showing skeletal myopathy, by electromyographic studies and by genetic analysis. The ECG is often more sensitive than cardiac ultrasound in detecting early cardiac involvement.

Causes of RVH

Any left-sided heart disease – especially hypertensive heart disease (although the ECG is often then dominated by ECG evidence of LVH). Mitral stenosis is a potent cause of RVH but is rare in the UK.

Chronic lung disease sufficiently severe to have caused pulmonary hypertension. The commonest lung disease to do this is severe chronic obstructive pulmonary disease, which usually has obvious clinical signs (hyperinflation, reduced air entry, wheeze, signs of CO_2 retention, especially bounding peripheral pulses and a 'metabolic' flap). Many other lung diseases can also cause pulmonary hypertension.

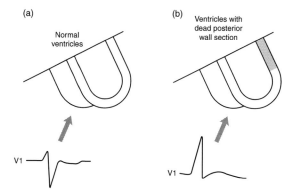

Figure 3.8
Mechanism of a dominant R wave in old posterior myocardial infarction. (a) The normal lead V1 QRS complex shows septal depolarization and prominent late negative deflection from the posterior wall. (b) Lead V1 QRS complex showing the effect of dead posterior wall section: septal depolarization not counterbalanced by any posterior wall depolarization.

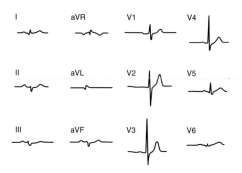

Figure 3.9
Established posterior wall mycardial infarction. There is a dominant R wave in lead V1 and loss of R wave height in the inferior leads (II, III, aVF) and lateral leads (V5, V6) indicating posterior, inferior and lateral infarction. One might expect LV function to be greatly impaired in this patient.

Thromboembolic lung disease.

Primary pulmonary hypertension. This is an exceptionally rare condition.

Unfortunately the ECG in many patients may not change (or may hardly change) despite massive elevations in right heart pressures. Thus if a raised right ventricular (RV) pressure is suspected the ECG must not be relied on to confirm this; noninvasive tests such as cardiac ultrasound should instead be used (RV pressure can be estimated by measuring the velocity of the

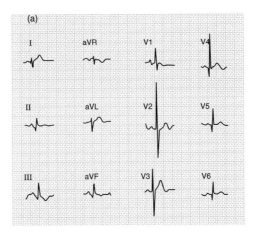

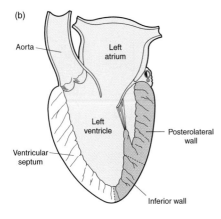

Figure 3.10
Duchenne muscular dystrophy. Despite the abnormal ECG (a), this young man had echocardiographically normal left ventricular function. The principle abnormality is the very tall R wave in lead V1; in addition, the QRS axis is shifted to the right. (b) The distribution of scar tissue in Duchenne muscular dystrophy explains the ECG findings, as the posterolateral wall is particularly heavily infiltrated with scar tissue (denoted by shading).

tricuspid regurgitant jet). If there is insufficient tricuspid regurgitation to calculate RV pressures accurately then invasive studies such as right heart catheterization should be considered.

Decreased R wave amplitude

Just as increased ventricular muscle mass can cause an increase in R wave amplitude, so a decrease in muscle mass can cause a decrease in R wave amplitude. Unfortunately it is not always easy to diagnose a reduced QRS amplitude. Experienced ECG readers become familiar over time with the normal range of QRS complex appearance (by reading several thousand tracings and comparing the ECG findings with the subsequent definitive diagnosis), and are able to spot deviations fairly readily. QRS voltages may be decreased locally (ie only in a few leads, usually reflecting the distribution of coronary arteries) or generally (ie throughout the ECG). The causes of these abnormalities are outlined below.

Local loss of R wave height

This is usually caused by loss of myocytes due to an old MI. Although there are several patterns, the easiest one to diagnose is loss of the anterior chest lead R wave. Instead of the normal steady increase in R wave size as one progresses across the chest leads (see Figure 1.4), leads V1 to V4 show no increase in the height of each succeeding R wave until there is a sudden 'jump' in R wave size. This is known as 'poor anterior R wave progression' (Figure 3.11) and raises the possibility of an old anterior wall MI; however, a late 'transition' point (see Figure 1.4) can also cause poor anterior R wave progression, ie anticlockwise rotation of the heart (a normal variant). In addition, severe LVH can also result in poor anteroseptal R wave

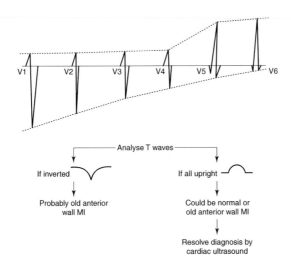

Figure 3.11
Poor anterior R wave progression due to anterior wall myocardial infarction (MI). There is little or no increase in R wave amplitude as one progresses from V1 to V4. Although discrimination from late transition due to anticlockwise rotation can be difficult, the presence or absence of other ECG abnormalities (eg T wave changes) can help make the diagnosis.

progression. When poor anterior R wave progression occurs the diagnosis should always be confirmed using cardiac ultrasound.

Other patterns of R wave loss can affect leads II, III and aVF, reflecting an old inferior wall MI, and leads V5 and V6, reflecting an old lateral wall MI.

Generalized loss of QRS amplitude

There are several causes of generalized loss of QRS amplitude. This usually reflects either generalized loss of ventricular muscle or an increase in the amount of tissue (eg in obesity) or fluid (eg in pericardial effusion) between the heart and the surface electrodes:

Decreased QRS complex amplitude due to generalized loss of ventricular myocytes occurs most commonly in ischaemic cardiomyopathy but may also be due to idiopathic dilated cardiomyopathy. This ECG pattern is usually associated with very poor left ventricular (LV) function. However, the reverse is not true – most patients with very poor LV function (ie ejection fraction ≤20–30%) have rather good R and S waves. Thus if a knowledge of LV function is important to decision-making (and this is usually the case) then it should be determined via cardiac ultrasound, radionucleotide ventriculography or cardiac catheterization.

Hypothyroidism can occasionally cause small QRS complexes. This may be due to myxoedema causing a pericardial effusion or to thyroxine deficiency inhibiting myocyte current generation.

Whenever small QRS complexes are seen it is wise to confirm the exact underlying pathology using clinical examination (especially looking for hypothyroidism, cardiac tamponade and heart failure) and cardiac ultrasound.

Q waves

Q waves occur when an electrode looks at the heart from the inside-out instead of from the usual outside-in perspective (see pp. 7 and 8 and Figure 1.9). Instead of 'seeing' the normal pattern of depolarization spreading towards the electrode from the endocardium to the epicardium (resulting in an R wave), the electrode sees depolarization spreading away from itself from the endocardium to the epicardium (resulting in a Q wave). Thus Q waves result when an electrically neutral 'window' into the middle of the heart exists, through which the electrode looks. Such a situation may have physiological or pathological causes.

Physiological Q waves

The aVR electrode is positioned to look through the atrioventricular valves (which are electrically inert fibrous structures) into the middle of the heart and in health it records deep Q waves. Small physiological Q waves are also found in the left-sided leads as a consequence of septal depolarization (see p. 12).

Pathological Q waves

Pathological Q waves result when an electrically inert area occurs in the ventricular myocardium (Figure 3.12). The commonest cause of this is an

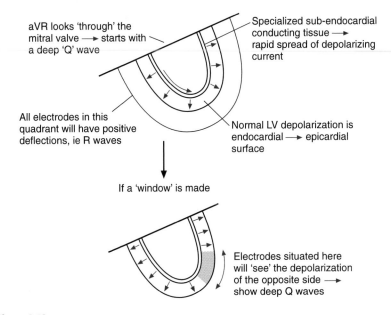

Figure 3.12
Genesis of pathological Q waves. An electrical 'window' (caused by MI-associated scar tissue) allows an electrode to 'see into' the heart and detect endocardial-to-epicardial depolarization of the opposite wall.

old, full-thickness MI. Other causes include myocyte death due to extensive cardiac fibrosis from a cardiomyopathic process, such as old viral myocarditis or idiopathic dilated cardiomyopathy. The pattern of Q waves reflects the pattern of myocardial damage. As an old MI is overwhelmingly the commonest cause, the Q wave pattern usually reflects the distribution of the affected coronary arteries (Figure 3.13), as follows.

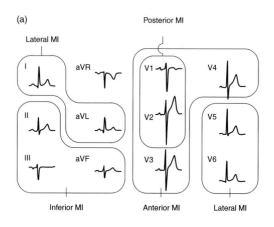

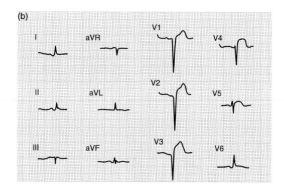

Figure 3.13
Patterns of Q waves found in myocardial infarctions (MIs) in different territories. (a) Distribution of basic patterns. Combinations of these patterns occur in inferolateral, inferoposterior and anterolateral MIs. (b) Anterior MI. There are Q waves from V1 to V3, and a deep S wave in lead V4. The anterior ST segments are still elevated; either this is early on in the course of the MI or there is persisting ST elevation associated with a persistently occluded 'infarct-related' artery and an increased risk of developing a left ventricular aneurysm (although most subjects with persisting ST elevation do not develop an aneurysm).

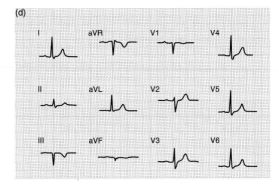

Figure 3.13 (continued)
(c) Inferolateral Q wave MI. There are deep Q waves in the inferior leads; inferiorly and laterally there is persisting ST segment elevation, suggesting that the MI is still relatively young, ie <24 hours or so. (d) A more established old inferior wall MI. There is a deep and pathological Q wave in leads III and aVF. There is no Q wave in lead II. [This pattern (ie Q waves in leads III and aVF but not in lead II) can sometimes be difficult to distinguish from the physiological deep Q wave sometimes seen at certain phases of the respiratory cycle in lead III. It is sometimes impossible on ECG grounds to determine if an old inferior wall MI is present, or whether the ECG is a variant of normal – the distinction could be made using cardiac ultrasound.]

V1 to V4: old anteroseptal MI, often caused by occlusion of one of the major branches of the left anterior descending (LAD) coronary artery such as the first septal perforator or occasionally the first diagonal; more rarely, occlusion of the mid LAD vessel itself.

V5 to V6: lateral MI, often caused by occlusion of a diagonal branch of the LAD; sometimes caused by occlusion of a large ventricular branch of the right coronary artery (RCA) or an obtuse marginal branch of the circumflex artery.

V1 to V5 or V6: often caused by proximal occlusion of the LAD and often associated with substantial impairment of LV function. (However, occasionally LV function in patients with this ECG pattern is found to be only mildly impaired. This illustrates the point that the ECG may suggest a differential diagnosis but only occasionally can it provide a 'cast-iron' diagnosis.)

II, III and aVF: old inferior wall MI, usually due to occlusion of the RCA. However, some 5% of the population have a 'dominant' left circulation (ie the posterior descending artery, which supplies blood to the inferior part of the interventricular septum, originates from the circumflex rather than from the RCA) and in these people Q waves in the inferior leads usually relate to an old circumflex artery occlusion (Figure 3.14).

Q waves from the posterior wall are seen as dominant R waves in lead V1 (Figure 3.15). A posterior wall MI is usually due to circumflex artery

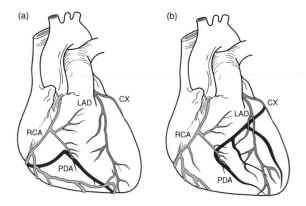

Figure 3.14
(a) Right-dominant and (b) left-dominant coronary artery circulations. The definition of right- or left-dominant circulation depends on whether the posterior descending coronary artery (PDA) arises from the right coronary artery (RCA) or the circumflex branch of the left coronary artery (CX). LAD, left anterior descending artery.

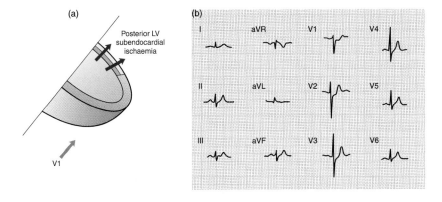

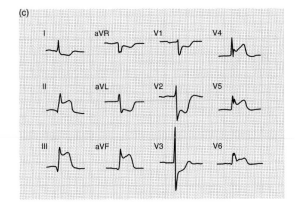

Figure 3.15
Acute posterior wall myocardial infarction (MI) resulting in ST depression in leads V1 and V2. (a) No electrode routinely used looks at the posterior wall from the outside. Thus the effect of a posterior wall MI on the opposing septal wall, which is mainly observed by leads V1 and V2, is used to make the diagnosis. If posterior wall subendocardial ischaemia occurs, a current will flow into the posterior wall subepicardium from the posterior wall subendocardium (so a lead adjacent to the posterior wall subepicardium would show ST elevation). The continuation of this current will flow through the septum, causing ST depression in leads V1 and V2. Lead V6, the most laterally placed lead, does not look at the posterior wall. However, leads extended around the chest to look at the posterior wall – V7, V8 and V9 – would show ST elevation in a posterior MI. (b) Acute posterior wall MI – there is ST depression in leads V1 to V3. This is often very difficult to differentiate from anterior wall ST depression, especially if, as here, there is no associated inferior wall MI. Often the true diagnosis only becomes apparent with time. The subsequent ECG (Figure 3.9) showed an established posterior wall MI, with a dominant R wave in lead V1. (c) Sometimes the ECG changes are so gross as to be patently obvious. This ECG shows an inferior, lateral and posterior wall MI due to a very large occlusion of the right coronary artery. Surprisingly, the patient survived their index admission with this electrocadiographically vast MI.

occlusion but occasionally is caused by blockage in a very dominant RCA. These two causes can be differentiated on ECG grounds: RCA occlusion often leads to an inferior wall MI (ie ST and Q waves in leads II, III and aVF) whereas a pure circumflex territory MI does not usually cause such changes.

The key to determining the cause of Q waves (in addition to history, examination, etc) is cardiac ultrasound. Demonstration of damage localized to certain areas of the heart usually (but not always) indicates coronary artery disease.

Chapter 4
ST segment and T wave abnormalities

ST segment changes

Characteristic changes occur to the ST segment in certain diseases [eg myocardial infarction (MI) and pericarditis]. These can be very useful in diagnosis and in following the response to treatment (eg thrombolytic efficacy in acute MI).

The normal ST segment

The ST segment is normally isoelectric with the baseline. This is because current flow between different parts of the heart is required to create movement in the ECG trace, and this only occurs when the ventricle is either partially depolarized or partially repolarized.

During the normal ST segment (which follow the QRS complex and lasts until the start of the T wave) the heart is fully depolarized, no current flows and the ECG trace is thus isoelectric with the baseline.

Likewise, when the heart is fully repolarized, as during the TP interval, no ECG signal is normally generated and the ECG signal is again isoelectric with the baseline.

Physiological ST segment elevation

For unclear reasons some 2–3% of the normal population have 'fixed' ST elevation in leads V2 and V3 throughout their life (Figure 4.1). This 'physiological' ST segment elevation is a normal variant and has no pathological significance (Figure 4.2a). This can occasionally cause diagnostic difficulties if such patients present to casualty departments with chest pain. The easiest way to determine if ST segment elevation is pathological or not is to compare the current ECG with an old one. Clearly this option is not always available, and in the absence of an old ECG other distinguishing features should be used: history (absence of ischaemic chest pain), demographics (low risk of epicardial coronary artery disease), physical examination (absence of a third heart sound S3), and the exact pattern of ECG changes may all help establish this completely benign diagnosis. If doubt remains, a cardiac ultrasound may help achieve a diagnosis (in ST segment elevation due to MI the affected territory moves less well than normal, or not at all). Another cause of ST segment elevation in leads V1 to V3 is the Brugada syndrome (Figure 4.2d: V1 trace), a rare inherited condition in which there is a predisposition to (lethal) ventricular arrhythmias (see p. 212). In Brugada syndrome the ST elevation is so bizarre that it cannot really be confused with 'physiological' ST elevation.

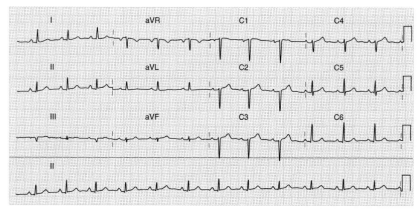

Figure 4.1
'Physiological' ST segment elevation – not always an easy diagnosis. Although this ECG does show physiological anterior lead ST segment elevation (V1, V2, V3), it also shows poor anterior R wave progression (due to a late 'transition' point). In this situation it is often difficult to know if the anterior ST segment elevation reflects myocardial ischaemia or is benign – a cardiac ultrasound often resolves the issue.

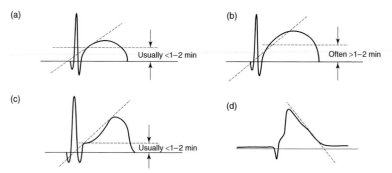

Figure 4.2
Different forms of ST segment elevation. (a) 'Physiological' ST segment elevation: 'concave downwards'; usually only found in leads V1 to V4; and usually a clear transition point. (b) Myocardial infarction: 'concave downwards'; can occur in any lead (follows distribution of coronary arteries); and often no clear transition point (ie no clear demarcation between the end of the QRS complex and the start of the ST segment). (c) Pericarditis: 'concave upwards'; usually in anterolateral leads; and can be very widespread. (d) Brugada syndrome: 'ski slope' appearance; usually only in leads V1 to V3; and often shows a 'terminal bump'.

Pathological ST segment changes

In disease the ST segment can change in several ways: ST elevation or depression can occur, as can 'ST flattening' (although the principal abnormality here is flattening of the T wave rather than any change to the ST segment itself). ST segment changes occur in the distribution of whatever part of the heart is damaged. The processes underlying ST segment changes are rather speculative, but the following presents the basic pathophysiological mechanisms.

ST segment elevation

ST segment elevation (Figure 4.3a, b) implies that when the heart is fully depolarized (ie just after the QRS complex) current continues to flow within the area of the damaged tissue from the endocardium to the epicardium (and then on towards the electrode). This occurs when the epicardium is less depolarized than the endocardium during this phase of the cardiac cycle. What can cause this? The initial depolarized membrane potential is largely set by the difference between the concentrations of sodium either side of the myocyte membrane (according to the Nernst equation). If the internal concentration of sodium rises (which it will if the cell is unhealthy and unable to expel sodium efficiently) the depolarized membrane potential is decreased: less Na^+ will enter the cell with each action potential, leaving more positive charge outside. Negative charge (as electrons) will flow into such an area. Thus if it is the epicardium that is less healthy than the endocardium then current will continue to flow towards the epicardium from the endocardium following depolarization. Furthermore the reverse will apply when the heart is repolarized: the resting membrane potential (determined by the difference between potassium concentrations on either side of the membrane) will be more positive (and less negative) than normal (as the cell will not be able to pump potassium back into itself), so current will flow in the reverse direction, ie from the epicardium to the endocardium. Thus the apparent isoelectric line will be depressed, exaggerating the amount of ST segment elevation seen after depolarization. Therefore ST segment elevation implies a sick epicardium, or at least an epicardium sicker than the endocardium.

ST segment 'flattening'

A flattened T wave is a nonspecific abnormality found in many conditions, including MI, cardiomyopathy and hyperventilation. Pathophysiologically,

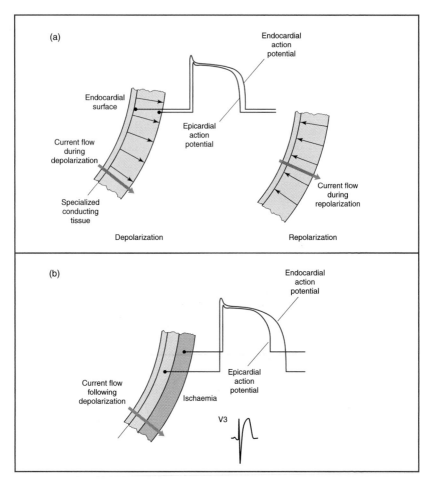

epi–endocardial differences in action potential duration have been minimized in this condition (see below). Thus there is no current flow between the different parts of the heart during repolarization and the resulting T wave is flat.

ST segment depression

The reverse of the explanation for ST segment elevation applies to ST segment depression (Figure 4.3c): ie following complete depolarization of the ventricle, current continues to flow from the epicardium to the endocardium (ie away from the observing electrode). This will occur if the myocardium adjacent to the endocardium is not as healthy as that adjacent

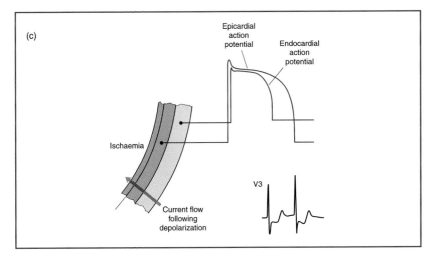

Figure 4.3

Mechanism of ST segment elevation and depression. (a) Normal spread of depolarization and repolarization. The direction of repolarization is epicardial-to-endocardial, as the epicardial action potential finishes earlier. As repolarization moves positive charge outside the cell, electrons (ie current) flow into the repolarized areas from yet-to-be repolarized areas, causing an upright T wave. (b) Mechanism of ST segment elevation in subepicardial myocardial ischaemia. In the ischaemic area less positive charge enters the cells with each action potential, creating an excess external positive charge outside the myocytes. Electrons (ie current) thus flow from the endo- to the epicardium, causing ST segment elevation. (c) Mechanism of ST segment depression in subendocardial myocardial ischaemia. Ischaemic cells at rest are partially depolarized, and so less positive charge enters the cell with each action potential, creating an excess of positive extracellular charge, so electrons (ie current) flow from the epi- to the endocardium, causing ST segment depression. As the endocardial action potentials shorten with ischaemia, repolarization proceeds from endo- to epicardium, so the T wave becomes inverted.

to the epicardium, so that the depolarized potential of the endocardial cells is less positive than the depolarized potential of the epicardial cells (such as occurs if endocardial cells are unable to extrude sodium as effectively as epicardial cells). In leads showing ST segment depression the T wave is also often inverted. The reason for this is as follows. Unhealthy cells usually have shortened action potentials. In health endocardial action potentials are longer than epicardial action potentials, thus accounting for the vector of the normal T wave. However, in disease endocardial action potentials become shorter than epicardial ones, the vector of repolarization reverses and the vector of the T wave reverses on the surface ECG. Thus in the leads in which ST segment depression occurs T wave inversion is also often seen.

Pathological causes of ST segment elevation

There are two principal pathological causes of acute ST segment elevation.

Acute full thickness MI (Figure 4.2b) due to occlusion of a major epicardial coronary artery. It is thought that during a full thickness MI the epicardium is sicker than the endocardium. Why this should be so is speculative; it may be that the epicardium is more ischaemic than the endocardium. It is important to realize that although many MIs cause ST segment elevation during the acute phase [ST segment elevation MIs (STEMIs)], there are many MIs that do not (so-called non-STEMIs). The consequences of this are outlined in Chapter 10.

Acute pericarditis (Figure 4.2c). In this situation the pathophysiology is easier to understand. Acute pericarditis results in damage to the myocardium immediately adjacent to the inflamed pericardium, ie damage to myocytes adjacent to the epicardial ventricular surface. Due to this damage, these myocytes lose their ability to expel sodium in a normal fashion. As the amount of depolarization is determined (according to the Nernst equation) by the difference between intra- and extracellular sodium concentrations, this means that 'sick' myocardial cells adjacent to the myocardium will, in their depolarized state following the QRS complex, be less depolarized than the more distant healthy endocardial cells. Current therefore flows into the epicardium from the endocardium throughout systole, and ST segment elevation results.

Unsurprisingly, the exact pattern of ST segment elevation in these two conditions differs: in acute MI the ST elevation is 'concave downwards' whereas in acute pericarditis it is 'concave upwards' ('saddle-shaped') (Figure 4.2b, c). This difference is not always present, however, and in establishing the diagnosis the clinical features (risk factors for coronary disease, nature of the chest pain, presence of a pericardial rub) are often as important as the exact pattern of ST segment elevation. If doubt remains then a cardiac ultrasound should be used to establish the diagnosis: in acute pericarditis left ventricular function is normal and there may be a small rim of pericardial fluid; in acute MI the affected territory moves poorly if at all.

Another useful way to distinguish the ST segment elevation of pericarditis from that of MI is the distribution of ECG changes (Figure 4.4): in acute pericarditis ST elevation often occurs in many ECG leads (eg more than six) and is relatively mild (ie usually ≤2 mm); whereas in acute MI (see below) the ST elevation is usually (but not always) more substantial (ie ≥2–3 mm) and is usually found in only a few leads (commonly four or less). If widespread ST segment elevation is due to an MI, the infarct is usually large and the patient is usually fairly 'sick', whereas in pericarditis with similarly extensive ECG changes the patient is usually fairly well.

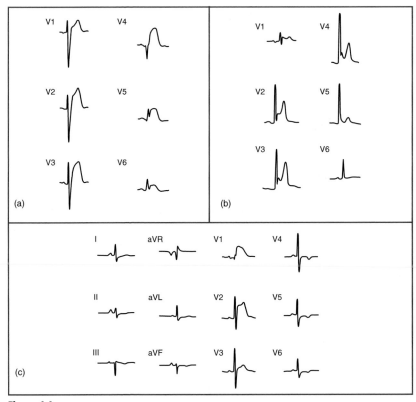

Figure 4.4
Different ECG patterns associated with different causes of ST segment elevation. (a) Anterior wall ST segment elevation myocardial infarction. (b) Pericarditis with 'concave-upwards' ST segment elevation. (c) Brugada syndrome. There is ST segment elevation in leads V1 to V3. (Unusually, there is also T wave inversion laterally – this was due to coincident ischaemia arising from a ruptured plaque in the mid-left anterior descending coronary artery.)

ST segment and T wave changes in myocardial infarction

Acute ST segment elevation myocardial infarction

The pattern of ST segment elevation in acute STEMI corresponds to which artery is occluded (Figure 4.5):

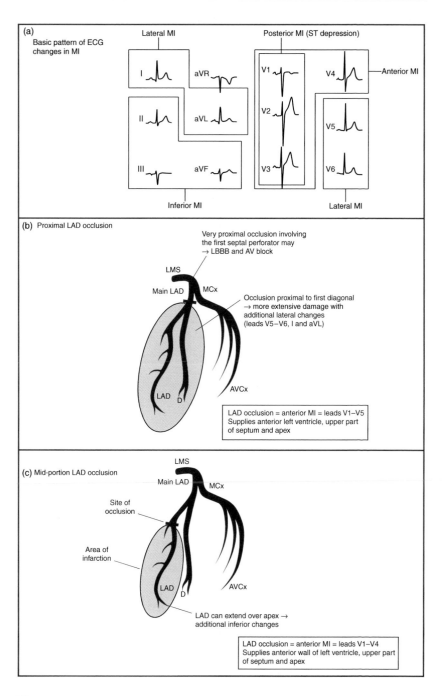

(a) Basic pattern of ECG changes in MI

Lateral MI

Posterior MI (ST depression)

I

aVR

V1

V4 ———Anterior MI

II

aVL

V2

V5

III

aVF

V3

V6

Inferior MI

Lateral MI

(b) Proximal LAD occlusion

Very proximal occlusion involving the first septal perforator may → LBBB and AV block

LMS

Main LAD   MCx

Occlusion proximal to first diagonal → more extensive damage with additional lateral changes (leads V5–V6, I and aVL)

AVCx

LAD D

LAD occlusion = anterior MI = leads V1–V5
Supplies anterior left ventricle, upper part of septum and apex

(c) Mid-portion LAD occlusion

LMS

Main LAD   MCx

Site of occlusion

Area of infarction

LAD D

AVCx

LAD can extend over apex → additional inferior changes

LAD occlusion = anterior MI = leads V1–V4
Supplies anterior wall of left ventricle, upper part of septum and apex

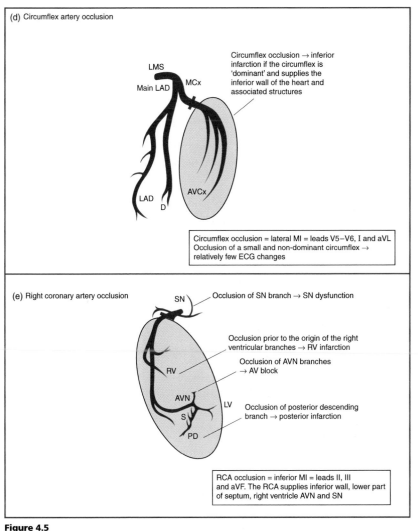

(d) Circumflex artery occlusion

LMS

Main LAD

MCx

Circumflex occlusion → inferior infarction if the circumflex is 'dominant' and supplies the inferior wall of the heart and associated structures

LAD

D

AVCx

Circumflex occlusion = lateral MI = leads V5–V6, I and aVL
Occlusion of a small and non-dominant circumflex → relatively few ECG changes

(e) Right coronary artery occlusion

SN

Occlusion of SN branch → SN dysfunction

Occlusion prior to the origin of the right ventricular branches → RV infarction

Occlusion of AVN branches → AV block

RV

AVN

LV

S

Occlusion of posterior descending branch → posterior infarction

PD

RCA occlusion = inferior MI = leads II, III and aVF. The RCA supplies inferior wall, lower part of septum, right ventricle AVN and SN

Figure 4.5

Pattern of ECG changes in myocardial infarcts (MIs) due to occlusion of different arteries. (a) Basic patterns. Combinations of these patterns occur in inferolateral, inferoposterior and anterolateral MIs. (b) ECG changes associated with proximal left anterior descending coronary artery (LAD) occlusion. (c) Pattern associated with mid LAD occlusion. (d) Pattern associated with circumflex artery occlusion. (e) Patterns associated with right coronary artery occlusion. SN, sinoatrial node; LBBB, left bundle branch block; AV, atrioventricular; LMS, left main stem; MCx, main circumflex coronary artery; D, first diagonal branch of LAD coronary artery; AVCx, atrioventricular circumflex coronary artery; RV, right ventricle; AVN, atrioventricular node; S, septal perforator; PD, posterior descending branch of right coronary artery; LV, left ventricle. Reprinted with permission from Davies C, Bashir Y. *Cardiovascular Emergencies*. London: BMJ, 2001.

V1 to V3: anteroseptal MI often due to the occlusion of the left anterior descending coronary artery (LAD; or one of its branches, eg the septal perforator or the first diagonal).

V1/V2 to V4, V5 or V6: anterolateral MI, due to occlusion of the proximal LAD.

V3 to V4: often due to occlusion of a diagonal branch of the LAD.

V4 to V6: lateral MI usually due to occlusion of a branch of the circumflex coronary artery or the left ventricular branch of the right coronary artery (RCA).

Leads II, III and aVF: inferior wall MI due to occlusion of the RCA (or, in the 2–3% of the population who have dominant circumflex coronary arteries, to occlusion of the circumflex coronary artery).

Posterior wall myocardial infarct

Like any infarct, a posterior wall MI causes ST elevation in those leads that 'look' at the heart from the outside, and the reverse (ie ST depression) in those leads that look at the heart from the inside. None of the standard leads looks at the posterior wall from the outside; thus in pure posterior wall MI no leads show ST elevation. However, leads V1 and often V2 look at the posterior wall from the inside, and thus show ST depression in a posterior wall MI.

The posterior wall of the left ventricle is supplied partly by the left ventricular branch of the RCA, which also supplies the inferior wall (thus posterior wall MI often occurs in conjunction with an inferior wall MI) and partly by the circumflex artery (thus a circumflex artery occlusion usually results in a posterior wall MI). Curiously, although the circumflex artery is nondominant in 95% of individuals (ie the posterior descending artery arises from the RCA), circumflex artery occlusion not infrequently results in inferior lead ST segment elevation. The clue that an inferior wall STEMI relates to circumflex artery occlusion is to be found in the exact pattern of inferior lead ST segment elevation: greater ST segment elevation in lead II than in lead III suggests RCA occlusion, whereas greater ST segment elevation in lead III than in lead II suggests circumflex artery occlusion. Many circumflex artery occlusions do not result in an inferior wall MI, but they may cause a 'pure' posterior wall MI (Figures 3.9 and 4.6).

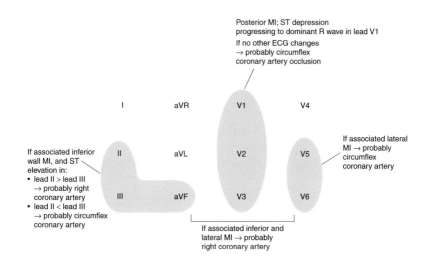

Posterior MI; ST depression progressing to dominant R wave in lead V1
If no other ECG changes → probably circumflex coronary artery occlusion

If associated lateral MI → probably circumflex coronary artery

If associated inferior wall MI, and ST elevation in:
• lead II > lead III → probably right coronary artery
• lead II < lead III → probably circumflex coronary artery

If associated inferior and lateral MI → probably right coronary artery

Figure 4.6
Different patterns of posterior wall myocardial infarction (MI) due to occlusion of the right or circumflex coronary artery.

Right ventricular myocardial infarct

Right ventricular (RV) infarcts are due to occlusion of the RV marginal branch of the RCA. A RV MI is seen electrocardiographically as ST segment elevation in the right-sided chest leads. These are not routinely used, but should be in every patient with an inferior wall MI.

There are two important consequences of RV infarction. First, affected patients need high 'filling' pressures and can rapidly go into a low-cardiac-output state with renal failure if 'over-diuresed and under-filled'. Second, as the RV marginal branch arises very early on in the course of the RCA, an RV MI is due to a proximal occlusion of the RCA and hence is usually associated with a large inferior wall MI (usually obvious electrocardiographically) with adverse long-term consequences.

Evolution of ECG changes in STEMI

The ECG changes sequentially as the MI evolves (Figure 4.7).

The ECG may initially be normal!

Although most patients with acute MI show some ECG changes at presentation, some 2–5% will have a normal ECG. A large trial examining the role of thrombolytic therapy in acute MI [the International Study of Infarct Survival (ISIS) 2] showed that these patients, like those with ST segment elevation MI, benefit from thrombolytic treatment (in this case streptokinase). Furthermore, MI patients who initially present with a normal ECG can have many of the standard complications of an MI, including acute phase ventricular arrhythmias, which are clearly lethal if not treated

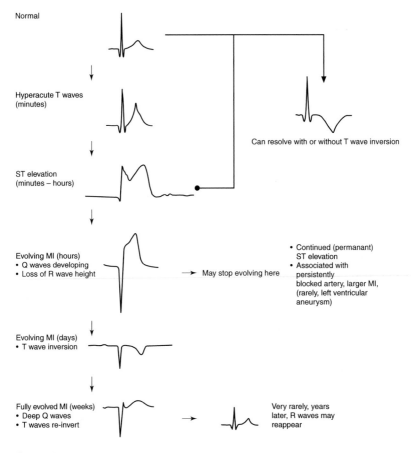

Normal

Hyperacute T waves
(minutes)

Can resolve with or without T wave inversion

ST elevation
(minutes – hours)

Evolving MI (hours)
• Q waves developing
• Loss of R wave height

May stop evolving here

• Continued (permanant)
  ST elevation
• Associated with
  persistently
  blocked artery, larger MI,
  (rarely, left ventricular
  aneurysm)

Evolving MI (days)
• T wave inversion

Fully evolved MI (weeks)
• Deep Q waves
• T waves re-invert

Very rarely, years
later, R waves may
reappear

Figure 4.7
Evolution of ECG changes following a myocardial infarction (MI).

promptly. Patients should thus not be discharged home from the emergency room solely on the basis that a normal ECG negates MI, as it clearly does not!

This again emphasizes the importance of history-taking in making a diagnosis. The ECG should be used to complement the clinical history, not as a definitive test considered in isolation from the clinical situation.

Early T wave changes

In the first few minutes after a coronary artery occlusion has commenced an MI, the T waves may become tall and peaked. The reasons for this are unclear; it may be that the earliest effect of myocardial ischaemia is to shorten the already short duration of the subepicardial cell action potential, increasing epi–endocardial differences and so increasing current flow during the repolarization phase of the cardiac cycle. These tall peaked T waves are often the very earliest ECG evidence of an MI and usually only occur very early on, resolving as the MI progresses; they are therefore termed 'hyperacute T wave changes'. They are rarely observed, probably because most patients present after this very acute phase.

ST segment elevation

After the first few minutes of a coronary artery occlusion, ST segment elevation occurs (as above), usually resolving over the next 6–18 hours. Resolution of ST segment elevation implies that the epi–endocardial potential differences have resolved, either because the infarct-related artery (IRA) has reopened (spontaneously or due to the effects of treatment) or, conversely, because the whole of the territory supplied by the IRA has died. These two radically different outcomes can be distinguished electrocardiographically by observing the state of the R wave and whether or not Q waves have appeared. Well-sized R waves and no Q waves imply early patency of the IRA and viability of the tissue in the area supplied by it. Conversely, poorly-sized R waves and/or new Q waves imply persistent occlusion and a substantial-sized infarct (see below).

Resolution of ST segment elevation

Studies have shown that the speed of resolution of ST segment elevation during an MI is related to the patency of the IRA. Techniques differ, but often the total amount of ST segment elevation in the one (or three) leads with the greatest ST elevation is measured: ≤50% decrease in the amount of ST segment elevation in the 90 minutes after giving a thrombolytic indicates a high chance of the IRA being persistently occluded; conversely a ≥50% resolution of ST segment elevation >90 minutes post thrombolysis is associated with IRA patency. Unsurprisingly, failure of the elevated ST segments to resolve in ≤90 minutes is associated with a larger infarct size and thus a higher mortality.

Failure of the ST segment to resolve implies continued occlusion of the IRA. Consequentially, it may be that more aggressive methods should be deployed to open the artery [eg further thrombolytic treatment (although the efficacy of this approach is unknown) or 'salvage' angioplasty]. Also, as the infarct is larger and more complete (ie more of the cells in the IRA territory have died), the development of a left ventricular aneurysm is more likely, particularly with an anterior MI (however, most patients with persistent ST segment elevation do not develop an aneurysm).

R wave amplitude decreases as the infarct progresses

This may occur fairly quickly (over minutes to hours) as the infarct progresses. The amount of loss of the R wave relates to the size of infarct: small infarcts show little or no loss of R wave; medium-sized infarcts show more substantial R wave loss; and in large infarcts Q waves usually develop and R waves disappear (see below).

However, like many ECG signs, loss of the R wave is not entirely reliable in determining infarct size, as occasionally quite large infarcts can have surprisingly little loss of R wave and vice versa. To reliably establish left ventricular function post MI, cardiac ultrasound should be used.

Q wave development

Q waves can appear in the infarcted territory, usually 12–36 hours after the onset of the MI. Infarcts associated with Q waves are termed, un-surprisingly, 'Q wave MIs' (sometimes 'full thickness MIs', a phrase implying the death of substantial numbers of myocytes). Q waves indicate a significant-sized MI, and benefit from angiotensin-converting enzyme inhibitor drugs, certainly in anterior MI and often in inferior MI. As no ECG lead looks at the posterior wall, a Q wave posterior wall MI cannot be seen directly. However, lead V1 looks, via the septum, at the posterior wall from the inside. Loss of the 'negative' current flow from the posterior wall will then allow the 'positive' septal current to dominate. Thus a Q wave posterior wall MI will result in a dominant R wave in V1 (see Figure 3.9).

Q waves usually indicate the permanent death of myocytes in the territory of the IRA. In most patients Q waves are permanent, but in a few they may disappear, over the course of many years. Indeed, occasionally the ECG can, to all intents and purposes, return to normal! This implies that the 'electrical window' on the heart caused by the infarct-related scar tissue has disappeared. The explanation for why Q waves can disappear is theoretical; one view is that the old infarct scar tissue becomes repopulated with significant numbers of healthy myocytes arising from hypertrophy within islands of cells remaining after the MI or (much more speculatively) from division of these cells or the migration of healthy cells from beyond the infarct into the infarct zone. Previously it had been believed that adult myocytes could not divide or move; an increasing body of work suggests that this old view is incorrect, and the disappearance of Q waves may provide indirect evidence to support this new theory.

T wave changes

Late T wave changes in Q wave MIs. As the initial ST segment elevation resolves, the T wave usually inverts, 12–36 hours after the onset of an MI. These inverted T waves usually return to their normal upright morphology 2–7 days after the onset of the MI. Persistent T wave inversion can occur; in a significantly sized infarct (ie in those with Q waves or substantial loss of R wave height) the significance of this is uncertain.

Deep T wave inversion with persistently good R waves: aborted or threatened MI. Transient ST segment elevation (≤30 min) without loss of R waves or the appearance of Q waves followed by deep T wave inversion is typical of an aborted (if thrombolytic treatment has been given) or threatened (no thrombolytic treatment given) infarct (Figure 4.7). The presence of persistent T wave inversion in this situation is associated with a high-grade stenosis (with superimposed thrombus) in the supplying artery and a high risk of early reinfarction. An aborted or threatened MI T wave inversion following transient ST segment elevation is thus conventionally taken as an indication for early coronary angiography.

ECG estimation of infarct size in ST segment elevation acute coronary syndromes

Several ECG features allow estimation of the size of the (threatened) STEMI:

- How widespread are ECG changes? The more leads showing ST segment elevation, the larger the MI.
- How much ST segment elevation is present? The greater the total amount of ST segment elevation, the larger the MI.
- Distribution: anterior MIs generally tend to be larger than inferior ones, which in turn are larger than circumflex territory MIs (see below). This reflects the size of the territory supplied by the different arteries.
- Degree of resolution of ST segment elevation with thrombolysis: the quicker the resolution, the more likely the infarct-related artery is to be patent and the less the degree of myocardial damage.
- The appearance of widespread and deep Q waves indicates a large infarct.

Non-ST segment elevation myocardial infarction

As previously stated, it is important to realize that 40–60% of MIs are not associated with ST segment elevation. Although the diagnosis of MI can often be made on clinical grounds, it is vital to differentiate STEMIs from non-STEMIs as the former benefit from thrombolytic therapy whereas the latter benefit from very aggressive antiplatelet therapy and often from early intervention. What ECG patterns may patients with non-STEMI show?

- The ECG may be normal – this is very unusual but possible.
- T wave flattening or inversion may occur (usually in the distribution of whichever coronary artery is affected).
- ST segment depression is a common finding.
- Intermittent, self-resolving ST segment elevation can also occur.

Why distinguish between STEMI and non-STEMI?

It is crucial to separate out these different groups as their treatment is radically different. STEMIs benefit from thrombolytic therapy but not from 'intensive' antiplatelet therapy (other than aspirin), while non-STEMIs do not benefit from thrombolytic therapy but do benefit from intensive antiplatelet therapy and early angiography with a view to revascularization.

Risk stratification in myocardial infarction

See pp. 232 and 234.

Causes of ST segment depression

ST segment depression is one of the commonest ECG abnormalities (Figure 4.8). The common causes include:

- myocardial ischaemia, including that due to atheromatous macrovascular coronary artery disease (a progressive and potentially lethal disease process) or to microvascular disease (syndrome X, or microvascular angina; often a benign process associated with a normal life span)
- left ventricular hypertrophy
- primary heart muscle disease (cardiomyopathy)
- drugs, especially digoxin
- hyperventilation
- unknown.

These diseases can also cause T wave abnormalities, including T wave flattening and inversion, instead of ST segment depression (see below). This illustrates a basic principle of using the ECG to evaluate cardiac disease (which can be quite frustrating to the newcomer): a particular ECG abnormality can have many causes and a particular disease process can cause many different ECG abnormalities. Thus, although the pattern of ST segment depression may

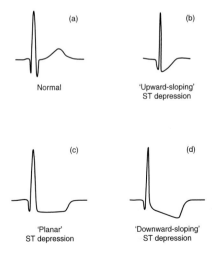

(a) Normal

(b) 'Upward-sloping' ST depression

(c) 'Planar' ST depression

(d) 'Downward-sloping' ST depression

Figure 4.8
Different patterns of ST segment depression associated with different disease processes.

differ between the different illnesses above, which can be useful diagnostically, no one pattern is associated exclusively with any one disease (Figure 4.8). Bearing this warning in mind, the pattern of ST segment depression can however be used to order one's differential diagnosis, but establishing the correct diagnosis relies ultimately on a comprehensive assessment of the clinical situation, not just on the ECG changes themselves.

Myocardial ischaemia and ST segment depression

Angina (due to coronary artery narrowing not occlusion) is held conventionally to cause more ischaemia to the endocardium than the epicardium, whereas infarction (due to total occlusion of a coronary artery) causes more ischaemia to the epicardium than the endocardium (Figure 4.3). Ischaemia interferes with cell function, raising the intracellular sodium concentration (which reduces the membrane potential following depolarization) and lowering the intracellular potassium concentration (which raises the resting membrane potential). If the resting potential is higher and the depolarized potential lower then fewer sodium ions will flow into the cell during depolarization, resulting in excess extracellular positive charge.

This basic pathophysiology of angina means that during episodes of ischaemia endocardial cells in their depolarized state have a lower positive potential than do epicardial cells. In other words, less positive charge has flowed into the endocardial cells, so there is an excess of positive charge external to them. Electrons from around the epicardial cells will thus flow towards the endocardial cells to neutralize this positive charge. This will be seen on the ECG as ST segment depression.

The amount of ST segment depression relates to the severity of endocardial ischaemia at the time the ECG was recorded and does not necessarily indicate how much ischaemia can potentially occur at other times. It is vital to understand that in coronary disease the amount of ST segment depression reflects active ischaemia (ie current, ongoing oxygen deprivation to the ventricular myocytes) and not the extent or severity of coronary disease *per se*. Thus a patient at rest, free of chest pain (ie with no angina and thus no myocardial ischaemia), may often have a completely normal ECG even in the presence of widespread (indeed critical) coronary disease. This is a key point: a normal ECG at rest does not rule out critical coronary disease. This greatly limits the value of the resting ECG in detecting coronary artery disease and is why the exercise ECG was developed (see Chapter 11).

ST segment changes with chest pain and angiographically normal coronary arteries

Some patients presenting with chest pain have ST segment depression on an exercise ECG but 'normal' coronary arteries on angiography. Several pathophysiological theories have been suggested, but most cardiologists consider that these patients fall into one of two groups.

Group I comprises patients who have a 'disorder of the coronary microcirculation', meaning they cannot 'relax' the resistance blood vessels in the coronary microcirculation during exercise. Thus coronary blood flow cannot increase with exercise, resulting in myocardial ischaemia with its symptoms and ECG changes. Some researchers have termed this condition 'microvascular angina' or 'syndrome X'. Most cardiologists consider that a diagnosis of 'microvascular angina' requires typical symptoms (ie a 'tight' or 'squeezing' retrosternal sensation, not present before exercise, provoked by effort and rapidly and totally relieved by rest) and typical ST segment changes as well as normal coronary arteries at angiography. Such cases do occur but they are rare.

Group II comprises those patients with ST segment depression and normal coronary arteries who do not have myocardial ischaemia but do have another benign cause for the ECG changes, such as hyperventilation (see below) or excess catecholamine release (from anxiety, physical deconditioning or both). These physiological changes are commonly found in anxious, depressed people with noncardiac chest pain and may be a more likely explanation for the ST segment changes in this group of patients than myocardial ischaemia. Many patients in this group have atypical features to their chest pain (eg unusual site or nature, unclear relationship to effort, or prolonged duration) and a paucity of risk factors for atheromatous coronary disease. Such cases are very common. Most cardiologists would not regard these patients as suffering from 'microvascular angina' and would rather diagnose them as having noncardiac chest pain.

Left ventricular hypertrophy and ST segment depression

ST segment depression is quite frequently caused by left ventricular hypertrophy (LVH). As the severity of LVH increases, the ST segment in the anterolateral chest leads (ie leads I, aVL and V4 to V6) changes: the amplitude of the T wave initially diminishes and subsequently the ST segment becomes depressed. ST segment depression in LVH was previously termed 'strain' (as in 'LVH with strain'); it is now termed a 'repolarization abnormality'. In LVH due to hypertension the presence of these repolarization abnormalities is associated with more severe hypertrophy and a dramatically worsened prognosis (Figure 4.9), implying that hypertension control has been poor and should be substantially improved.

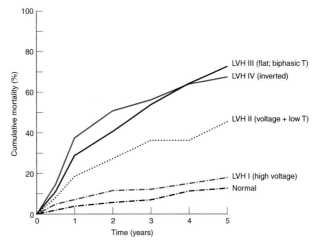

Figure 4.9
Prognosis in hypertension relating to the resting 12-lead ECG. Relationship between degree of electrocardiographic left ventricular hypertrophy and outcome in the premodern treatment era. Adapted with permission from Sokolow M, Perloff D. The prognosis of essential hypertension treated conservatively. *Circulation* 1961; **23**: 697.

ST segment changes in cardiomyopathy

Cardiomyopathy ('primary disease of heart muscle') very commonly causes both ST segment flattening and depression. However, these changes are often very nonspecific and the differential diagnosis is wide. Clues indicating cardiomyopathy as the cause of ST segment changes include the following.

The symptoms are characteristic of cardiomyopathy (especially breathlessness) rather than of coronary disease (ie chest pain), and there is a very different clinical picture (eg the patient may be young and known to have a skeletal myopathic process or a high alcohol intake).

There are very widespread ST segment changes that do not follow the distribution of a particular coronary artery. In dilated cardiomyopathy it is not uncommon to see ST segment changes in all the precordial leads. However, such widespread ST segment changes are unfortunately not exclusively found in cardiomyopathy; they may occur in extensive coronary disease (eg multiple previous acute coronary syndromes in different territories) or previous pericarditis.

Q waves are rare in most cardiomyopathies but common in coronary disease.

Clearly one cannot diagnose most cardiomyopathies confidently from the ECG alone; the best way to establish the diagnosis is cardiac ultrasound.

Drugs affecting the ST segment

Many drugs can affect the ST segment; the most archetypal is digoxin, which classically causes anterolateral ST segment depression (in a 'downward tick' pattern; see Figure 4.8d), although this is not found in all patients. The distribution of ST segment depression mimics that found in LVH, being in leads I, II, aVL and V4 to V6. Clues that digoxin is the cause of these changes come from:

- drug history
- presence of atrial fibrillation; if sinus rhythm is found then digoxin has usually been prescribed for chronic heart failure and patients have relevant symptoms (breathlessness, effort intolerance, possibly weight loss) and an ECG compatible with heart failure (see Chapter 6)
- distribution of ECG changes (see above)
- morphology of the ST segment (digoxin often causes a 'reversed tick' pattern of ST depression; however this ST pattern can also be caused by LVH and coronary disease – the history and clinical examination will enable differentiation).

Many other drugs can also cause ST changes, especially ST depression, including:

- antiarrhythmics, particularly class I drugs
- psychotropics, including antidepressants and antipsychotics
- antihistamines.

ST segment changes are more marked when drugs are taken in high dose or in overdose.

ST segment changes in hyperventilation

The ST segment can be dramatically affected by hyperventilation (Figure 4.10). Indeed, hyperventilation is an extraordinarily common and much under-diagnosed cause of ST segment depression; this is true both in health and in disease.

In healthy volunteers who overbreathe, deep, downsloping ST segment depression can occur, exactly mimicking ST segment changes due to coronary disease. Although overt (and thus obvious) overbreathing is rare, covert overbreathing is relatively common – it is a normal physiological response to pain. Thus 'false-positive' ST segment depression (ie ST depression in a normal heart) may occur in some patients due to subclinical hyperventilation.

Unfortunately, hyperventilation-induced ST segment changes are most common in the very situation where the ECG is most needed, ie in the emergency room. Patients typically present with noncardiac chest pain that has provoked great anxiety and in turn hyperventilation. This hyperventilation is usually not accompanied by obvious tachypnoea. The diagnosis is usually made from the history rather than the ECG, where ST segment depression can dramatically mimic that of coronary disease. Sometimes the diagnosis is obvious (eg in young women with classic noncardiac chest pain), but more often it involves a difficult process of exclusion. The unwary can fall into the trap of informing the patient on the basis of the ECG changes alone that they have severe heart disease, causing enormous difficulties when the true diagnosis is established. Again, the ECG must be used in conjunction with the clinical features to make a diagnosis, never in isolation.

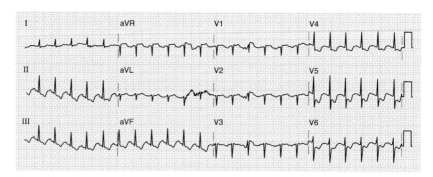

Figure 4.10
Hyperventilation. This patient had frequent panic attacks, during one of which this ECG was recorded. There was no evidence of any coronary artery disease, despite the very dramatic ST segment depression. Once her anxiety had subsided, the ECG returned to normal.

In subjects known to have coronary artery disease, voluntary overbreathing leads to significant ST segment changes in about 25%, changes that may be ameliorated by β-blockers.

Given such diagnosic difficulty, further investigations to exclude coronary disease may well be appropriate in patients presenting with ECG changes suspected as being due to hyperventilation.

Differential diagnosis of anterolateral ST segment depression (Table 4.1)

Table 4.1 Causes of anterolateral ST depression

Condition	ECG clues
	Usually dynamic ST depression i.e. 'comes and goes'
Ischaemia	ST changes usually 'come and go' but can less commonly be 'fixed'. Usually associated with typical ischaemic chest pain. Often raised troponin.
Hyperventilation	ECG changes can be very widespread. Dynamic. Symptoms usually atypical for myocardial ischaemia. Increased ventilation may or may not be obvious.
	Usually 'fixed' ST depression
Digoxin	Usually only causes ST depression in leads V (4), 5 and 6. Patient often in AF. History usually diagnostic.
Left ventricular hypertrophy	Usually ST depression only in leads V5 and 6. LV voltages usually increased.
Cardiomyopathy	Often widespread ECG changes, including decreased QRS voltages. Patient often breathless, sometimes signs of heart failure.
Pericardial disease	Usually found in the chronic phase, so patient often asymptomatic. Not common.

AF, atrial fibrillation; LV, left ventricular

Left ventricular hypertrophy (see above). This is usually obvious as QRS complexes are increased in size and fulfil the voltage criteria for LVH (see Chapter 3). However, occasionally the QRS voltages are not increased and the only indication of LVH is the presence of anterolateral ST segment depression. QRS complexes may not be increased in LVH occurring in those with a high body mass index (as chest fat diminishes the transmission of electricity from the heart to the skin surface) or in the elderly (in whom LVH may be associated with smaller increases in cardiac voltages and hence smaller increases in extracardiac current flow). Any doubt as to the presence or otherwise of LVH can be clarified by cardiac ultrasound.

Myocardial ischaemia. This can often be determined from the history. The ST segment depression often fluctuates with time (ie over hours or days), unlike the fixed ST segment depression of LVH. The QRS complexes are usually not increased (unless coincident hypertension is present). Sometimes the distribution of the ST segment depression is more extensive than that due to LVH. In particular, ST segment depression seen to involve leads V3 to V6 (as opposed to involving only chest leads V4 to V6) is almost always due to myocardial ischaemia. The extra involvement of lead V3 in this setting is therefore a fairly reliable sign of ischaemia, as ST segment inversion in lead V3 is almost never due to acquired LVH (although, confusingly, it may be found in the very rare, genetically determined hypertrophic cardiomyopathy).

Digoxin therapy. This is usually obvious. The distribution of the ST segment changes are identical to those due to LVH; thus if ST segment depression is found in lead V3 in a patient on digoxin, the cause is less likely to be the digoxin itself and is most likely to be myocardial ischaemia.

T wave changes

The normal T wave

The T wave is generated by the repolarization of myocardial cells. In health epicardial cells repolarize first and endocardial cells repolarize last, so the direction of repolarization is in the opposite direction to that of depolarization, in which endocardial cells depolarize first and epicardial cells depolarize last (Figure 4.3). However, as the current flow in repolarization is the reverse of the current flow in depolarization, the vector of the T wave is usually much the same as the vector of the QRS complex (the 'two negatives' cancel each other out), so wherever there is a significant-sized R wave, the T wave will be upright.

T wave abnormalities (Figure 4.11)

T wave changes are very common. The principal abnormalities are:

- Mild T wave flattening or inversion – this can be localized or generalized (see below).
- Localized severe T wave inversion, often due to a process that regionally affects the heart – by far the most common is coronary artery disease.

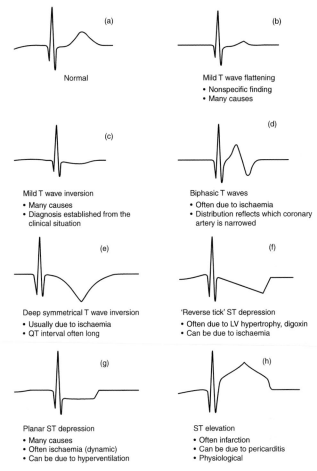

(a) Normal

(b) Mild T wave flattening
- Nonspecific finding
- Many causes

(c) Mild T wave inversion
- Many causes
- Diagnosis established from the clinical situation

(d) Biphasic T waves
- Often due to ischaemia
- Distribution reflects which coronary artery is narrowed

(e) Deep symmetrical T wave inversion
- Usually due to ischaemia
- QT interval often long

(f) 'Reverse tick' ST depression
- Often due to LV hypertrophy, digoxin
- Can be due to ischaemia

(g) Planar ST depression
- Many causes
- Often ischaemia (dynamic)
- Can be due to hyperventilation

(h) ST elevation
- Often infarction
- Can be due to pericarditis
- Physiological

Figure 4.11
Different patterns of repolarization abnormalities and their causes.

- Generalized severe T wave inversion, often due to severe proximal coronary disease, especially a high-grade stenosis in the proximal segment of the LAD.

For other causes, see below.

Mild T wave changes

Mild T wave flattening or inversion is a very nonspecific sign, and a diagnosis of the underlying disease process often cannot be readily made from the ECG alone. In essence almost any cardiac disease process, as well as many noncardiac diseases, can cause these changes. The following are particularly common causes of T wave flattening and/or mild inversion:

- Coronary disease: T wave changes are often (but not always) restricted to the affected territory.
- Pericarditis, typically late on in the recovery period; ECG changes may be quite widespread.
- Hypokalaemia: all the T waves are usually flat and return to normal once the potassium concentration is normalized.
- Cardiomyopathy: this often causes widespread changes; it can be distinguished from old pericarditis by the clinical picture (breathlessness and signs of heart failure); cardiac ultrasound is diagnostic.
- Hyperventilation (see above).
- Mitral valve prolapse: physical examination should be diagnostic.
- Post-tachycardia T wave changes: T wave flattening and inversion, often affecting the anterior chest leads (although all leads can be affected) is quite common after a tachyarrhythmia, even in the absence of coronary artery disease. Occasionally these T wave changes can be quite dramatic.
- Post-pacing T wave changes: flattened or inverted T waves are quite common following ventricular pacing.

Substantial T wave changes

Occasionally T wave changes occur that are highly specific for a single disease process (usually coronary disease), eg deep symmetrical T wave inversion affecting the precordial leads (Figure 4.12; so-called 'pan-anterior' T wave inversion). By far the commonest cause of this abnormality is a high-grade stenosis in the LAD, often in the proximal segment. As revascularization in those with high-grade stenosis of the proximal portion of the LAD improves the prognosis of symptomatic patients, the finding of a 'proximal LAD syndrome ECG' is taken as an indication for angiography in those with chest pain. Other causes of deep pan-anterior T wave inversion include:

- Post-tachycardia: usually either a supraventricular tachycardia (most commonly atrioventricular nodal reentrant tachycardia) or atrial fibrillation. T wave changes can be dramatic or minimal (see above).
- Post-pacing: occasionally dramatic T wave changes occur.
- Cerebrovascular disease: patients with subarachnoid haemorrhage (SAH) can subsequently develop deep, pan-anterior T wave inversion. The

conventional explanation is that an SAH results in a substantial systemic release of catecholamines, which causes coronary vasospasm and myocardial ischaemia. The diagnosis is usually obvious from the clinical setting.

- Cardiomyopathy: especially if due to hypertrophic cardiomyopathy, can produce gross T wave inversion (see Figure 3.3b).

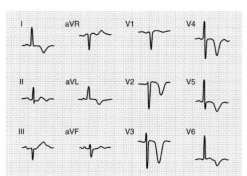

Figure 4.12
'Pan-anterior' T wave inversion due to a high-grade lesion in the proximal portion of the left anterior descending coronary artery. There is widespread anterior lead T wave inversion, and this is deep and symmetrical. The QT interval is prolonged.

ST segment and T wave changes in pericarditis

Pericarditis has been reported as changing the ECG in a characteristic sequence:

- stage I: ST segment elevation (see above), 'concave-up' occurs initially
- stage II: the ST segment becomes isoelectric and (in most cases) T wave flattening starts to occur
- stage III: subsequently T wave inversion develops
- stage IV: the ECG returns to normal.

Some 90% of patients presenting with acute pericarditis show this sequence of ECG changes. The sequence can, however, become 'arrested' at any stage; the ECG sometimes does not return fully to normal and some (usually mild) T wave changes may persist. In some patients the diagnosis of pericarditis can then be made retrospectively from these persisting T wave abnormalities; careful review of the clinical history sometimes reveals a history of pain consistent with pericarditis, eg during a 'flu epidemic.

Summary: diagnosing the cause of ST segment and T wave abnormalities

As there is a wide range of causes of ST segment and T wave abnormalities it is important to have a systematic approach to diagnosis. As ever, the best approach is one that amalgamates clinical and ECG information. The following scheme may be useful.

*First, establish what the most likely diagnosis is on clinical grounds.*The most important question is usually whether or not coronary disease is present [assessed on the basis of risk factors, the nature of the chest pain, and (in chronic stable angina) provocation by effort and rapid, total relief by rest]. Valvular heart disease, hypertension and heart failure (although not always LV dysfunction) are usually readily detected by clinical examination. A full drug history can be very helpful.

Second, establish the clinical differential diagnosis. Order the possible diagnoses by probability, according to the clinical features and (importantly) the patient's demographics (ie age, sex, and risk factors for coronary and other heart disease).

Third, examine the ECG and determine whether this alters your differential diagnosis.

- Do the ECG changes follow a 'regional' pattern (ie localized to a few leads)? This suggests coronary disease; check the risk factors and concentrate on the history.
- Are the changes generalized (ie present in all the leads)? This raises the possibility of severe coronary disease (usually clear from the risk factors and history), cardiomyopathy, or a 'metabolic' problem such as drugs (diagnosis is established from the history), hypokalaemia or hyperventilation.
- Is the ECG diagnostically abnormal? This is rare, but can 'clinch' the diagnosis. (eg the deep anterior T wave inversion very frequently due to a high-grade stenosis in the proximal portion of the LAD).

If ECG changes are mild and nondiagnostic they add little to the diagnosis. Accept this, and use the clinical features to guide what should be done next.

Chapter 5
The ECG in chest pain

Chest pain is a common clinical problem. The ECG has a crucial role in its diagnosis and in following the response to treatment.

General diagnostic approach to chest pain

'The history establishes the diagnosis in 80% of cases, examination in 10% and investigations in a further 10%', so the saying goes, and this is certainly true for chest pain. Perhaps more so than for any other condition, to avoid diagnostic error it is crucial to establish a working clinical diagnosis for chest pain before investigations are examined; failure to do this can easily lead to serious error. Diagnosis of the cause of chest pain requires an understanding of which structures can give rise to pain and what pathology can affect these structures. A working diagnosis is established by obtaining (and understanding!) the clinical history and physical examination; it is then tested using appropriate investigations, including an ECG.

The following is an approach to the diagnosis of chest pain.

First, take a full history and perform a clinical examination. This gives a good idea of the most likely diagnosis and what other diagnoses should be excluded (Figure 5.1).

Second, assess the resting ECG.

Third, perform investigations that if positive will establish the most likely diagnosis. For example, if the likely diagnosis is aortic dissection then a chest and abdomen computed tomography (CT) scan can 'clinch' the diagnosis. If the likely diagnosis is chronic obstructive pulmonary disease (COPD) then lung function tests can be diagnostic. Ask whether the diagnostic test establishes the diagnosis beyond doubt. If not, perform the definitive test (or if this is not available or appropriate, keep your differential diagnosis open).

Fourth, actively exclude ischaemic heart disease (IHD) by the most appropriate method unless you are 100% certain of an alternative diagnosis,

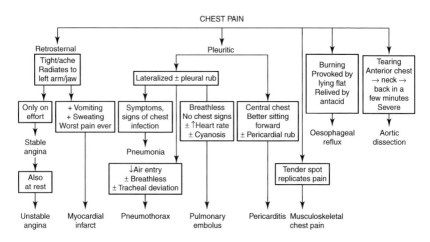

Figure 5.1

Algorithm for diagnosing the cause of chest pain. Reproduced with permission from Davey P. *Medicine at a Glance*. Oxford: Blackwell Science.

or the risk of coronary disease is so low as to be irrelevant. As IHD is such an important and common diagnosis, all patients presenting with chest pain must at least have their coronary risk factors established [age, sex, smoking (status, family history of premature coronary artery disease (CAD), history of hypertension and diabetes, cholesterol levels] and a resting ECG performed (even though this is unlikely to be abnormal, even in the presence of severe CAD). If chest pain occurs at rest, a troponin level may be required. Many patients need an exercise ECG and some will need coronary angiography.

Fifth, remember that all tests have a false-positive and false-negative rate. Thus some tests can 'falsely' reassure. The resting and exercise ECG can both mislead, and even coronary angiography, the 'gold standard', can mislead [eg some patients with unambiguous myocardial infarction (MI) have fairly normal coronary arteries angiographically]. Thus test results must always be analysed in their clinical context.

Finally, keep an open mind about the diagnosis, and if progress is not as expected then be prepared to review the original diagnosis.

Structures causing chest pain

In considering causes of chest pain it is helpful to work initially from an anatomical perspective, as different pathologies affecting the same part of the same organ often cause identical symptoms (Figure 5.2). Whether

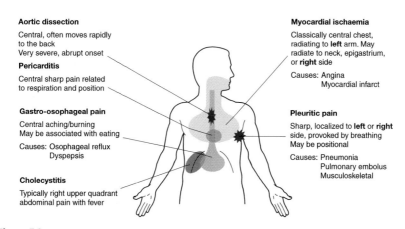

Aortic dissection

Central, often moves rapidly
to the back
Very severe, abrupt onset

Pericarditis

Central sharp pain related
to respiration and position

Gastro-osophageal pain

Central aching/burning
May be associated with eating

Causes: Osophageal reflux
        Dyspepsis

Cholecystitis

Typically right upper quadrant
abdominal pain with fever

Myocardial ischaemia

Classically central chest,
radiating to **left** arm. May
radiate to neck, epigastrium,
or **right** side

Causes: Angina
        Myocardial infarct

Pleuritic pain

Sharp, localized to **left** or **right**
side, provoked by breathing
May be positional

Causes: Pneumonia
        Pulmonary embolus
        Musculoskeletal

Figure 5.2
Structures giving rise to chest pain. Reproduced with permission from Davey P. *Medicine at a Glance*. Oxford: Blackwell Science.

structures in and around the chest can or cannot give pain depends on the nature of their sensory innervation:

Heart. Damage to the endocardium, whatever the cause, does not produce pain. Some insults to the myocardium cause pain (eg ischaemia) while others do not (eg inflammation resulting in myocarditis, toxic damage due to iron overload). Pericardial inflammation usually causes pain.

Great vessels. Inflammation of the aorta (eg due to atheroma, vasculitis or syphilis) does not cause pain, whereas splitting of the various layers of the wall of the aorta (as in dissection) does. Spontaneous damage to the great veins is extraordinarily rare and probably causes pain similar to aortic dissection.

Lungs. Damage to the lung parenchyma, by whatever pathology, causes little or no pain, whereas inflammation of the pleural lining of the lungs is painful.

Oesophagus. Inflammation of the lining of the oesophagus or spasm of the muscle in the wall of the oesophagus gives pain. Pain from oesophageal spasm is due to smooth muscle ischaemia.

Musculoskeletal system. Arthritis of the various joints in the chest wall and injury to the ligaments and muscles themselves are a common cause of chest pain. Pain can infrequently arise from rib pathology, eg fractures or (much more rarely) malignant deposits.

Structures of the back. Vertebral collapse and arthritis of the joints of the back are common causes of pain, as is bony pathology impinging on nerves exiting the intervertebral foramina, causing neuralgia via extrinsic compression (eg osteoarthritis). Herpetic infection of a peripheral nerve is another cause of neuralgia.

Structures below the diaphragm. Pathology in the abdomen can sometimes give rise to chest pain, although in practice this is most unusual. Gallbladder disease is occasionally felt as chest pain.

It is often most helpful to diagnose from the clinical history which structure is involved in producing the pain, then to determine what pathology is responsible. Characteristic histories are given below.

Clinical evaluation of patients with chest pain

Understanding the clinical features gives most of the clues necessary to establishing the diagnosis.

Clinical history in chest pain

The aim of the clinical history (nature of the pain, duration, provoking and relieving factors) is to classify the chest pain into one of several patterns (see below), which can then give a strong indication to the diagnosis. However, these clinical features can on occasion mislead and should not be relied on exclusively.

One should also evaluate the following: presence of associated symptoms in other parts of the body (eg constitutional symptoms, abdominal pain, depression); demographics (age, sex, comorbid illness); risk factors for the various causes of chest pain (eg smoking); and prevalence of the various causes of chest pain in the local community (eg CAD, influenza epidemic). Previous medical history can be highly informative.

Patterns of chest pain

Although many pathologies cause rather nonspecific pain, some disease processes give rise to well-recognized patterns of pain.

Ischaemic chest pain. In most (but not all) patients it is possible to make a presumptive diagnosis of myocardial ischaemia, atypical angina or non-cardiac chest pain on the basis of clinical features alone. Ischaemic chest pain is a 'blanket' term referring to a brief (less than a few minutes in stable angina, up to 20 minutes in unstable angina) retrosternal ache, often described as a 'heavy' sensation or a 'tight' pain, which may radiate to the neck or the arm (usually left, sometimes right as well). If this pain has been present for more than 3–4 weeks it will have a strong relationship with effort: pain will be absent before exercise, will be reliably provoked by walking too far or too fast, and will be totally relieved (within a few minutes) by rest. These features are characteristic of typical angina. In stable angina the amount of effort required to provoke the pain is fairly constant (and the strong relationship with exercise and rapid relief with rest is more diagnostically useful than the exact location or character of the pain). Thus atypically located chest pain (eg left shoulder pain), reliably effort provoked and rest-relieved, is likely to be anginal in origin, whereas if long-standing (ie present for more than 5–6 weeks) 'typical' ischaemic chest pain (ie retrosternal 'aching', 'tightness') occurs and is unrelated to effort, it is unlikely to be due to myocardial ischaemia. The more symptoms differ from this, the less likely epicardial CAD is to be present. Beware, however, as if anginal pains have been present for less than 2–3 weeks (ie if unstable angina is present) for unknown reasons there may not be a close relationship to effort. Chest pain with some typical but other atypical features of classic angina is termed atypical angina. Noncardiac chest pain has none of the features of typical angina.

Infarction-type chest pain. This has the same quality as ischaemic-type chest pain (ie central, retrosternal, 'heavy', or 'tight', radiating to the jaw or arms) but is much more severe (eg 'an elephant on my chest', 'the worst pain ever', 'I thought I was going to die', 'I was very frightened by how severe the pain was'). Sweating or vomiting are commonly associated with myocardial infarction – their occurrence in patients with ischaemic chest pain increases the likelihood that an MI has occurred.

Pleuritic chest pain. When chest pains are provoked or substantially exacerbated by deep inspiration they are termed 'pleuritic'. Pleuritic pains can be so painful that deep breaths are consciously avoided, resulting in shallow respiration. They can result from inflammation of the pleura (pleurisy) or inflammation of the pericardium (pericarditis).

Neuralgic pain. The typical symptoms arising from damage to the peripheral sensory nerves are pain of a peculiarly unpleasant quality, in the distribution of a dermatome.

Oesophageal pain. This is felt as a retrosternal 'burning' discomfort, provoked by eating or lying flat, and relieved by antacids. Oesophageal spasm can cause a pain identical to that of myocardial ischaemia.

Musculoskeletal chest pain. This is often felt as a localized pain (an 'ache') lasting many hours. There may be point tenderness to the chest wall, which exactly replicates the pain. Occasionally the pain is exacerbated by effort, but many hours' rest is required for its relief.

Nonspecific chest pain. This pain has characteristics that do not allow one to place patients into any of the categories above.

Physical examination in chest pain

Physical examination has a definite role in establishing the diagnosis, although diagnostic clinical signs are rare. The commonest features sought are:

Nonspecific responses to severe pain (tachycardia, hypertension, sweating). These usually (but not always) indicate a serious cause for the pain.

Third heart sound (S3). In patients with ischaemic heart disease a third heart sound is present during ischaemic chest pain but not between anginal attacks. This sign can be useful in the emergency room assessment of chest pain occurring at rest.

Signs of aortic stenosis. These are a slowly rising carotid pulse (not an easy sign to elicit), a quiet second heart sound and (especially) a loud ejection systolic murmur (in severe aortic stenosis this murmur can be quiet, but only where there is significant impairment of left ventricular function).

Signs of heart failure. These are a third heart sound, bibasal crepitations, raised jugular venous pressure and ankle oedema. An apical, pansystolic mitral regurgitation murmur is common in many cases of heart failure.

Pleural or pericardial rubs.

Pulse asymmetry. Absent or reduced arm, neck or leg pulses raise the possibility of aortic dissection.

Cyanosis. This should be confirmed by detecting arterial hypoxaemia from arterial blood gases. It occurs in pulmonary embolism (PE).

Signs of cardiogenic shock. These are tachycardia, low blood pressure, raised jugular venous pressure and evidence of organ malperfusion (eg cool skin, oliguria, confusion). Cardiogenic shock is found in many conditions, including MI and massive PE (where cyanosis will also be evident).

Chest wall tenderness that exactly reproduces the pain. It is crucially important to realize that both IHD and chest wall pain are common diagnoses, and many patients with symptomatic IHD can also have chest wall pain.

Most patients with chest pain have a normal physical examination, regardless of whether or not serious pathology is present.

Investigations in chest pain

Routinely useful investigations for the assessment of chest pain include:

- An ECG at rest and during exercise (see Chapters 10 and 11).
- Biochemical markers of myocardial damage (in those with chest pain at rest), including 'conventional' cardiac enzymes (eg aspartate aminotransferase and creatine kinase) and the new 'sensitive' markers of myocardial damage (troponins T and I).
- Laboratory tests, including haemoglobin, white cell count (in suspected infection), lipid profile, and renal and thyroid function tests.

Radiological investigations in chest pain

Transthoracic cardiac ultrasound at rest (in those with valvar heart disease and heart failure) and with stress (for suspected myocardial ischaemia), and *transoesophageal ultrasound* in suspected aortic dissection.

Chest X-ray is particularly useful in pneumothorax, heart failure, pleural effusion and pneumonia. It is less useful in ruling out aortic dissection and almost always unhelpful in angina. A chest X-ray should always be considered in those with 'rib' pain, musculoskeletal chest pain or 'atypical angina' to rule out metastatic disease. *CT scan* and *magnetic resonance imaging (MRI)* are particularly useful in the diagnosis of aortic disease.

Scintigraphic lung scanning ('ventilation–perfusion' scan) is useful in suspected PE. CT or conventional pulmonary angiography can also be useful if this diagnosis is suspected.

Nuclear cardiac imaging, mainly using isotopes taken up by healthy but not by ischaemic or dead myocardial tissue (see p. 266).

Coronary angiography is an appropriate test in many patients with chest pain. It is the gold standard in deciding whether CAD is present. The main indications for this are:

- Limiting angina or angina associated with an early positive exercise test (symptoms and/or ST segment depression ≥2 mm before stage III of the Bruce protocol).
- Angina in diabetics and others with extensive risk factors for CAD.
- Post-MI angina and angina associated with impaired left ventricular function (ejection fraction ≤40%).
- Unstable angina with ongoing symptoms or high-risk features (see p. 234).
- Intrusive chest pain that may not have many of the characteristics of angina but that is worrying the patient significantly, where noninvasive tests have not clearly excluded angina.
- Suspected congenital coronary anomalies, which can give rise to angina in young patients.

Dealing with diagnostic uncertainty in chest pain

The history, examination and investigations usually establish a clear diagnosis. What should one do if this is not the case? There are many reasons for diagnostic uncertainty; however, for most patients there are two key questions:

- First, is CAD present?
- Second, if CAD is present, what is the prognosis of medical therapy?

The first question can be clarified via a coronary angiogram. However, whether this is the best way to proceed depends on the answer to the second question. The second question can be answered largely by determining:

- exercise capacity and the nature of ECG changes during exercise
- left ventricular function.

If exercise capacity and left ventricular function are good then the outlook, even if CAD is present, is likely to be good. Thus many patients in this situation can be managed 'expectantly' with medical therapy (aspirin, statins, angiotensin-converting enzyme inhibitors, etc), and further investigations (including angiography) are not needed.

If exercise capacity is poor then severe underlying CAD may be a possibility, with a poor outcome on medical therapy. In this situation the best way to proceed depends on the probability of CAD being present, which is established from the history and demographics. If the probability is low or medium then a noninvasive study (eg stress myoview or ultrasound) should be considered; if this is abnormal then a coronary angiogram may be appropriate. If the probability of CAD is medium to high then it is often appropriate to undertake a coronary angiogram.

If the coronary angiogram is normal, two possibilities arise. The first is that the patient has noncardiac chest pain – this is the usual interpretation. The other is that the patient has syndrome X, a very rare (and much overdiagnosed) condition (see p. 67 for pathophysiology and ECG changes). To make this diagnosis the patient must have typical anginal symptoms, an exercise test showing ST segment depression plus these symptoms, and angiographically normal coronary arteries. Unsurprisingly, very few patients fulfil this strict definition.

If the coronary angiogram is abnormal there are several possibilities. First, mild to moderate CAD may be demonstrated, and on retaking the history and reviewing the ECG and other evidence one can believe that this is responsible for the symptoms; one should then proceed conventionally. Second, on reevaluating the data one may be certain that CAD is not responsible for the symptoms; one should then proceed according to the nature of the CAD, revascularizing if appropriate on prognostic grounds. Third, if one is uncertain as to whether the CAD is responsible for symptoms or not then a trial of anti-ischaemic therapy (preferably medical) is appropriate, but if this is unsuccessful then it may be justifiable to proceed to percutaneous or even surgical revascularization. If symptoms are relieved it can sometimes be difficult to know if this is due to the very powerful placebo effect of angioplasty or surgery or to a genuine mechanical relief of symptomatic atypical angina. If critical CAD is found (ie left main disease or three-vessel CAD involving the proximal portion of the left anterior descending coronary artery) then in practice no test will help one decide if the patient's symptoms arise from this, and it is conventional to revascularize the patient. It is crucially important to explain to the patient that revascularization may not relieve symptoms.

Specific disease processes causing chest pain

Stable effort angina

The causes of effort angina (ie typical ischaemic chest pain occurring only on effort, and rapidly and totally relieved by rest) are as follows.

Atherosclerotic disease of epicardial coronary arteries

This is by far the commonest cause of effort angina. Patients usually have significant risk factors for CAD. The resting ECG in stable angina occurring only on effort is usually normal, unless patients have previously experienced an MI, in which case Q waves, loss of R waves or ST segment flattening may be seen. The exercise test (see Chapter 11) may show ST segment depression, with the workload at which this occurs relating moderately well to CAD severity and prognosis. However, one should be aware that the exercise test may show no changes at all, even in those with severe CAD!

'Microvascular' angina

This condition is probably much less diagnosed than talked about. A prerequisite for the diagnosis is angiographically normal coronary arteries; the syndrome may relate to an inadequate 'vasodilator reserve' (ie an inability to vasodilate the coronary arteries in response to exercise). It may be more prevalent in middle-aged women. Conversely, similar symptoms can occur in those with hypertension or hypercholesterolaemia in the absence of any angiographic evidence of CAD. Exercise test findings can mimic those for CAD.

Aortic stenosis

This is a common cause of effort-induced chest pain. It does not cause angina at rest – rest pains in aortic stenosis are usually due to concomitant IHD. The clinical examination in aortic stenosis is usually diagnostic. ECG evidence of left ventricular hypertrophy (LVH) is almost universal, although the elderly may not show classic increases in LV voltages but instead lateral lead T wave changes only. Hypertrophic obstructive cardiomyopathy (HOCM), the clinical signs of which can (despite what is written in textbooks) be confused with those of aortic stenosis, may cause LV outflow tract obstruction, increasingly severe during exercise, but only rarely causes effort-dependent chest pain. The ECG in HOCM is usually (not always) dramatically abnormal, with increased voltages and widespread T wave inversion throughout the precordial leads.

Pulmonary hypertension

Pulmonary hypertension, especially if primary, is an unusual (but not rare) cause of effort-dependent chest pain. (For causes of pulmonary hypertension see p. 38). The diagnosis is suspected from the clinical examination (right parasternal lift, loud P2 heart sound, with or without a high venous pressure, ankle oedema and hepatomegaly) and confirmed by cardiac ultrasound or, if this is unhelpful, by direct invasive measurement of the pulmonary artery pressure at cardiac catheterization. The ECG is unreliable in the diagnosis of pulmonary hypertension and may or may not show right ventricular hypertrophy (RVH) regardless of how elevated is the pulmonary artery pressure. A normal or near-normal ECG does not rule out severe pulmonary hypertension.

Other causes of effort-related chest pain

Musculoskeletal problems

Musculoskeletal problems can also cause effort-dependent chest pain, although the clinical features usually differ markedly from angina: pain is usually present before exercise and takes 20 minutes or more to improve afterwards (and patients are often left with some abnormal sensation for many hours, compared with the complete relief within a few minutes of rest experienced in angina). The character of musculoskeletal pain can be quite variable, being variously described as 'sharp' or 'aching', but rarely as 'tightness'. It is often felt laterally, most often on the left side of the chest (as pains here give rise to concern). Chest wall tenderness may be present and movement of the left arm (eg carrying objects, using tools) may exacerbate symptoms. The ECG is usually normal, although associated anxiety can induce changes including ST segment depression (see p. 254), especially if hyperventilation is present (see p. 69). For the same reason, the exercise ECG is usually (but not always) normal.

Oesophageal reflux or spasm

This is a rare cause of effort-dependent chest pain (see below). Oesophageal reflux or spasm can be exceptionally difficult to distinguish clinically from angina as the quality of the pain may be similar and rest may promptly relieve both forms of pain. Associated dyspeptic symptoms may point towards oesophageal aetiology; however, dyspepsia is unfortunately also common in those with angina. It is therefore best to regard effort-induced chest tightness promptly relieved by rest as being due to angina (due to 'straightforward' CAD), at least until appropriate investigations have been carried out. The ECG is usually normal, although pain can induce mild changes (see p. 67).

Asthma and chronic obstructive airways disease

Both asthma and COPD frequently cause effort-induced chest 'tightness' rapidly relieved by rest. The feature distinguishing airways disease from angina is that wheezing and breathlessness are often marked and occur reliably in association with the chest discomfort. The diagnosis of airways obstruction is established from lung function tests (variable airflow obstruction in asthma, 'fixed' obstructive pattern in COPD).

Occasionally airways disease causes chest tightness but no wheezing, which can then be very difficult to distinguish from angina on the history alone. Full 'anginal' investigations are then usually appropriate.

The resting ECG is usually normal in asthma and in mild to moderate COPD, although RVH can occur in severe COPD (see p. 37). Most patients with COPD are or have been smokers, so IHD and hypertension are commonly also present, and these may result in mild T wave changes or increased LV voltages. Occasionally it is important to rule out IHD more definitely, using an exercise ECG. However, standard exercise testing is often not possible due to breathlessness, or produces equivocal results. In this situation it is often best to establish the diagnosis from a pharmacological 'stress' nuclear perfusion scan or cardiac ultrasound, or (more reliably) from coronary angiography.

Causes of resting 'ischaemic-type' chest pain

The causes of ischaemic-type chest pain (ie retrosternal 'heaviness', 'pressure', 'tightness', possibly radiating to the jaw or left arm) occurring at rest include the following:

Unstable angina, typically causes episodes of chest pain at rest lasting between a few minutes and half an hour. Pain lasting much longer than this is usually either due to MI (a diagnosis easily confirmed from the ECG) or is not from the heart at all (eg oesophageal spasm). ECG findings in unstable angina are described on p. 227 and are summarized in Figure 5.3.

Myocardial infarction (see below) gives a pain that has the same quality as typical angina but is usually more severe ('the worst pain ever'), and prolonged (usually lasting ≥20 minutes), often associated with vomiting, sweating and a feeling of impending doom. Patients may look grey and clammy and may show signs of pain (tachycardia, hypertension, hyperventilation) or haemodynamic upset (tachycardia, hypotension, signs of heart failure).

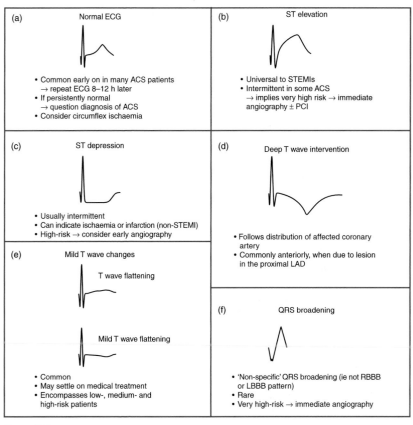

Figure 5.3
ECG changes in acute coronary syndromes (ACS). STEMI, ST segment elevation myocardial infarction; non-STEMI, non-ST elevation myocardial infarction; LAD, left anterior descending coronary artery; PCI, percutaneous coronary intervention; RBBB, right bundle branch block; LBBB, left bundle branch block.

Oesophageal spasm can give rise to pain identical to that of myocardial ischaemia. The ECG and troponin levels usually allow differentiation between these diagnoses.

Other dyspeptic syndromes (eg stomach or duodenal mucosal pathology, hiatus hernia) are occasionally responsible for tight retrosternal chest pains occurring at rest.

Chest wall pain of musculoskeletal origin can occasionally mimic 'ischaemic' chest pain.

Neuralgia can very occasionally be confused with ischaemic chest pain, especially when due to herpes zoster infection.

Pleuritic chest pain

Pleurisy is felt laterally and is often (but not always) associated with a 'rub' heard with the stethoscope over the area of maximum pain during deep inspiration. The causes of pleurisy include the following:

Infection, which is usually viral; bacterial lung infection is a rare but much more serious cause of pleuritic chest pain. Systemic upset, fever and productive cough are vital clues to the diagnosis; 'bronchial breathing' may be heard over the affected lung, and the chest X-ray and blood cultures are often diagnostic. A raised white cell count and C-reactive protein are commonly found. The ECG is clearly not helpful diagnostically but may show a sinus tachycardia. Nonspecific T wave flattening may occur. Atrial fibrillation can complicate pneumonia and is associated with more severe infection and higher in-hospital mortality. The incidence of acute MI is raised threefold over baseline in the few weeks following a respiratory tract infection.

Acute pulmonary embolus provokes pleuritic pain by causing pulmonary infarcts. The patient usually (but not always) volunteers that they have suddenly become breathless. The absence of breathlessness in those with pleuritic chest pain significantly decreases the probability of PE. In large or massive PE there may be haemodynamic upset (tachycardia, decreased blood pressure) with a raised venous pressure. Most (but not all) PEs result in intrapulmonary arteriovenous shunting and thus arterial hypoxaemia (only partially responding to supplementary oxygen). Fibrinogen breakdown products are raised (eg D-dimers). Ventilation–perfusion technetium scinti-scanning, spiral CT scanning or pulmonary angiography can be diagnostic. The ECG is unremarkable in most PEs and thus cannot be used to rule in or rule out the diagnosis. The larger the PE, the more likely sinus tachycardia and 'acute right heart strain' (manifest as a rightward shift of the QRS axis) are to occur. This is sometimes seen as a prominent S wave in lead V1, with a large Q wave and inverted T in lead III – the so-called $S_1Q_3T_3$ pattern. Very rarely the right heart strain results in acute right bundle branch block – this usually indicates a very large PE that will be quite obvious clinically. Atrial fibrillation can occur with PEs of any size.

Pneumothorax. The clinical signs are often not easy to elicit unless a tension pneumothorax is present, in which case haemodynamic collapse with tracheal deviation occurs. The ECG is unhelpful diagnostically. Tachycardia and nonspecific ST changes may occur.

Trauma, with blood in the pleural space. The ECG is usually unremarkable.

Malignancy, involving the pleura (originating in either the lung or the ribs) is a rare cause of pleuritic chest pain.

Autoimmune disease, particularly systemic lupus erythematosus (SLE). It is exceptionally rare for the presenting feature of SLE to be pleuritic chest pain; pleurisy usually occurs only in those with previously diagnosed SLE. The ECG is usually normal, although associated pericarditis (which may or may not be symptomatic) may give rise to changes (see below).

Pleural effusion. Although pleural effusion may complicate most diseases that can cause pleural inflammation, most pleural effusions are not painful (probably because they are transudates rather than exudates). However, if the pleural fluid has become infected (ie it is an empyema) then pleuritic pain may occur. The ECG is usually normal in those with pleural effusions, reflecting only the coincidental pathology.

Pericardial chest pain

Pericardial pain is felt centrally as a retrosternal sensation, usually 'sharp', exacerbated by deep inspiration and often position-dependent (usually relieved by sitting forward, exacerbated by lying down flat). It may be associated with a 'pericardial rub', a 'scratchy' position-dependent sound heard only at certain phases of the cardiac cycle. Pericarditis can be caused by:

Infection. The commonest cause of pericarditis is viral infection, eg influenza or coxsackievirus. With all pericarditis there is some inflammation of the adjacent myocardium (responsible for the ECG changes; see below). If myocarditis is extensive, heart failure can develop. Thus myocarditis associated with pericarditis can cause pleuritic chest pain. (However, interestingly, most patients who present with heart failure due to myocarditis do not have associated pericarditis and so usually do not have pericardial pain.)

Trauma. Surgical (eg following cardiac surgery) or accidental trauma are common causes of pericarditis. Blood in the pericardium is intensely irritating.

Vasculitis and autoimmune disease. Rheumatoid arthritis and SLE can infrequently cause isolated pericarditis. Following an MI or any cardiac operation that involves cutting through the pericardium ('pericardotomy'), autoantibodies against the pericardium may develop, provoking pericardial inflammation and pain. Dressler syndrome is the name given to post-MI autoimmune pericardial inflammation. This is usually a self-limiting illness causing retrosternal pleuritic chest pain, sometimes shoulder pains and occasionally systemic upset (malaise, anorexia and fever). It usually responds to nonsteroidal anti-inflammatory drugs, although very occasionally steroids are required.

Malignancy is an exceptionally rare cause of pericardial pain, although it can cause painless pericardial effusion and tamponade. Occasionally a very large pericardial effusion causes a dull, continuous retrosternal chest ache due to stretching of the pericardium. However, in this situation features other than chest pain often dominate the clinical situation (preceding weight loss, malaise, and signs of tamponade including low blood pressure, pulsus paradoxus, raised venous pressure and progressive renal failure).

The ECG may be completely normal in those with pericardial pain or may show the classic changes of pericarditis, with 'concave–upwards' ST segment elevation often occurring in many leads (Figure 5.4). Over time (several days to weeks) the ST segments first flatten, then the T wave inverts, followed by return of the ECG to normal. The ECG changes may become 'arrested' at any stage in this process. In addition to these changes, the ECG may show changes relevant to any other ongoing disease process (eg Q waves in peri- or post-MI pericarditis).

Large pericardial effusions classically cause two abnormalities: first a decrease in the size of the ECG complexes; and second 'electrical alternans', wherein alternate beats vary dramatically in size or axis, as the heart swings around within the pericardial sac (Figure 5.5).

Oesophageal chest pain

Pathology of the oesophagus can cause two quite distinct pains:

Reflux pain occurs when the oesophageal mucosa is damaged and acid irritates the submucosal nerves. It is felt as a retrosternal burning ('heartburn'), often worse lying flat, usually unrelated to effort and often lasting many hours. Abdominal obesity is a potent predisposing factor. Milk and other fluids may relieve symptoms. Belching may accompany the pains,

(a)

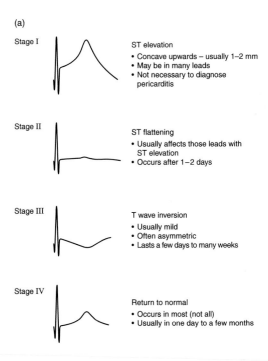

Stage I

ST elevation
- Concave upwards – usually 1–2 mm
- May be in many leads
- Not necessary to diagnose pericarditis

Stage II

ST flattening
- Usually affects those leads with ST elevation
- Occurs after 1–2 days

Stage III

T wave inversion
- Usually mild
- Often asymmetric
- Lasts a few days to many weeks

Stage IV

Return to normal
- Occurs in most (not all)
- Usually in one day to a few months

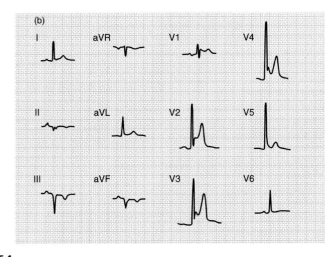

Figure 5.4
(a) Sequential ECG changes in pericardial disease. (b) Q wave inferior wall myocardial infarct with anterior lead ST elevation due to complicating pericarditis.

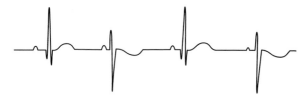

Figure 5.5
Electrical alternans (also termed 'cardiac nystagmus') in pericardial effusion. The QRS (± T wave) direction and amplitude may alternate with every heart beat (as here) or may change more slowly over every three to four beats, due to dramatic shifts in heart position within the fluid-filled pericardial sac. However, note that less than 10% of patients with cardiac tamponade show electrical alternans.

but this may also occur in myocardial ischaemia. Likewise, the relationship to effort does not always discriminate between the two, as oesophageal reflux (as well as spasm) can sometimes be provoked by exercise, which relaxes the oesophagogastric sphincter; however, pains often take a long time to resolve after effort. The ECG is normal.

Oesophageal spasm can very easily be confused with myocardial ischaemia as both pains are due to ischaemia in structures within the mediastinum (the smooth muscle of the oesophageal wall and the heart respectively). Acid reflux induces the smooth muscle in the oesophageal wall to go into spasm, generating a pressure greater than that of the arterioles contained within it, so interfering with its blood supply and provoking oesophageal ischaemia. This results in a 'tight' pain, which is often very uncomfortable (the patient tries numerous positions to seek relief, whereas in myocardial ischaemia the patient often – but not always – sits quietly). The pain may be severe. As it is caused by acid refluxing from the stomach into the oesophagus, factors that promote acid reflux (obesity, especially abdominal, or lying down) promote symptoms, which are often relieved by antacids. The ECG is usually normal but pain and anxiety can induce ST segment changes (see p. 69).

If oesophageal pain is a serious possibility a trial of a proton pump inhibitor (PPI) may be diagnostic. Endoscopy has a role in a small number of PPI-resistant patients, and oesophageal pH monitoring has a role in an even smaller number of patients. Most patients with oesophageal pain have normal resting ECG and exercise tests. However, recent data show that in a very small number of patients oesophageal pain can, through an oesophagocardiac reflex, cause coronary vasoconstriction and thus exercise-induced ST segment depression in the absence of atherosclerotic CAD.

Aortic pain

Aortic pathology (aortic dissection and aortic aneurysm) gives rise to two different sorts of pain.

Aortic aneurysm

Exceptionally rarely, a massive aortic aneurysm can give rise to chest pain; this is usually due to the aorta compressing adjacent structures (ribs, vertebra, etc) that carry somatic innervation rather than arising from the aorta itself.

Aortic dissection

By far the most important cause of aortic pain is aortic dissection (Figure 5.6). This pain has a number of key features:

- It is often 'tearing' or 'sharp' in quality. Many patients find the quality of the pain difficult to articulate.
- It is severe, often exceptionally so, and requires frequent opiates for relief.
- The pain usually (but not always) lasts for many hours. Thus transient severe chest pain (eg less than few minutes) is usually not due to dissection.
- The site where the pain is felt depends on which part of the aorta is dissected.
- Ascending aortic pain is felt in the anterior chest, aortic arch pain is felt in the neck, and descending aortic pain is felt in the back.
- The fact that a dissection propagates rapidly (within a few minutes) distally from its entry point is reflected in the symptoms. In a type A dissection (originating in the ascending aorta) pain classically starts in the anterior chest then moves rapidly into the neck and then into the back, whereas in a type B dissection (originating below the origin of the left subclavian artery) pain starts in the middle of the back and may propagate more distally as the dissection travels down the abdominal aorta.

Examination shows a patient in obvious pain (which may itself cause tachycardia). Hypertension is common. Pulses may be lost (typically in the left arm and also the femoral arteries, although any pulse can be affected). Carotid or spinal artery damage may cause neurological damage (stroke or paraparesis). In proximal aortic dissection the tear tracks back, rupturing into the pericardium and resulting in tamponade and death, usually within a number of hours. Occasionally proximal tracking of the dissection 'tears' a

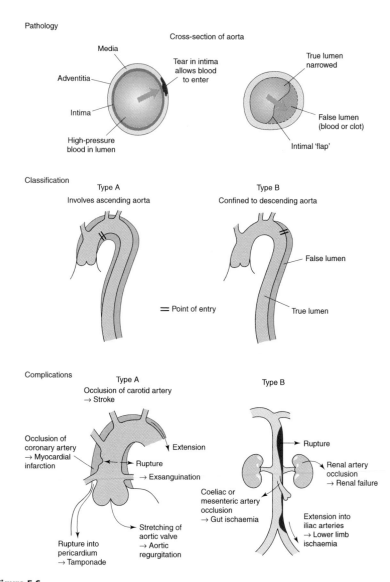

Figure 5.6
Consequences of aortic dissection. Reproduced with permission from Davey P. *Medicine at a Glance*. Oxford: Blackwell Science.

coronary artery away from its origin, causing MI. Disruption of the left main stem by dissection is usually fatal immediately, whereas disruption to the right coronary artery may result in an inferior wall MI from which the patient survives at least sufficiently long to present to hospital.

The diagnosis in aortic dissection is made radiologically. The best approach in the UK is a CT scan with contrast; next best is MRI where available. Although much promoted, the use of transoesophageal echocardiography (TOE) is best avoided outside cardiothoracic centres, as the blood pressure surge caused by inserting the TOE probe can cause aortic rupture and immediate death.

The ECG in aortic dissection may show:

- nothing abnormal
- LVH from long-standing hypertension – a potent risk factor for dissection
- nonspecific T wave changes from the catecholamine release accompanying acute severe illness
- an inferior wall MI (see above)
- ECG signs of tamponade (small ECG complexes, perhaps T wave changes; electrical alternans is not seen, as this requires a very large pericardial effusion and in tamponade from aortic dissection the pericardial effusion is usually fairly small).

When the dissection involves the ascending aorta the hourly mortality rate is about 1–2%. So, although aortic pain from an aortic dissection is a very rare cause of chest pain, when it does occur it constitutes the highest level of medical emergency, mandating immediate radiological diagnosis and definitive therapy (aortic surgery in ascending aortic dissection) and meticulous blood pressure control for all dissections regardless of anatomy.

Neurological, rheumatological and infectious disease causing chest pain

Arthritic disease of the vertebra, leading to compression of the nerve as it passes through the intervertebral foramina. Often the patient has widespread degenerative disease of the vertebral column, with chronic back pain. Back movements may exacerbate the symptoms.

Inflammatory disease affecting the ribs, particularly the costochondral junctions, such as is found in some viral infections (eg coxsackie).

Intervertebral disc prolapse, compressing the nerve.

Herpes zoster, in which the pain often builds up over a few days and can be quite excruciating. Very rarely the pain can start very rapidly, within a few minutes; when it affects a left-sided chest dermatome it can be confused with MI pain. The typical rash appears a few days after pain starts.

The ECG in these conditions is unremarkable, except that as these diseases are common in the elderly there may be incidental cardiac pathology reflected in the ECG.

Pain felt in the chest arising from pathology below the diaphragm

It is consistently taught in textbooks that subdiaphragmatic pathology can cause chest symptoms. Although strictly speaking this is correct, it is important to realize that subdiaphragmatic pathology is in clinical practice an exceptionally rare cause of chest pain, and if it does occur it is usually not difficult to diagnose the true cause.

Biliary disease: biliary colic, although it is typically felt in the epigastric region, may occasionally be felt retrosternally. Cholecystitis can cause pain in the lower right chest, usually pleuritic in nature.

Peptic ulcer pain may be felt low down in the central chest. It usually lasts for many hours and is unrelated to effort.

Pancreatic pain is almost always felt in the epigastrium and radiates through to the back; occasionally it is felt higher up.

Clearly the ECG in these conditions should be normal unless there is coincidental cardiac pathology.

Chapter 6
The ECG in breathlessness and heart failure

General diagnostic approach to breathlessness

In diagnosing the cause of breathlessness, the usual approach is:

- First, develop some diagnostic suspicions based on the patient demographics (age, sex, smoking status, exposure to noxious substances, eg fibrogenic dusts, etc) and the previous medical history.
- Second, develop a differential diagnosis based on the history.
- Third, refine that differential diagnosis from the physical examination, producing hopefully a single diagnosis or at least a shortlist of possible diagnoses.
- Fourth, confirm the most likely diagnosis using the minimum of tests, also useful to exclude other possible diagnoses.

This is usually done by: taking a full history, conducting a full physical examination and performing basic bedside investigations (resting ECG and peak flow). This approach will lead to a definitive diagnosis in most patients, which can be confirmed by 'targeted' investigations. If the diagnosis remains unclear then undertake further investigations, including:

- respiratory tests, including a chest X-ray and full lung function tests (ie all lung volumes, flow-volume loops and gas transfer rates)
- cardiac tests, especially a cardiac ultrasound
- a ventilation–perfusion $\dot{V}/\dot{Q}$ scan should be considered to exclude pulmonary emboli (PE).

These investigations will diagnose many of the outstanding patients.

If the patient is still undiagnosed then consider performing an exercise test, as this allows exercise capacity to be determined formally. If the patient's symptoms are out of proportion to the objective findings then psychological rather than medical causes are likely. An exercise ECG will also detect 'occult' ischaemia by showing ST segment depression. Occult ischaemia is a relatively rare but important cause of breathlessness, particularly prevalent in diabetics and in heart transplant recipients (conditions in which there is some denervation of the heart sensory supply); it may also be more common in the elderly.

If the diagnosis remains in doubt, consider ordering a high-resolution computed tomography (CT) scan of the chest. This may reveal occult lung disease (eg interstitial lung disease such as sarcoidosis) or increase suspicion of pericardial constriction. If this approach is not diagnostic and one is still convinced that breathlessness has an organic origin then cardiac catheterization is sometimes indicated. This enables definitive detection of coronary artery disease (CAD) and also measurement of intracardiac pressures, which will confirm or deny many cardiac aetiologies for the breathlessness (pericardial constriction in particular, although the clues are usually already clear: raised venous pressure and ascites rather than peripheral oedema).

Clinical history in breathlessness

Patient demographics

Young adults are more likely to have asthma, pneumothorax and psychogenic breathlessness whereas older patients are more likely to have chronic obstructive pulmonary disease (COPD), heart failure, bronchial cancer and other malignancies. 'Angina-equivalent' breathlessness is commoner in the elderly and in diabetics. Pneumonia is common regardless of age (though the organism varies). Obesity and physical deconditioning are usually fairly obvious causes of breathlessness. Exposure to industrial or organic dusts predisposes to many respiratory illnesses. Smoking increases the probability of COPD, malignancy and CAD with consequent heart failure.

Specific symptoms

Speed of onset, wheezing and other associated symptoms, particularly chest pain and fevers, are all important and should specifically be asked about.

Speed of onset

See Table 6.1.

Table 6.1 Aetiology of breathlessness according to speed of onset

Causes	Acute onset	Recurrent	Breathlessness relentlessly progressive over:	
			Weeks/months	Years
Respiratory	Asthma Pneumothorax Respiratory infection	Asthma Exacerbation of COPD	Pleural effusion Pulmonary fibrosis and other interstitial lung disease Lung cancer	COPD Pneumoconiosis
Cardiac	Pulmonary oedema Acute pulmonary embolism	Pulmonary oedema CHF	CHF Recurrent pulmonary emboli Angina-equivalent breathlessness	CHF
Other	Fever Metabolic acidosis Psychogenic Guillain–Barré syndrome	Psychogenic	Anaemia Physical deconditioning (from any illness) Neuromuscular diseases	Obesity

COPD, chronic obstructive pulmonary disease; CHF, chronic heart failure.

Wheezing

Wheezing suggests asthma (with normal breathing between attacks), COPD (never normal breathing) and (rarely) heart failure ('cardiac asthma'; usually clear predisposing factors and marked orthopnoea).

Breathlessness with chest pain

Chest pain can be an important clue to the cause of breathlessness and may be due to:

Angina. Effort-induced retrosternal chest 'tightness' or 'heaviness', rapidly relieved by rest, raises the possibility of CAD or aortic stenosis. The CAD usually needs to be severe or associated with previous myocardial infarction (MI) to cause breathlessness. Severe pulmonary hypertension (usually primary, occasionally secondary) can also cause angina, although this is a rare illness.

Pleuritic chest pain. This is 'sharp' or 'knife-like' pain, made much worse by deep inspiration. If situated centrally, it suggests pericarditis (in which it may be position-dependent, characteristically improved by sitting forward). If situated laterally, it suggests pleurisy, for which there is a wide differential diagnosis, including pneumonia, pulmonary infarction and pneumothorax.

Musculoskeletal pain. This is localized, lasts for hours at a time or longer, is worse with coughing or chest movement, and is sometimes accompanied by 'point' tenderness. Musculoskeletal pain is common and usually does not have a specific aetiology, but occasionally is caused by coughing (where it may reflect chronic lung disease, especially COPD), arthritis (if rheumatoid, be aware of the associated interstitial lung disease) and rarely by metastatic malignancy (breathlessness may relate to anaemia, pleural effusion or lymphangiitis carcinomatosis). Anyone with musculoskeletal chest wall pain should therefore have a chest X-ray, blood count and biochemical screen [including the inflammatory markers erythrocyte sedimentation rate and C-reactive protein] to exclude the very remote possibility of malignancy.

Breathlessness with fever

Fever usually suggests infection, either of the airways (upper respiratory tract infection can underlie an acute asthmatic attack or exacerbation of COPD) or of the lung parenchyma itself (pneumonia). Pneumonia is commonly caused by bacterial pathogens (including streptococci, *Haemophilus influenzae*, legionella and myocoplasma), tuberculosis and numerous other organisms in the immunocompromised.

Rarely, fever relates to infective endocarditis, in which breathlessness arises from heart failure and/or anaemia. Patients with pulmonary malignancy can also have a marked fever. Occasionally fever relates to recurrent PE. Rarely fever relates to adverse drug reactions and very rarely to pulmonary vasculitis.

Physical examination in breathlessness

Particularly helpful clues to the diagnosis from the physical examination include:

- General appearance: in acute breathlessness a 'cold and clammy' appearance suggests acute left heart failure (rarely, acute massive PE); a warm and vasodilated appearance suggests either pneumonia or COPD with CO_2 retention.
- Bibasal crepitations and a third heart sound suggest LVF.
- Raised venous pressure and ankle oedema suggest right heart failure. The commonest cause of this is left heart failure; however, COPD and other lung diseases (especially end-stage pulmonary fibrosis) also commonly cause right heart failure, as do PE especially if chronic or repeated.
- Wheeze is a common finding in asthma and COPD. It can, however, also occur in left heart failure, usually but not always in association with bibasal crepitations, in which case a chest X-ray is usually diagnostic.
- 'Obvious' hyperventilation may well be psychological in origin, but one should be very wary in making this diagnosis as many patients with organic causes of breathlessness can appear to have disproportionate anxiety.
- Obesity is an important and common cause of breathlessness; the body mass index (BMI; weight in kg/height in m^2) is usually ≥ 30. Extreme obesity (BMI ≥ 40) can cause type II respiratory failure.

Investigations in breathlessness

The resting ECG

A key question is how the ECG changes in breathlessness, and whether the ECG can be used to confirm or refute any diagnosis. Each of the major causes of breathlessness [asthma, exacerbation of COPD, left ventricular failure (LVF), pneumonia, acute PE and pneumothorax] has distinctive clinical features and definitive diagnostic tests (see below) – the ECG is usually supplementary to these in making the right diagnosis. However, there are some ECG patterns that point to certain diagnoses (Table 6.2).

If the ECG is completely normal, breathlessness may be due to asthma, COPD (although often the ECG is rather nonspecifically abnormal), dysfunctional breathing (previously termed 'hyperventillation'; many patients have fluctuating ST segment changes), obesity (although the QRS complexes are rather small) or physical deconditioning.

Very rarely, patients with critical CAD present with breathlessness. The ECG at rest may be normal. Usually patients are not only breathless but they also experience typical or atypical angina. However, breathlessness as an 'angina-equivalent' symptom does occur as a consequence of critical multivessel CAD in those with (relative) cardiac denervation. This is found in diabetics, the elderly and heart transplant recipients, amongst others. If the diagnosis of 'angina-equivalent' breathlessness is suspected then the exercise ECG usually shows ST segment depression at a low workload (but bear in mind the usual limitations to this test).

Exercise ECG

The exercise ECG has a small but definite role in the evaluation of breathlessness:

Supplying objective data on exercise capacity. This is probably its most useful role. Some patients complain bitterly of breathlessness yet no abnormality can be found on standard investigation. Before going on to more complex and invasive testing, objective evidence that work capacity is truly impaired can be very useful. A helpful although rarely available refinement of standard exercise testing is to obtain data on resting and exercise gas exchange (ie O_2 uptake and CO_2 excretion), as this provides data on fitness, peak effort capacity, etc.

Exclusion of 'angina-equivalent' breathlessness. This again can be very useful in selected patients (diabetics, the elderly, etc) – but bear in mind that the same strengths and weaknesses of the exercise test apply, and that many breathless patients hyperventilate, which can alter the ST segment response regardless of the presence or absence of underlying CAD.

Table 6.2 ECG patterns assisting diagnosis of breathlessness

	Normal	Mild 'nonspecific' ST changes	ST elevation	Q waves	Prominent left-sided voltages	Dominant R wave in V1	Small QRS complexes	Left bundle branch block
Interpretation	LV dysfunction unlikely	Nondiagnostic ECG	MI	Myocyte necrosis unless very small Qs, when physiological	LVH	RVH	Very few functioning myocytes, or increased electrical insulation of heart	Damage to left bundle, ie LBBB
Most likely diagnosis	Respiratory disease (eg asthma) or psychogenic breathlessness	Any	Pulmonary oedema	Heart failure due to previous MI	Heart failure due to aortic stenosis or end-stage hypertension	Pulmonary hypertension due to COPD	Obesity (normal ST/T) Extensive myocardial damage (abnormal ST/T)	Many causes, heart disease possible
Cardiac disease	Unlikely 'Angina-equivalent' breathlessness	Possible IHD, DCM Valvular heart disease	Acute MI Pericardial disease	Previous MI DCM	As above Aortic regurgitation Mitral regurgitation	Mitral stenosis Cardiomyopathy (eg with Duchenne muscular dystrophy)	Poor LV function Pericardial effusion	Poor LV function Aortic stenosis IHD Hypertension
Respiratory disease	Asthma Dysfunctional breathing	Possible asthma COPD Interstitial lung disease	Unlikely	Unlikely unless due to comorbid disease	Unlikely	Chronic fibrotic lung disease Chronic PEs	COPD (occasionally)	COPD
Other	Physical deconditioning Neurological disease	Neuromuscular disease			Thin patient Physical deconditioning	Obesity	Hypothyroidism	Any systemic disease (eg vasculitis)

LV, left ventricular; MI, myocardial infarction; LVH, left ventricular hypertrophy; RVH, right ventricular hypertrophy; COPD, chronic obstructive pulmonary disease; IHD, ischaemic heart disease; DCM, dilated cardiomyopathy; PE, pulmonary emboli; LBBB, left bundle branch block.

Exclusion of effort-induced arrhythmias. Although most patients with effort-induced breathlessness with palpitations are physically unfit, a small number have effort-provoked arrhythmias that can be diagnosed from the exercise ECG.

Other investigations in breathlessness

There are several other investigations that are routinely useful in the diagnosis of breathlessness.

Chest X-ray is useful in excluding many diagnoses (eg pneumothorax and ongoing left heart failure) – but bear in mind that there are limitations to this investigation. For example, many patients with severe left ventricular systolic dysfunction have normally sized cardiac silhouettes (ie a cardiothoracic ratio less than 50%), so the chest X-ray often cannnot exclude heart disease. Equally, obese individuals can have apparent radiological cardiomegaly (due to pericardial fat deposition) despite normal cardiac function. In addition, due to the way that X-rays are attenuated as they pass through obese subjects, radiologists not infrequently report the chest X-rays of obese subjects as showing 'upper lobe blood diversion, consistent with early LVF', despite left heart pressures being normal and there being no excess fluid in the lungs. Thus the chest X-ray has both a false-positive and a false-negative rate.

Lung function tests can be extremely useful, particularly in the diagnosis of 'fixed' abnormalities, eg in COPD and pulmonary fibrosis (Figure 6.1). These tests are less useful in the diagnosis of asthma as they may be normal between attacks.

Cardiac ultrasound is often useful in the diagnosis of heart failure or pulmonary hypertension. However, a normal or near-normal cardiac ultrasound does not necessarily rule out heart failure due to critical coronary ischaemia, pericardial disease or diastolic failure (the latter being a relatively common cause of heart failure in the elderly).

Arterial blood gases are useful both in diagnosing the cause of breathlessness (eg in PE) and in assessing the response to treatment (eg in asthma, COPD and severe LVF).

Chest CT is useful in suspected interstitial lung disease, lung cancer and PE. Other imaging techniques for the detection of PE include ventilation–perfusion nuclear isotope imaging and CT pulmonary angiography (especially useful in PE). Occasionally leg venography can help when tests for PE are ambiguous.

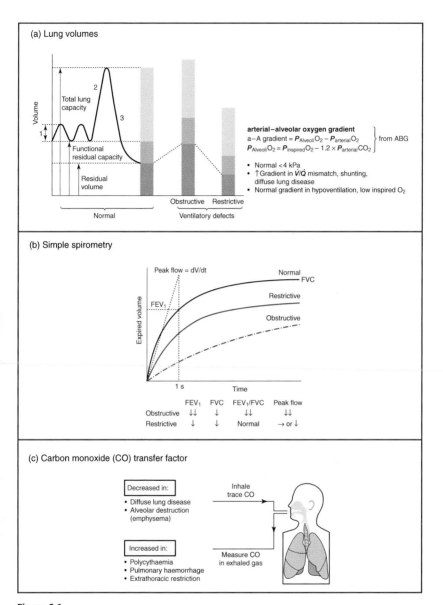

Figure 6.1

Lung function tests. (a) Normal lung volumes and changes in obstructive and restrictive ventilatory defects. 1, Tidal volume; 2, forced inspiration; 3, forced expiration. (b) Simple spirometry. (c) Carbon monoxide transfer factor. ABC, arterial blood gases; $\dot{V}$, ventilitation; $\dot{Q}$, perfusion; FEV$_1$, forced expiratory volume in 1 second; FVC, forced vital capacity. Reprinted with permission from Davey P. *Medicine at a Glance*. Oxford: Blackwell Science.

Bronchoscopy is useful in suspected malignancy and infection in immunocompromised individuals.

Coronary arteriography can be useful if breathlessness is felt to be 'angina-equivalent' (ie due to critical CAD in the presence of normal or near-normal LV systolic function).

Specific diseases causing breathlessness

Asthma

Asthma is difficult to define, but clinicians recognize it as 'symptoms (cough, wheeze and/or breathlessness) due to reversible narrowings of the airways'. Inflammation of the airways is an important part of the pathophysiology and explains the response to steroids.

Characteristic symptoms

Asthma is characterized by intermittent wheezing and/or breathlessness, occurring either spontaneously or on exercise, seasonal or nocturnal, and relieved by inhaled bronchodilators. Patients should be asymptomatic between attacks – if not, another complicating disease process should be considered, usually a respiratory one such as COPD or bronchiectasis. Nocturnal cough is another characteristic symptom; marked orthopnoea raises the possibility of heart failure rather than asthma.

Physical examination

The physical examination is normal between attacks. The hallmark of the acute asthma attack is wheezing. As the severity of the attack increases, the heart and respiratory rates increase, as does the wheezing. Peak flow decreases along with the ability to talk. Confusion, cyanosis despite 100% oxygen, a 'silent' chest (ie no audible wheezing) and inability to talk are ominous signs indicating impending death; immediate intensive care assessment is indicated with a view to mechanical ventilation.

Diagnosis

Diagnosis of asthma is usually not difficult and is made from the clinical features (attacks of breathlessness associated with wheezing, separated by complete normality with normal lung function tests), demonstration of variable airflow obstruction on peak flow recordings; and positive response to inhaled bronchodilators.

ECG in asthma

Between asthma attacks the ECG is not diagnostically helpful. In an acute attack:

- Sinus tachycardia is common, and is proportional to the severity of the attack (and the amount of β-agonists given).
- Nonspecific ST segment changes are commonly found, including ST segment flattening and occasionally ST segment depression, even in the absence of coexisting CAD.
- Arrhythmias occasionally occur, due either to hypoxaemia or to β-agonists. The commonest are atrial fibrillation and atrioventricular node reentrant tachycardias.
- Bradycardia due to arterial hypoxaemia can occur in severe (preterminal) asthma. This is a very ominous sign – immediate ventilation is required.

Chronic obstructive pulmonary disease

COPD is characterized by airflow limitation (reduced peak flow and forced expiratory volume in 1 second, FEV_1) due to hypertrophy of the mucosal glands of the bronchial tree and destruction of the structures that support the airways. The principal cause of COPD is cigarette smoking; other factors (industrial pollution, adverse climate, genetic) have a smaller role.

Characteristic symptoms

Typical symptoms of COPD include:

- Those of chronic bronchitis: early morning productive cough for 3 or more months per year for 2 or more years in succession. These symptoms often predate COPD by many years.
- Gradually increasing breathlessness over many years with gradual decline in exercise capacity. Breathlessness is associated with a wheeze and sometimes a 'tight' chest (particularly on effort – this can be difficult to differentiate clinically from angina).
- Exacerbations during which breathlessness rapidly becomes much worse (over a few days to a week or so), often occurring at rest. Exacerbations

are often triggered by viral or bacterial infection and are due to a temporary increase in airways resistance.

Physical examination

Clinical examination for COPD may show the signs of:

- air trapping – decreased ratio of sternal angle to cricoid cartilage distance, causing a 'barrel-chested' appearance
- airway obstruction with wheezing
- right heart hypertrophy (with a left parasternal lift) and failure (raised venous pressure, peripheral oedema)
- respiratory failure in advanced COPD – hypoxaemia classically leads to agitation, and confusion, whereas hypercapnoea leads to a warm, vasodilated periphery, sleepiness and coma
- cachexia – frequently found in advanced COPD.

Diagnosis

The diagnosis of COPD is made from the clinical features and lung function tests, with spirometry showing an obstructive picture. A chest X-ray should be performed to exclude other smoking-related disease (particularly lung cancer) and, in those breathless at rest, concomitant heart failure or chest infection.

ECG in COPD

The ECG in COPD may show a number of changes.

The most important abnormalities to look for are right axis deviation and/or a dominant R wave in lead V1, both indicative of pulmonary hypertension. Pulmonary hypertension is associated with a worse outlook, especially if there is complicating right ventricular failure, and is therefore a key finding. Early signs of right ventricular hypertrophy (RVH), such as right axis deviation of the QRS complex, are suggestive but can have other explanations (eg conducting tissue disease). Likewise, the sign of advanced RVH, a dominant R wave in V1, is neither sensitive nor specific for pulmonary hypertension; many patients with COPD-related pulmonary hypertension do not have this sign and many patients with this sign do not have pulmonary hypertension (they may have an old posterior wall MI). The best approach to diagnosing pulmonary hypertension in this setting is by cardiac ultrasound [the velocity of the jet of tricuspid regurgitation is in many patients a good, noninvasive measure of pulmonary arterial pressure (PAP)].

The ECG is often nonspecifically abnormal, showing mild lateral lead T wave changes (eg T wave flattening). The significance of such changes is very uncertain – they should probably have no influence on subsequent management.

Hypertension is common in those with COPD and the ECG may reflect this in showing left ventricular hypertrophy (LVH). Clearly, unless the prognosis from the COPD is extremely poor, any hypertension associated with LVH should be vigorously treated.

Coronary artery disease is common in this group and may be seen on the ECG, either as evidence of previous infarction (old Q waves or more commonly ST flattening, or T wave inversion following previous non-Q wave MI) or as ST changes (see below).

Patients may demonstrate ST depression during an exacerbation, often without any chest pain; this is often due to a combination of CAD, arterial hypoxaemia and inhaled β_1-agonists (used as bronchodilators to improve any reversible component to airways obstruction) increasing cardiac contractility, cardiac workload and oxygen demand. How asymptomatic ST depression during an acute episode should be managed is unclear – minimizing cardiac workload (eg via 'heart rate-slowing' drugs such as diltiazem) seems sensible. Further investigations designed to confirm or exclude ischaemic heart disease (IHD) may be appropriate following the acute episode (including exercise ECG, pharmacological stress nuclear imaging, cardiac ultrasound and, rarely, coronary angiography).

Heart failure

See below.

Pulmonary emboli

PE is a potent cause of breathlessness, and it is vital to rapidly establish the diagnosis and start treatment. PE give rise to three different clinical syndromes.

Small pulmonary emboli

Small PE cause mild breathlessness and/or pleuritic chest pain. The physical examination is usually normal although there may be evidence of calf deep vein thrombosis. Arterial hypoxaemia increases suspicion, and the diagnosis is established from nuclear $\dot{V}/\dot{Q}$ scanning or CT (or conventional) pulmonary angiography. The ECG is usually unremarkable.

Massive pulmonary emboli

Massive PE cause severe breathlessness, sudden collapse (sometimes with syncope) and shock. The patient is obviously unwell with (marked) tachypnoea and signs of low cardiac output: pallor, cool and sweaty skin, tachycardia (heart rate often ≥120 bpm) and hypotension (systolic blood pressure ≤80–90 mmHg). The jugular venous pressure is raised. The diagnosis is usually obvious clinically but can be confirmed by cardiac ultrasound, which often shows acute right heart strain, a dilated poorly functioning right ventricle, and evidence of raised PAP (high-velocity tricuspid regurgitant jet on cardiac Doppler ultrasound). Free-floating right atrial thrombi can sometimes be seen. The ECG in massive PE is often dramatically abnormal, with extreme rightward axis shift (seen as R wave height decreased in lead I and increased in lead III). Acute right heart strain may interfere with right bundle function; right bundle branch block (RBBB) is therefore not uncommon in massive PE. Once the PE has been successfully treated (usually with thrombolytic therapy, occasionally by surgical removal), the right heart strain resolves and the ECG returns to normal.

Chronic pulmonary emboli

Chronic thromboembolic lung disease is a rare syndrome but an important diagnosis as treatment can be life-saving. Patients have repeated PE over several months but none large enough to cause severe symptoms warranting hospitalization. Patients become progressively more breathless over time and effort capacity falls. Physical examination shows a patient who becomes breathless easily. There may be signs of right heart strain or failure, manifest as a left parasternal lift (from RVH) and a raised jugular venous pressure, both are consequences of a dramatically elevated PAP which may be supra-systemic! The chest X-ray is usually normal although there may be some cardiomegaly (with a right ventricular outline pattern). The ECG in chronic thromboembolic lung disease is often (but not always) rather dramatically abnormal, with RVH manifest as a dominant (and narrow) R wave in lead V1 along with rightward QRS axis shift. Conversely the ECG may be virtually normal, showing only trivial changes. Do not rely on the ECG to accurately reflect PAP! The diagnosis of chronic thromboembolic lung disease is confirmed by $\dot{V}/\dot{Q}$ scanning, although a CT pulmonary angiogram should be undertaken as this outlines how much thrombus has become endothelialized in the main pulmonary arteries and thus whether pulmonary thrombendarterectomy can be performed.

Once the diagnosis of chronic PE is established immediate anticoagulation is indicated. The PAP often falls with prolonged warfarin therapy; as this happens, the magnitude of the R wave in V1 will diminish. If, despite prolonged warfarin anticoagulation, symptoms remain unacceptable or the PAP remains above 50 mmHg, pulmonary thrombendarterectomy may be indicated. Although the ECG gives some guide to the success or otherwise of treatment, cardiac ultrasound-derived measures of PAP are much more reliable.

Pleural effusion

This is a relatively common cause of breathlessness. Symptoms arise either from the effusion itself (although this needs to be quite large to cause breathlessness) or from the underlying disease process. If the effusion is due to malignancy then anaemia may be a major contributor to breathlessness, whereas if heart failure is the cause then adverse haemodynamics will be responsible.

The ECG does not change in pleural effusion, but may show changes from any underlying disease process.

Inflammatory and fibrotic lung diseases

Inflammatory and fibrotic lung diseases are rare but important causes of breathlessness.

Clinical history

The clinical history often provides some clues to the presence of inflammatory or fibrotic lung disease, ie progressive breathlessness without wheeze or orthopnoea, often with rather marked extrapulmonary features or with predisposing diseases such as rheumatoid arthritis or sytemic lupus erythematosus (SLE) being present. However, the real clue to their presence is often obtained from the chest X-ray (which shows diffuse–nodular 'infiltration' or 'honeycombing') and lung function tests (which show a restrictive defect).

Investigations

The diagnosis is usually established from high-resolution CT scan of the lungs, often aided by various blood tests [eg antibody assays (antineutrophil cytoplasmic antibody assay or antinuclear antibody), rheumatoid factor, and precipitins against organic dusts or microbes] and sometimes by lung biopsy. These diseases all interfere with the flow of blood through the lung and, as a consequence, cause the PAP to rise; the cardiac ultrasound therefore often shows a normal left heart with a raised tricuspid regurgitant jet velocity indicative of pulmonary hypertension.

The pulmonary hypertension found in inflammatory and fibrotic lung disease causes characteristic ECG changes of right axis deviation, with a dominant R wave in lead V1. There are typically rather small elevations in PAP with inflammatory lung diseases (such as acute sarcoidosis), greater increases in PAP with acute adult respiratory distress (now more commonly known as acute lung injury) and much more impressive increases in PAP with fibrotic lung disease (eg chronic sarcoidosis or cryptogenic fibrosing alveolitis). Therefore the more marked the R wave in V1 is, the more likely fibrosis is to be present and the poorer the response to treatment will be. As inflammatory lung disease tends to respond rather well to therapy, whereas fibrotic lung disease tends to respond rather poorly, the presence of a dominant R wave in lead V1 in these conditions is associated with a worse prognosis.

Obesity

Obesity, now referred to by the pseudonym 'high BMI', is a common cause of breathlessness. Dyspnoea in this situation is due to a number of mechanisms, including increased cardiorespiratory work from carrying the extra body mass and 'splinting' of the diaphragm causing a restrictive-type of lung defect.

ECG changes

Obesity changes the QRS axis, typically in a rightward direction, and, more frequently, diminishes QRS complex height (as chest tissue interferes with the flow of electricity to the ECG electrodes). The differential diagnosis of small QRS complexes includes very poor LV function due to substantial (and usually permanent) myocyte damage. In the clinic it is sometimes difficult to know if the patient is 'just obese' or if they have heart disease as well. Other than the obvious clues from the physical examination, high-BMI subjects without heart disease tend to have small QRS complexes in an otherwise unremarkable ECG, whereas in patients with LV dysfunction the small QRS complexes are associated with ST and T wave changes.

Obstructive sleep apnoea

Obstructive sleep apnoea (OSA) is a common complication of obesity. During sleep the upper airway recurrently 'blocks off' (causing initially loud snoring then apnoea), resulting in arousal and sleep disturbance (and so excess daytime tiredness, which can be quantified by a standardized, questionnaire-based scoring system). The PAP increases so the changes of pulmonary hypertension may occur on the ECG (rightward QRS axis shift, dominant R wave in V1). Occasionally frank right heart failure occurs. Hypertension is common in the obese, especially if OSA is present, and this may be seen on the ECG as LVH.

Dysfunctional breathing

Hyperventilation (also termed 'psychogenic breathlessness') is now referred to by the more modern term of dysfunctional breathing, is an extraordinarily common cause of breathlessness.

Clinical history

Dysfunctional breathing tends to produce breathlessness at rest. Although dysfunctional breathing can cause effort-related dyspnoea, this is rather rare, and breathlessness that occurs reliably at the same level of exercise is most likely to have an underlying organic cause. Patients may have associated symptoms due to 'functional' hypocalcaemia (circumoral parasthaesia, and tingling in the hands and feet) and may or may not be visibly tachypnoeic.

Investigations and treatment

If available, measurement of arterial blood gases in dysfunctional breathing shows supranormal O_2 levels and depressed CO_2 levels. The ECG is often not normal – there may be quite substantial ST segment and T wave changes – but these should revert to normal after the episode. Psychological treatments for dysfunctional breathing may prove highly effective.

Heart failure

Heart failure is an extremely common cause of breathlessness. It is a syndrome primarily caused by an abnormality in the heart that causes cardiac, renal and skeletal muscle dysfunction. It can be defined and quantified by:

Impact on exercise capacity (via New York Heart Association grade): grade I = no limitation; grade II = symptoms on moderate effort (eg walking one-quarter to one-half of a mile); grade III = symptoms on mild effort (eg walking less than a few hundred yards); grade IV = symptoms at rest.

Aetiology. See below.

Time course and symptomatology: acute heart failure is usually synonymous with pulmonary oedema (causing acute, severe breathlessness; pink, frothy sputum if severe; tachycardia; cold, clammy skin; and bibasal pulmonary crepitations), and chronic heart failure (causing effort intolerance due to breathlessness and/or fatigue, lethargy, and eventually weight loss) is synonymous with right heart failure (raised venous pressure, peripheral oedema and hepatomegaly), although left heart failure can also occur. Combined left and right heart failure is sometimes called 'congestive heart failure'.

Abnormal haemodynamics: impaired LV systolic or diastolic performance, decreased cardiac output and increased cardiac filling pressures.

Changes in neurohormonal function: raised concentrations of catecholamines, antidiuretic hormone, endothelin and cytokines (including tumour necrosis factor α) together with activation of the renin–angiotensin axis all contribute to the pathophysiology.

Characteristic symptoms

The most common symptom of heart failure is breathlessness, occurring only on substantial effort initially but requiring less effort as the condition advances and eventually occurring at rest. In congestive heart failure fluid accumulates in the legs during the day, where it may or may not give rise to noticeable oedema. At night horizontal posture allows the fluid to move from the legs into the central circulation and then into the lungs. Nocturnal LVF results, waking the patient up typically at two to three a.m., very breathless and frightened. Patients in this situation 'need to get more fresh air' and so get up to throw the windows open. Assuming an upright posture improves the breathing over 15–20 minutes.

Other common symptoms of heart failure include effort intolerance for nonspecific reasons, tiredness and lassitude, weakness, and occasionally weight loss (an ominous sign).

Physical examination

Physical examination reveals signs specific to the cause of the heart failure, especially in valvular heart disease. Signs general to patients with significant established cardiac dysfunction are also found. In most (but not all) patients with heart failure cardiac enlargement occurs, detected clinically as a displaced apex beat. Mitral regurgitation (MR) occurs as a consequence of LV dilatation; it often improves as heart failure is treated and so may be used as a guide to treatment success.

Signs of fluid retention are also seen with heart failure, specifically bibasal crepitations in those with left heart failure and a raised jugular venous pressure, with or without ankle oedema, in those with right heart failure.

Unfortunately many patients breathless from heart failure have a fairly unremarkable clinical examination, so this cannot be relied on for the diagnosis.

Causes of heart failure

Ischaemic heart disease

Pre-MI causes of heart failure. In the setting of critical proximal multivessel CAD, heart failure can occur either when LV function is normal or near-normal (and thus the resting ECG can be completely normal) or when 'hibernation' is present (ie the ECG is usually diffusely abnormal); see Box 6.1. Hibernation occurs when myocardial ischaemia is sufficiently severe to cause myocyte contractile function to 'switch off' but insufficient to actually

117

Box 6.1 Premyocardial infarction causes of heart failure*

(A) Acute left ventricular failure (good LV function on cardiac ultrasound once LVF is treated

- Critical proximal multivessel disease
  - Often no (or only short) history of preceding angina
  - LV function good (once pulmonary oedema treated)
  - Resting ECG often unremarkable although minor ST/T wave changes may occur
  - Exercise ECG may show ST segment depression
  - Angiography diagnostic
- Arrhythmias
  - AF most common
  - Often 'stiff' heart (eg LVH) also present
  - Usually (not always) arrhythmia still present at hospital presentation
- Papillary muscle dysfunction
  - Causes acute MR
  - Murmur not heard during acute LVF (too much lung noise) or afterwards (papillary muscle no longer ischaemic so little MR)
  - Resting ECG shows dominant T wave in V1
  - Angiography shows circumflex artery disease
- Renal artery stenosis
  - Very rare
  - Can cause 'flash' pulmonary oedema
  - Suspect when all other causes excluded
  - Renal angiography diagnostic

- Beware – the troponin level is often raised in acute LVH regardless of cause

(B) Chronic (or subacute) heart failure (>1 week; poor LV function on cardiac US)

- Hibernation
  - ECG: ST/T wave change only; good 'volts' (ie good R waves)
  - Echocardiography: dilated, poor LV function; normal wall thickness
  - 'Stress' echocardiography: global and regional LV function improves
  - Nuclear studies: late pick-up of isotope
  - Good response to revascularization
- Old 'silent' MI
  - ECG: Q waves, small complexes
  - Echocardiography: dilated, poor LV function; thin walls
  - 'Stress' echocardiography: no improvement in LV function
  - Nuclear studies: no isotope pick-up
  - No response to revascularization

*No previous myocardial infarction (MI), valvular disease or other cause. LV, left ventricular; LVF, left ventricular failure; AF, atrial fibrillation; LVH, left ventricular hypertrophy; MR, mitral regurgitation; US, ultrasound.

cause myocyte necrosis; ie the cells remain viable. Hibernation can last for many months, indeed until formal revascularization occurs. However, after years of hibernation viable cells are replaced with scar tissue (thus at this point revascularization will have no beneficial impact). The phenomenon of 'hibernation' is important to diagnose, as revascularization early on can result in a dramatic improvement in LV function, reduced symptoms and prolonged life.

Hibernation is suspected when a patient presents with heart failure and is found to have both substantial impairment of LV function and critical CAD, without evidence of previous infarction. It is crucial to differentiate this from a patient who has irreversible myocyte cell death as a consequence of MI, as the former will benefit (dramatically) from revascularization whereas the latter probably will not. The presence of hibernation is established via:

- the presence of angina, indicating viable cells in ischaemic territory
- the resting ECG: the presence of good-sized R waves and the absence of Q waves indicate substantial numbers of viable myocytes within ischaemic territory
- isotope studies: isotopes that are taken up by metabolically active cells, are injected intravenously. If areas of the heart that contract poorly or not at all 'pick up' significant amounts of tracer, it is concluded that they contain substantial numbers of viable cells
- stress studies, especially stress echo: increasing the inotropic state of myocytes improves the contractile function of all viable myocytes, including those in hibernation.

Peri-MI causes of heart failure. Heart failure in this setting is usually (Figure 6.2) due to loss of contractile tissue from within the area of the infarct. See p. 225 for ECG changes of MI. The larger the infarct, the more likely it is that heart failure will develop. Some idea of the size of the MI can be gained from the ECG. Infarcts with the following characteristics are particularly likely to result in heart failure:

- where substantial ST segment elevation is present
- where ST segment elevation affects many leads
- with anterior ST segment elevation
- where thrombolysis fails to resolve ST segment elevation, and where Q waves develop.

Sometimes myocyte function in the peri-infarct area is reversibly impaired and improves in the days following the MI. These cells are referred to as 'stunned'.

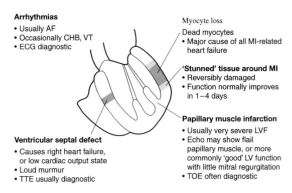

Arrhythmias
- Usually AF
- Occasionally CHB, VT
- ECG diagnostic

Myocyte loss
Dead myocytes
- Major cause of all MI-related heart failure

'Stunned' tissue around MI
- Reversibly damaged
- Function normally improves in 1–4 days

Papillary muscle infarction
- Usually very severe LVF
- Echo may show flail papillary muscle, or more commonly 'good' LV function with little mitral regurgitation
- TOE often diagnostic

Ventricular septal defect
- Causes right heart failure, or low cardiac output state
- Loud murmur
- TTE usually diagnostic

Figure 6.2
Peri-myocardial infarction (MI) causes of heart failure. AF, atrial fibrillation; CHB, complete heart bock; VT, ventricular tachycardia; TTE, transthoracic echocardiography; LVF, left ventricular failure; Echo, echocardiography; TOE, transoesophageal echocardiography.

There are two other important causes of peri-MI heart failure: acute MR and acute ventricular septal defect (VSD). Patients with acute ischaemic MR usually develop sudden and extraordinarily severe pulmonary oedema. They sit bolt upright, are very breathless, produce pink frothy sputum, are tachycardic and have lungs full of crepitations. The MR murmur can be very quiet or absent. Medical treatment is often unsuccessful; in those salvaged by diuretics and mechanical ventilation immediate valve replacement surgery is indicated. Many (but not all) patients with acute MR complicating an MI have circumflex coronary artery territory ischaemia or infarction causing either a ruptured papillary muscle or reversible papillary muscle ischaemia. Thus the ECG commonly shows changes in leads V1 to V3, ST segment depression for a posterior MI, evolving to a dominant R wave in lead V1 (see p. 58).

Patients with acute VSD usually present with predominant right heart failure or symptoms and signs of a low cardiac output (cool skin, oliguria). The diagnosis is usually easy (loud pansystolic murmur at the base of the left sternal edge, with typical echo appearances). Surgical (or perhaps percutaneous) closure for VSDs associated with anterior wall MIs can be life-saving. However, VSDs associated with inferior wall MIs still have a near 100% mortality even if treated surgically. The ECG in ischaemic VSD shows the acute MI but little else that is pathognomonic of the condition.

Box 6.2 Cardiac ultrasound findings in the heart failure syndrome following an MI

- Aneurysm at site of MI, remaining LV function good
  - Suspect when persisting ST segment elevation
  - Consider aneurysmectomy
- Akinetic wall at MI site, good remaining LV function
  - Consider that ischaemia to viable tissue underlies heart failure
  - Undertake coronary angiography
- Akinetic MI site, poor remaining LV function
  - Adverse LV remodelling is the most common cause
  - Hibernation to distant (non-MI) tissue rare but important
  - Consider coronary angiography ± stress echocardiography ± nuclear studies to distinguish hibernation from adverse remodeling

---

Box 6.3 Exacerbating factors in heart failure

- Anaemia
- Atrial fibrillation
- Thyrotoxicosis
- Sepsis
- New valve lesion, especially aortic stenosis

Post-MI heart failure. Heart failure post MI can have a number of aetiologies (Boxes 6.2 and 6.3). The most important cause is loss of myocytes at the time of the MI, leading to dilatation of the LV ('adverse LV remodelling'). Cardiac enlargement is mechanically disadvantageous, according to the law of Laplace. Thus, following even relatively mild cardiac enlargement, the heart enlarges further, becoming even less efficient, which causes further enlargement, etc. The ECG is usually very abnormal, with loss of R waves and/or pathological Q waves along with ST segment and T wave changes.

However, in addition to adverse LV remodelling, two other causes must be considered as potentially contributing to heart failure in the post-MI patient (just as in the pre-MI patient): hibernation (see above) and critical CAD (supplying areas that remain conventionally viable).

It is often very difficult to ascertain how much tissue is permanently dead and how much is not. Angiography is often a good first step in clarifying this: if there is no flow-limiting stenosis then there is no hibernation, whereas if there are flow-limiting stenoses then, if the supplied territory is hypo- or akinetic, the possibility of hibernation arises. In this situation the presence of angina should be taken to indicate viability and revascularization should be performed. If no angina is present then functional studies (ie nuclear or stress cardiac ultrasound) may be needed for clarification.

Cardiomyopathies

Cardiomyopathies are common causes of heart failure and are separated into three classes on the basis of their cardiac ultrasound appearance (Figure 6.3).

Dilated cardiomyopathy (DCM). This is the commonest cardiomyopathy, wherein left (often right as well) ventricular systolic function is dramatically reduced and the heart dilates as a consequence. The left ventricle is therefore enlarged echocardiographically and has poor systolic function. The wall is often thinned. These ultrasound appearances are usually not difficult to see. Heart failure and arrhythmias [atrial fibrillation (AF) and not infrequently lethal ventricular arrhythmias] are common. DCM is most commonly an autoimmune disease (anticardiac myocyte antibodies are found) with a substantial genetic predisposition (50–60% of patients have similarly affected family members). Some patients with apparent idiopathic DCM are in fact suffering from the late consequences of undiagnosed viral myocarditis. Excess alcohol, thyrotoxicosis and iron overload (genetic, environmental or due to multiple blood transfusions) can also cause DCM (Box 6.4).

The ECG in idiopathic DCM is usually very abnormal. The rhythm is often AF; nonsustained or sustained ventricular arrhythmias may also be present. Broadening of the QRS complex proceeding to full left bundle branch block (LBBB) is common and RBBB is not rare. If bundle branch block does not occur, two alternative and rather paradoxical patterns may be seen: loss of R wave amplitude, often with very abnormal ST segments and T waves (the commonest pattern; Q waves occasionally occur); and LVH (commoner in younger patients), particularly with the more 'inflammatory' forms of DCM (eg postviral myocarditis LV dysfunction).

Hypertrophic cardiomyopathy. This is a rare, genetically mediated disease. Only relatively few cases are complicated by heart failure; arrhythmias are a much more common problem (AF, ventricular tachycardia and ventricular fibrillation). Cardiac ultrasound appearances are usually typical. In some (but not most) families genetic diagnosis is possible. The ECG often (but not always) shows LVH (see p. 33) and (often widespread) T wave inversion throughout the anterolateral leads. Sometimes only T wave inversion is seen. Disturbingly, in about 5% of cases the ECG may show surprisingly few abnormalities.

(a)

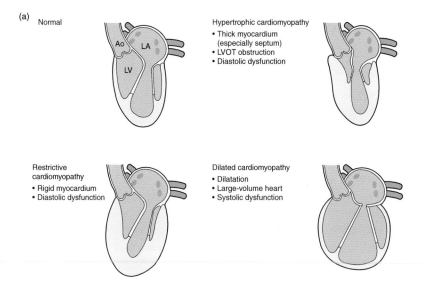

(b)

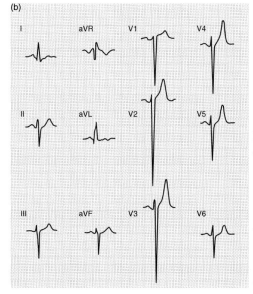

Figure 6.3

(a) Different forms of cardiomyopathy. Ao, aorta; LA, left atrium; LV, left ventricle; LVOT, left ventricular outflow tract. Reprinted with permission from Davey P. *Medicine at a Glance*. Oxford: Blackwell Science. (b) ECG from a patient with hypertrophic obstructive cardiomyopathy and an outflow tract gradient at rest of 4 m/s (64 mmHg). The patient was asymptomatic and the diagnosis was made on screening. This ECG shows left atrial enlargement, left axis deviation and increased chest lead voltages (indicating LVH).

123

Box 6.4 Some common causes of dilated cardiomyopathy

- Toxins
  - Alcohol
  - Drugs (anthracyclines)
- Endocrine
  - Hypothroidism
  - Thyrotoxicosis
  - Phaeochromocytoma
- Infection
  - Viruses (coxsackie)
  - *Trypanosoma* species (Chagas' disease)
- Dietary
  - Beri-beri (thiamine deficiency)
- Infiltrative
  - Sarcoid
  - Iron overload (haemochromatosis, excess blood transfusions)
- Genetic
  - Familial dilated cardiomyopathy
  - Muscular dystrophies (Duchenne, myotonic, mitochondrial)

Reprinted with permission from Davey, P. *Medicine at a Glance*. Oxford: Blackwell Science, 2002

Restrictive cardiomyopathy. This is extraordinarily rare; it is caused by amyloidosis and various tropical hypereosinophilic syndromes. Ultrasound diagnosis can be easy but often is not, and it may be confused sometimes with constrictive pericarditis. The ECG often shows LVH and/or RVH, with or without widespread nonspecific ST segment changes.

Valvular heart disease

A not infrequent cause of heart failure is valvular heart disease, especially aortic valve disease (Figure 6.4a, b; aortic stenosis is very common in the elderly) but also mitral valve disease (Figure 6.4c, d), mainly MR. In patients with significant aortic stenosis the ECG usually (but not always) shows LVH. The same is true for patients with aortic regurgitation. However, surprisingly, LVH is not seen on the ECG in many patients with significant MR. Virtually all mitral stenosis is the consequence of rheumatic fever, and this is now very rare in the developed world. The ECG signs of mitral stenosis are left atrial enlargement, AF and RVH.

Myocarditis

Myocarditis is an unusual (but not infrequent) cause of heart failure. It can present 'late' as an apparent DCM (see above) or more rarely during the acute illness, when typically patients present with breathlessness progressive

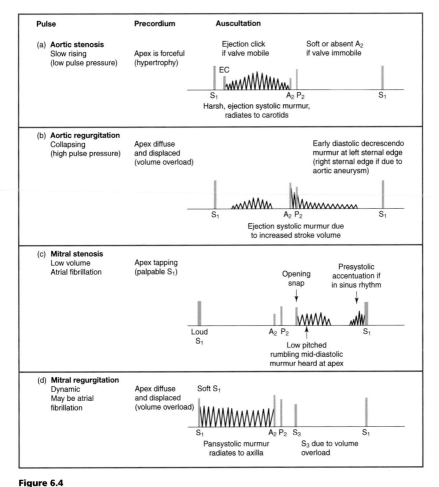

Figure 6.4
Clinical features of (a) aortic stenosis, (b) aortic regurgitation, (c) mitral stenosis and (d) mitral regurgitation. Reprinted with permission from Davey, P. *Medicine at a Glance*. Oxford: Blackwell Science, 2002.

over a few weeks (occasionally a few days). Examination shows the signs of right and left heart failure but the heart rate is usually much higher than would be predicted from the severity of the heart failure – this is a key clue that myocarditis is present.

Troponin concentrations are often raised and the ECG is usually nonspecifically abnormal, showing ST segment and T wave changes. Rarely, acute myocarditis presents in a fulminating fashion, with an ECG showing ST segment elevation (which can be confused with ST segment elevation MI due to standard atherosclerotic heart disease. If the condition is long-standing, LVH may occur. Conducting tissue disease such as a bundle branch block or prolonged PR interval can occur. The cardiac ultrasound shows decreased left (and often right) ventricular function, sometimes with hypertrophy. The condition may be caused by:

- viruses
- peripartum cardiomyopathy
- remote bacterial infection (eg rheumatic fever caused by streptococcal sore throat)
- Lyme disease (*Borrelia burgdorferi)* and Chagas' disease (*Trypanosoma cruzii)*
- autoimmune disease (eg scleroderma, SLE or polymyositis).

There is no specific therapy (immunosuppressive therapy helps in autoimmune disease). Often patients respond to standard heart failure treatment. If not, LV-assist devices can be life-saving until the condition spontaneously improves with viral clearing. Heart transplantation is a final option.

Pericardial disease

Pericardial constriction is a rare cause of heart failure. It is suspected when a heart failure syndrome develops and the examination shows major ascites but little or no leg oedema. The diagnosis is made from CT or magnetic resonance imaging of the pericardium and from invasively measured haemodynamics. The ECG usually shows only mild ST changes (flattening or inversion); R waves are usually well preserved but may be diminished in size.

Other factors exacerbating heart failure

Anaemia, infection and nonsteroidal anti-inflammatory drugs can all provoke a deterioration in those with cardiac dysfunction. These have no ECG consequences. Atrial fibrillation is a relatively common cause of deterioration. Heart block is a rare cause of deterioration.

The ECG in heart failure

The ECG in specific disease processes causing heart failure is detailed elsewhere. This section summarizes the ECG changes that may be found in an acutely or chronically breathless patient in whom the syndrome of acute or chronic heart failure is suspected (or confirmed) but the aetiology is still obscure.

ECG in acute heart failure (pulmonary oedema)

A *sinus tachycardia* may be the most obvious ECG manifestation of acute heart failure. It is proportional to the severity of the pulmonary oedema and is a good guide to the success or otherwise of treatment.

Acute MI may underlie LVF: either full-thickness [ie ST segment elevation MI (STEMI)] or non-STEMI (see p. 223). Signs of an old MI may be seen – usually Q waves or loss of R waves in the territory of the affected coronary.

Left ventricular hypertrophy is a good clue that heart failure is either the consequence of hypertensive heart disease or (more likely in the UK) of aortic stenosis. Some patients with cardiomyopathy initially present with pulmonary oedema and it is not uncommon to find LVH on the ECG. Very rarely patients with a phaeochromocytoma present with heart failure and an ECG usually shows LVH (hypertension may not be present if LV dysfunction is sufficiently severe; all patients with unexplained heart failure should therefore be screened for a phaeochromocytoma).

Left bundle branch block is common to many diseases, including CAD, aortic stenosis and cardiomyopathy, and advanced LVH often 'converts' into LBBB. Its presence does not aid diagnosis.

If none of the above are present (ie R waves are a good size, no Q waves are present and only mild T wave changes are seen) a number of other causes should be considered, including critical CAD and the extraordinarily rare 'flash' pulmonary oedema due to renal artery stenosis.

Rhythm abnormalities. Arrhythmias may be present in acute heart failure and the most common is AF. Excess ventricular ectopy is not rare. Primary bradyarrhythmias such as complete heart block are very occasionally seen.

The ECG in chronic heart failure

Rarely the ECG may be normal in chronic heart failure (CHF); however, most patients have some ECG abnormalities (albeit occasionally subtle); see Figure 6.5.

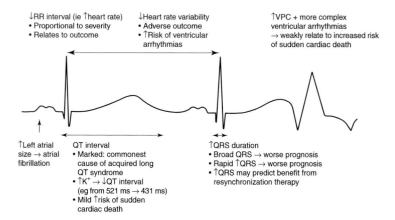

↓RR interval (ie ↑heart rate)
• Proportional to severity
• Relates to outcome

↓Heart rate variability
• Adverse outcome
• ↑Risk of ventricular arrhythmias

↑VPC + more complex ventricular arrhythmias
→ weakly relate to increased risk of sudden cardiac death

↑Left atrial size → atrial fibrillation

QT interval
• Marked: commonest cause of acquired long QT syndrome
• ↑K⁺ → ↓QT interval (eg from 521 ms → 431 ms)
• Mild ↑risk of sudden cardiac death

↑QRS duration
• Broad QRS → worse prognosis
• Rapid ↑QRS → worse prognosis
• ↑QRS may predict benefit from resynchronization therapy

Figure 6.5
ECG changes in chronic heart failure. VPC, ventricular premature contraction; HRV, heart rate variability.

QRS duration. QRS duration prolongation (progressing all the way to full LBBB) is common in heart failure of any cause, and is to some extent proportional to the severity of the LV dysfunction. The broader the QRS complex, the worse the outlook. Furthermore, rapidly increasing QRS durations confer the worst outlook (Figure 6.6). Conversely patients with broad QRS complexes may benefit substantially from multisite ventricular pacing. Although the relationship between QRS duration and prognosis is useful, other prognostic factors (Table 6.3) are more important in assessing outcome for most patients.

Q waves. Old Q waves, especially in the anterior chest leads, suggest a diagnosis of IHD, but patients with DCM can also (rarely) show Q waves – Q waves are thus not diagnostic of IHD.

Left ventricular hypertrophy. ECG evidence of LVH is frequently found in chronic heart failure as aortic stenosis and hypertension underlie many cases of CHF.

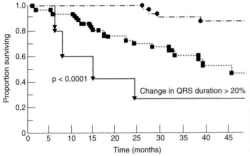

Figure 6.6
Relationship between change in QRS duration and outlook in chronic heart failure. Reproduced with permission from Shamin W, Yousufuddin M, Cicona M *et al. Heart* 2002; **88**: 47–51.

Table 6.3 Prognostic factors in heart failure

Prognostic factor	Worse outcome if:
Left ventricular EF	Low EF; treatment or spontaneous improvement in EF ≥5% associated with improved outcome
Exercise capacity, as per NYHA class	Poor exercise capacity or high NYHA class
Oxygen uptake at peak exercise	Low oxygen uptake
Serum [Na⁺]	Low [Na⁺]
Syncope	Presence (see Chapter 8)
Plasma neurohormones (catecholamines, including noradrenaline) and cytokines	Raised levels
Nonsustained VT	Presence
Duration and stability of disease	Shorter duration and inability to stabilize with treatment
Aetiology	IHD DCM worse than idiopathic DCM
Heart rate	Persistent sinus tachycardia
Heart rate variability	Low

EF, ejection fraction; NYHA, New York Heart Association; VT, ventricular tachycardia; IHD, ischaemic heart disease; DCM, dilated cardiomyopathy.

T wave changes. A pattern of nonspecific T wave changes only is common to many causes of heart failure, particularly DCM. Likewise, many cases of hibernation show only mild T wave changes.

Arrhythmias are very common in CHF, particularly AF. As the left ventricle is stiffer in LVF, atrial systole makes a greater contribution to overall cardiac output (around 20–40%) than in normal subjects (about 10%). Thus the loss of atrial systole in AF can lead to dramatic worsening of heart failure symptoms. Ventricular arrhythmias are also very common, including ectopy, couplets, and nonsustained and sustained tachycardias [the latter both monomorphic and polymorphic ('torsade-de-pointes') type ventricular tachycardias (VTs)]. Polymorphic VT often presents as 'sudden cardiac death'. The incidence of low-grade (ie isolated monomorphic ventricular premature contractions) and intermediate-grade (ie couplets, triplets and nonsustained VT) ventricular arrhythmias does bear some relationship to the subsequent development of high-grade ventricular arrhythmias. Implantable cardioverter defibrillators (ICDs) are an effective prophylaxis and treatment for high-grade, haemodynamically unstable ventricular arrhythmias. Accordingly, patients with heart failure should be screened for the presence of ventricular arrhythmias using 24-hour Holter ECG monitors; if they are found to be at higher risk, appropriate preventive therapy should be given. Current evidence suggests that those with an ejection fraction ≤30% are at high risk of developing high-grade, life-threatening ventricular arrhythmias and should receive an ICD regardless of whether or not they have frequent lower-grade arrhythmias. Patients with an intermediate ejection fraction (30–40%) should receive an ICD if nonsustained ventricular arrhythmias occur.

QT interval prolongation. Heart failure is a very potent and common cause of QT interval prolongation, proportionate to impairment of LV systolic function (although this is not sufficiently reliable to be used instead of cardiac ultrasound). QT interval prolongation in heart failure probably slightly increases the chance of sudden cardiac death. It can be minimized by maintaining an optimal K^+ concentration (ie 4.5–5.0 mmol/l).

Can the ECG be a substitute for a cardiac ultrasound in heart failure? Although a cardiac ultrasound is the definitive means of assessing cardiac function it is sometimes not available. Can the ECG be used to diagnose heart failure? The short answer is 'no', as many of the abnormalities seen in heart failure are also seen in other disease processes. However, the ECG is moderately helpful in ruling out heart failure; a normal ECG in a breathless patient (who has no diagnostic murmurs or other evidence of a cardiac problem on clinical examination) implies that the diagnosis is almost certainly not heart failure.

Other investigations in suspected heart failure

Other investigations usually performed in suspected heart failure include the following:

Chest X-ray. Many (but not all) causes of heart failure are associated with cardiac enlargement, which may be reflected in cardiomegaly on the chest X-ray. High left atrial pressures may be seen early on as 'upper lobe blood diversion' and later as frank pulmonary oedema (with interstitial fluid, pleural effusions, etc).

Cardiac ultrasound is the key investigation for heart failure, although it has significant false-positive and false-negative rates (see below).

Cardiac catheterization is indicated in those with heart failure and known valvular heart disease (as a prelude to surgery, mainly to exclude concomitant CAD), those with heart failure and known CAD (as part of the work-up to assess benefit from revascularization), and those with heart failure of unknown aetiology, to determine the contribution of CAD to the pathophysiology.

Biochemical measures of neuroendocrine activation, especially of the renin–angiotensin system (reflected as raised angiotensin II levels), and other neurohormones (eg brain natriuretic peptide) are useful in 'ruling out' symptomatic heart failure. However, they are less useful in diagnosing the heart failure syndrome.

Cardiac ultrasound

The key investigation in suspected heart failure is cardiac ultrasound, used to confirm the diagnosis (by demonstrating either significant impairment of left ventricular function and/or valvular heart disease) and estimate prognosis. Prognosis in CHF relates to many factors (Table 6.3) – ejection fraction is one key independent variable and can be estimated from the cardiac ultrasound.

An ultrasound scan is an indispensable aspect of the work-up of many breathless patients and of all those suspected of heart failure. However, it has limitations, and a normal or near-normal scan does not exclude the diagnosis. A (near) normal scan can occur in those with heart failure due to:

Predominant LV diastolic dysfunction. The usual clue to this is that the LV wall thickness is increased, often due to long-standing hypertension. There are, however, some patients who have substantial LV diastolic failure and very little LVH, and the diagnosis of diastolic heart failure can be a particularly difficult one to make in such circumstances.

Critical CAD. In this situation the presentation is typically with an episode of 'flash' pulmonary oedema. An ultrasound performed once the patient has improved shows good or normal LV function. The mechanism for heart failure in this situation is that in the presence of critical CAD myocardial ischaemia (ie cardiac oxygen demand greater than oxygen supply) can be easily provoked. Even mild ischaemia results in LV dysfunction, mild LVF and early pulmonary oedema. Breathlessness occurs, which provokes anxiety, increased blood pressure and so a greater cardiac workload, greater mismatch between oxygen demand and supply, more ischaemia, more LV dysfunction, etc, all of which results in life-threatening pulmonary oedema. Angina may or may not occur as well.

An intermittent problem, such as arrhythmias or mechanical valve malfunction, usually present along with (at least) mild LV dysfunction.

Pericardial disease, which may underlie symptoms.

Operator error, ie the amount of damage to the heart may have been inadvertently underestimated. This is not difficult to do, as in practice the assessment of LV function is one of the most difficult roles for the cardiac ultrasound assessor (despite what may be written in textbooks and journals).

For all these reasons, it is preferable that before ordering the cardiac ultrasound one is certain as to whether or not heart failure is likely to be present. If this is the case then one can 'ignore' a normal ultrasound report and so avoid dismissing a diagnosis of heart failure, with possibly disastrous consequences. Clearly there are frequent occasions when it is not possible to make a diagnosis before the ultrasound on clinical grounds alone. One will then have to rely on one's judgement as to whether or not the cardiac ultrasound is accurate!

Chapter 7
The ECG and palpitations

Palpitations are an extraordinarily common symptom, responsible for 10–20% of general cardiology referrals. The key to diagnosis is to obtain an ECG during an 'attack'. However, a very good idea of the diagnosis can be gained from the history alone (Table 7.1) – sufficient in most patients to classify the cause as either a stronger than normal appreciation of the normal heartbeat or an arrhythmia.

Diagnosis of palpitations

A diagnosis can generally be established by taking a full clinical history and physical examination and obtaining an ECG between (see below) and during an attack.

Table 7.1 Differences between arrhythmic and non-arrhythmic palpitations

	Appreciation of the normal heart beat	Arrhythmias
Speed of onset	Slow – many minutes	Instantaneous
Speed of offset	Slowly dies away	Sudden or slow
Anxiety	Before palpitations	After onset
Tired afterwards	Yes	Yes
Breathlessness	Due to hyperventilation – circumoral/finger paraesthesia	Due to heart failure, ie often symptoms on effort unrelated to palpitations
Syncope	Very rare (vasomotor)	Rare and dangerous
Structural heart disease	Very rare	More common
Frequency	Often very frequent	Often fairly infrequent
Duration	Hours–days	Seconds–minutes
Regularity	Regular	Regular or irregular
Speed	≤100 bpm	Often ≥140 bpm
Valsalva manoevre	Very rarely helpful	More frequently useful (SVTs)

SVT, supraventricular tachycardia

Obtain a 12-lead ECG between attacks

An ECG should be performed in everyone with palpitations, between attacks. One of several patterns may be shown.

Normal

A normal ECG between attacks greatly decreases the likelihood of a ventricular arrhythmia being the cause of palpitations but does not rule out most supraventricular arrhythmias. A near-normal ECG does not rule out fascicular tachycardia, although this is usually not dangerous, nor does it exclude many cases of right ventricular outflow tract tachycardia, which can be dangerous but are rare. In other words, a normal ECG makes a dangerous arrhythmia unlikely but does not exclude an arrhythmia as the cause of the symptoms.

Left ventricular hypertrophy

Left ventricular hypertrophy (LVH; Figure 7.1) increases the chance that symptoms are due to ventricular premature contractions (VPCs; irregular, slow palpitations), nonsustained ventricular tachycardia (VT; short bursts of regular, fast palpitations) or atrial fibrillation (AF; irregular, fast palpitations). Sustained ventricular arrhythmias relating to LVH alone are surprisingly rare in most clinical practices (surprising as substantial data show that LVH is a powerful substrate for ventricular arrhythmias).

Old myocardial infarct

An old myocardial infarction (MI; Figure 7.2) increases the chance that symptoms are due to isolated VPCs, AF or VT. Palpitations occurring for the first time following an MI should be aggressively investigated as they may relate to a ventricular arrhythmia. If no (pre)syncope is present then 24-hour monitoring, external loop recording (see below) or internal loop recording (see below) is often indicated to obtain an ECG during an attack. If near or actual blackouts have occurred then invasive electrophysiological studies (EPSs) are usually required (see p. 293).

Wolff–Parkinson–White syndrome

The Wolff–Parkinson–White (WPW) syndrome can give rise to atrio-ventricular reentrant arrhythmias (sustained palpitation) or atrial fibrillation (irregularly irregular palpitations). The heart rate in AF due to WPW syndrome can be very high and blackouts can occur. See Figure 7.3.

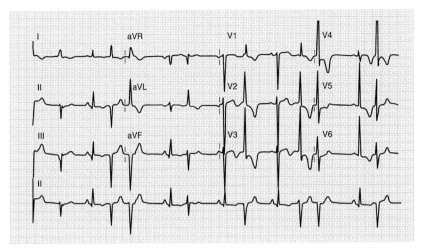

Figure 7.1

Left ventricular hypertrophy, with lateral lead repolarization changes, and frequent ventricular ectopy. In these situations it can sometimes be difficult to determine which beat in the 12-lead ECG is the sinus one. The best approach is to look at the rhythm strip, where the lead with the best developed P wave is displayed. One can then look above to the standard 12-lead ECG, to find the corresponding sinus beat.

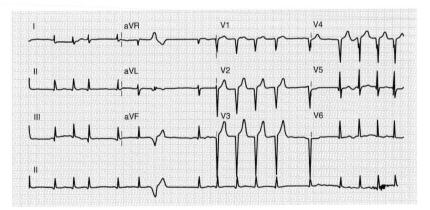

Figure 7.2

Remote anterior wall Q wave myocardial infarct, atrial fibrillation (AF), and frequent ventricular ectopy. Palpitations in this patient may be due to ventricular premature contractions (VPCs), to AF or to ventricular tachycardia (VT). This emphasizes the importance of the history – slow irregular palpitations are probably from VPC, faster irregular palpitations from AF, and fast regular palpitations probably from VT. If the history does not establish the diagnosis, or cannot exclude VT, then one should investigate this patient aggressively. 24-hour ECGs may establish the diagnosis; if not then loop recorders may. One should have a low threshold for ordering a ventricular stimulation study.

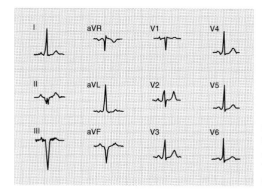

Figure 7.3
Wolff–Parkinson–White (WPW) syndrome. The delta wave is easily seen. The apparent inferior lead Q waves are an artifact, due to the WPW syndrome.

QT interval prolongation

QT interval prolongation commonly relates to drugs and/or LV dysfunction. It often predisposes to ventricular arrhythmias and raises the possibility of polymorphic VT (See Figure 7.4 and p. 201).

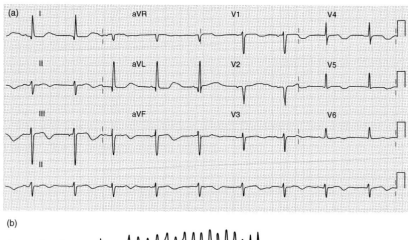

Figure 7.4
(a) Long QT syndrome, in this case acquired due to erythromycin. The patient was being treated with erythromycin for a chest infection, when she complained of palpitations, and subsequently syncope. This ECG was recorded, which shows dramatic prolongation of the QT interval. (b) The rhythm strip, recorded during symptoms, shows a run of polymorphic ventricular tachycardia. There is the classic 'short, long, short' interval between beats preceding the arrhythmia.

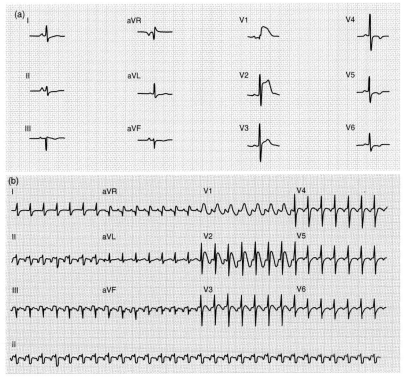

Figure 7.5
Brugada syndrome. (a) This shows the classic Brugada syndrome ECG, with ST segment elevation in leads V1, V2 and V3. Laterally there is T wave inversion, not a classic finding, and in this case due to concomitant LAD territory ischaemia. (b) Not all palpitations in Brugada syndrome are due to ventricular tachycardia. This ECG shows the same patient as in part (a), who developed palpitations. These are due to a supraventricular arrhythmia, probably an atrial tachycardia.

Fixed ST segment elevation in leads V1 to V3

This pattern may be due to the extraordinarily rare Brugada syndrome (Figure 7.5). However, the pattern is usually 'physiological' (see p. 49).

How to obtain an ECG during an attack of palpitations

The definitive diagnosis of palpitations rests on obtaining an ECG during an attack. Sometimes this is very easy, but on occasions can be quite difficult. How it is done varies, mainly according to how long and frequent are the attacks.

A standard ECG is an appropriate means of diagnosis if attacks are prolonged (ie lasting ≥30–45 minutes), as patients have time to seek medical attention, but it is difficult if attacks are of shorter duration.

A 24-hour Holter monitor is useful if attacks are relatively frequent (ie occur every 2–3 days). Even if attacks are less frequent, it is often worth carrying out a 24-hour ECG in the hope (rather than the expectation!) that a diagnostic ECG can be recorded or that presumptive evidence of causation can be found (eg sinus node disease).

If attacks are less frequent, a variety of devices are available for more prolonged home monitoring, external loop and event recorders being the most common (see Chapter 12).

If attacks are very disabling but defy diagnosis it may be appropriate to implant a loop recorder. This is also justified if attacks are felt to have a dangerous cause such as a ventricular arrhythmia, or more rarely a brady-arrhythmia due to atrioventricular (AV) block, or if syncope occurs.

What if an ECG cannot be obtained during palpitations?

In the presence of 'alarm' symptoms (eg palpitations post MI) or syncope and structural heart disease, urgent investigations are appropriate. These include defining the exact nature of the structural heart disease [cardiac ultrasound to define LV function and structure, and coronary angiography to ascertain the nature of any coronary artery disease (CAD)]. Often it is appropriate to undertake invasive EPS (see Chapter 13) and/or to implant a loop recorder.

If there are no 'alarm' features and syncope is not present, or if syncope occurs in the absence of structural heart disease and does not result in injury (ie is likely to be vasomotor in origin), an 'expectant' course may be followed. The commonest cause of palpitations in this situation is a heightened appreciation of sinus tachycardia (ie no rhythm disturbance is present). Some patients with these symptoms will have an arrhythmia but often one that is rather low-grade, which even if diagnosed would not require specific treatment. Examples include infrequent attacks of atrioventricular nodal reentrant tachycardia (AVNRT).

If symptoms have defied ECG diagnosis but are intrusive, a clinical judgement needs to be made. If there is suspicion that a dangerous rhythm disturbance underlies symptoms, it may be justified to implant a loop recorder. However, this is rarely the case, and in most situations it is appropriate to advise the patient that a serious cause of their symptoms is unlikely. If patients demand relief, empirical treatment with β-blockers can help; these are useful for heightened appreciation of both sinus tachycardia and reciprocating arrhythmias involving the AV node [AVNRT and atrioventricular reentrant tachycardia (AVRT)].

Causes of palpitations

Heightened appreciation of the normal heartbeat

When palpitations are due to a heightened appreciation of the normal sinus heartbeat they start gradually, often over many minutes or longer (unlike arrhythmic symptoms, which usually start instantaneously). Palpitations are felt as a 'heavy', regular beating of the heart, and if the heart rhythm is tapped out the rate is usually fairly slow, almost always ≤90–100 bpm. Symptoms can last for many hours. Patients may have associated symptoms such as anxiety (which often but not always starts before the attack) and breathlessness (along with circumoral or limb parasthesia due to dysfunctional breathing). Patients may be quite tired during the attack or afterwards. They may notice attacks more when they are under emotional stress (although this does not reliably discriminate from arrhythmic palpitations) and they may have other somatic manifestations of psychological distress, including irritable bowel symptoms. An indirect but moderately reliable sign is that some patients complain bitterly of intrusive symptoms occurring many times a day, yet when a 24-hour ECG is undertaken they are remarkably symptom-free or have only a 'minor' or atypical attack. Physical examination is normal and there is no evidence of structural heart disease (eg CAD, cardiomyopathy or hypertensive heart disease). The diagnosis is established by demonstrating normal sinus rhythm on an ECG at the time of symptoms.

Causes of heightened appreciation of the normal heartbeat

The cause of heightened appreciation of the normal sinus beat is almost always anxiety or another form of psychological distress, but occasionally organic disease presents in this fashion.

Thyrotoxicosis usually presents with a myriad of symptoms but occasionally palpitations are the most prominent. Sometimes these are due to AF but more often they are due to the catecholamine-enhancing effects of thyroxine increasing the strength of heart contraction. Therefore all patients with palpitations should have thyroid function tests performed. Treatment is with antithyroid medication, sometimes surgery and β-blockers.

Phaeochromocytoma is an exceptionally rare and usually benign tumour of adrenal medullary chromafin cells, which secretes large amounts of catecholamines, often but not always in 'bursts'. Typical symptoms comprise attacks of sweating, palpitations and great anxiety. Patients have extraordinarily high blood pressures during attacks and many are hypertensive outside attacks too. The diagnosis is made from measuring urinary catecholamine (metabolite) concentrations, along with abdominal computed tomography and/or magnetic resonance imaging. Treatment is combined α- and β-adrenergic blockade, then (usually laparoscopic) surgery.

Physical deconditioning (although perhaps not an illness!) can present as marked palpitations, often on effort. This is common in depression, chronic fatigue syndromes and anorexia nervosa. However, as some arrhythmias can also be effort-dependent, it is important to exclude genuine arrhythmias by appropriate ECG monitoring. If lack of physical fitness underlies palpitations then physical reconditioning can dramatically relieve symptoms.

Weight loss and fever (eg due to chronic infections or cancer) may cause palpitations. It is difficult to know if symptoms relate to the normal anxiety of the situation, to the fever or to a thin chest wall (due to weight loss) making the normal heart beat easier to appreciate. If necessary β-blockers can improve symptoms.

Arrhythmia

Almost all arrhythmic palpitations are due to tachyarrhythmias or ectopic beats – it is exceptionally rare for bradyarrhythmias to cause palpitations. A number of generic symptoms can occur with arrhythmic palpitations [including sudden onset and sometimes sudden offset of symptoms (although infrequent), and an easily remembered time duration of symptoms] as well as symptoms specific to the particular arrhythmia.

There are usually no manifestations of psychological distress in arrythmia; if anxiety is a prominent feature, it usually occurs only after palpitations have started, not before. Marked anxiety raises the possibility of 'panic attacks'. It is, however, important to bear in mind that many psychologically distressed people experience genuine arrhythmias.

Ectopic beats

Patients either feel the ectopic beat (described as an 'irregular' heart beat, 'like a car engine misfiring'; often at a fairly normal rate) or they feel the gap between the ectopic and the postectopic beat (so that they feel the heart 'stops, then restarts with a thud'). Anxiety is often provoked by these symptoms, which increases sympathetic outflow, increasing the frequency of ectopics and thus escalating the symptoms. For this reason patients may experience ectopic symptoms for many minutes, sometimes hours. Ventricular ectopics are more likely to be felt than atrial ectopics. Some ventricular ectopics are dependent on a long QT interval (often physiologically long rather than pathologically long). As the QT interval prolongs at low heart rates and at night, symptoms may be more marked when the patient rests during the day or at night. The diagnosis is suspected from the history and is made by demonstrating ectopics at the time symptoms occur.

LV dysfunction increases the chance of ventricular ectopy; if ectopics are frequent a cardiac ultrasound should be considered to exclude structural heart disease. Although a normal ECG makes heart failure (ie breathlessness due to cardiac disease) unlikely, patients who have LV dysfunction but are not breathless (ie do not have heart failure) can have a virtually normal ECG. Thus a normal or near-normal ECG in this situation does not preclude the need for cardiac ultrasound.

Supraventricular tachyarrhythmias

Patients with supraventricular tachyarrhythmias feel sudden-onset, fast, regular palpitations and tap out a heart rate of 150–180 bpm. Patients often have discovered for themselves that 'vagal' manoeuvres can relieve symptoms. There is often a long history extending back to their teens. Demographically the most likely arrhythmia giving these symptoms is AVNRT, which is associated with a completely normal ECG between attacks; however, AVRT due to WPW syndrome is also possible and is usually obvious from the resting ECG (see Chapter 9).

Atrial fibrillation

Patients can suffer palpitations caused by AF at any age, although it is more common in the elderly. Sufferers describe sudden-onset, fast, irregular palpitations, often associated with fatigue and effort intolerance during the attack and occasionally associated with angina if ischaemic heart disease (IHD) is present. If LV dysfunction or valvular heart disease is present (both of which make AF more likely) then breathlessness (due to heart failure) can be a prominent symptom. Patients may be known to have structural heart disease or hypertension or to drink heavily, although many do not fall into any of these categories. Occasionally (and unfortunately) the first manifestation of AF can be a stroke or limb or gut embolus. The differential diagnosis of irregular palpitations includes multiple ectopic beats.

During an attack of AF the ECG will show characteristic changes. At other times the ECG may be normal, or abnormalities of the P wave may occur (eg electrocardiographic left atrial enlargement, prolonged interatrial conduction time, or low-voltage P waves), reflecting intrinsic atrial pathology. As LV dysfunction is a potent cause of AF, QRS, ST segment and T wave abnormalities may also occur. For this reason all patients with AF should have a cardiac ultrasound.

Ventricular tachycardia

Patients with VT describe sudden-onset, regular, moderately (sometimes very) fast palpitations. Consciousness may be unaltered or depressed, sometimes to the point of syncope. Sometimes the first presentation of VT is 'sudden cardiac death'. Often (but not always) patients are known to have heart disease, particularly an old MI. New, regular palpitations following an MI should be assumed to be due to VT until proven otherwise, and in this situation one should go to extreme lengths to record an episode of palpitations, via either a 24-hour ECG or more prolonged recording. If attacks are difficult to record then consideration should be given to invasive EPS (see Chapter 13) or use of an implantable 'loop' recorder (see Chapter 12).

Syncope and palpitations

The presence of syncope with palpitations increases the possibility of additional or more serious disease. Possible diagnoses include:

Vasomotor syncope. Palpitations are felt, but are usually due to a heightened appreciation of the normal heartbeat, and often follow the syncopal event rather than precede it.

Sinus arrest following AF [a consequence of sinoatrial node (SN) disease]. The patient experiences typical AF symptoms (sudden-onset, fast, irregular palpitations) then blacks out when AF terminates. The reason is that during AF high-frequency atrial impulses continually bombard the SN and so suppress its intrinsic pacemaker function. When the AF terminates in those with a healthy SN, pacemaker function returns promptly, within 1–1.5 seconds. However, in those with SN disease this return of SN pacemaker function can take 3–5 seconds. During this period there is no SN activity (ie there is SN arrest) and unless a 'lower-order' pacemaker takes over promptly there is no cardiac electrical activity, no mechanical activity and thus no cardiac output. The more prolonged the sinus pause, the more likely the patient is to blackout. Permanent pacemaker implantation is indicated as this not only prevents the sinus pause but also, by increasing the heart rate and so reducing the dispersal of atrial 'refractoriness' (ie suppressing the substrate for AF), reduces or prevents episodes of AF.

Syncopal bradyarrhythmias. It is very rare indeed for high-grade AV block to present with palpitations but this does happen occasionally. Syncope can occur in SN disease due to sinus arrest, and these patients may also have inappropriate sinus tachycardias that can be felt as palpitations. However, these palpitations often occur at times quite remote from the syncope. The diagnosis of syncope due to SN disease is made from the 24-hour ECG.

Syncopal ventricular tachyarrhythmias. Palpitations are fast and regular and precede the blackout. Structural heart disease is usually known to be present, or the patient is taking a drug known to prolong the QT interval [eg nonsedating antihistamines, macrolide antibiotics such as erythromycin, cisapride (now withdrawn)], predisposing to polymorphic VT.

'Pre-excited' AF (ie AF in the setting of WPW syndrome). Fast, irregular palpitations precede the blackout. The ECG is usually diagnostic (see p. 205).

Presyncope (the feeling of being about to blackout, without proceeding to complete loss of consciousness) with palpitations is very common, and does not necessarily indicate a serious cause or indeed a genuine arrhythmia (unless other 'alarm' features are present, ie the presence of known heart disease). Key ECG features indicating danger are abnormal QRST complexes (reflecting structural heart disease or conducting tissue disease), long QT intervals, WPW syndrome and the extraordinarily rare Brugada syndrome.

Chapter 8
The ECG in syncope

Syncope and near-syncope are exceptionally common symptoms. There are a myriad of possible causes (Figure 8.1a) varying from the completely benign to those that kill within a few weeks. In almost no other clinical area is it so important to diagnose the cause rapidly and accurately. Although the diagnosis will on many occasions be obvious, there are times when it is quite unclear, and the physician and patient will have to live with some uncertainty, which both may find frustrating.

Syncope is defined as loss of consciousness along with loss of postural reflexes. Thus patients blackout and fall over (if standing) or slump down (if sitting). Patients who feel they blackout but have preserved postural reflexes do not have syncope as defined here.

Diagnostic approach to syncope

The clinical approach to syncope is the same as for other diseases, ie be aware of what diagnoses are possible, and with this in mind take a full history, perform a full physical examination (including postural blood pressure and neurological examination) and then undertake appropriate investigations guided by the working diagnosis.

The various possible diagnoses and the key points that allow some differentiation between them are outlined below.

Clinical history

Demographics

Young age and female gender make vasovagal syncope much more likely, whereas older age makes 'serious' causes [eg intermittent high-grade atrioventricular (AV) block] more likely.

Symptoms suggesting cardiovascular aetiology

- An 'aura' lasting from a few seconds to a minute or so, comprising a feeling 'as if about to black out'. More complex auras involving visual, auditory, olfactory or sensory symptoms suggest epilepsy.
- Brief duration (less than a few minutes). Syncope due to a cardiovascular cause may rarely be complicated by 'secondary' 'hypoxic' seizures (eg if patients with vasomotor syncope are propped up rather than allowed to lie flat). In this situation the duration of syncope can be quite long. However, more prolonged unconsciousness usually suggests either epilepsy or hyperventilation.
- Appearance during the episode 'as if dead' suggests a loss of cardiac output, ie a cardiac cause for the syncope. Witnesses should be specifically asked about this.
- Postsyncopal sweating.
- Immediate recovery of all faculties – a prolonged period of confusion (ie many hours) suggests either epilepsy or a cardiac cause complicated by 'secondary' seizure.
- Known cardiac disease, especially a previous myocardial infarction (MI) makes ventricular tachycardia (VT) much more likely, particularly if symptoms have only been present since the MI.
- Syncope with injury (eg 'black eye' or broken bones) suggests a more serious cause than repeated syncope without any injury. It increases the chance of a cardiovascular cause but does not rule out other pathologies.

Symptoms suggesting neurologic aetiology

- A complex aura involving visual, auditory, olfactory or sensory symptoms suggests epilepsy.
- A clear description of tonic–clonic seizure activity by a witness.
- Prolonged unconsciousness.
- Prolonged confusion lasting for several hours following the event.
- Previous stroke (provided cardiac disease is not also present) makes epilepsy more likely.

Symptoms that do not reliably differentiate between cardiovascular and neurologic aetiologies

- Minor 'twitching' and 'jerking' (all manifestations of seizure activity) all occur with epilepsy but can also occur when the blood pressure falls very low [eg with profound vasovagal reactions, syncopal VT or with asystole associated with onset of complete heart block (ie secondary 'hypoxic' seizure)].

- An 'aura' (ie a warning of some description that an attack is coming) is possible both with vasovagal syncope ('the blood drains away', 'I feel faint before blacking out') and with epilepsy (in which the aura may be quite complex, involving unusual moods, feelings, sensations, or auditory or visual hallucinations).

'Alarm' symptoms in syncope

Syncope is very common; some 7–10% of the population will black out at some stage in their lives (Figure 8.1b). Although most blackouts are due to vasomotor syncope (with a very benign prognosis), many are not and some of these have a very malignant prognosis (Figure 8.2). It is therefore vital to spot dangerous syncope and to investigate this early and aggressively. 'Alarm' features suggestive of a poor outcome include:

Family history of premature sudden (cardiac) death. This raises the possibility of hereditary long QT interval prolongation, Brugada syndrome or another genetic disease.

Post-MI syncope. New blackouts developing after an MI are a high-level alarm symptom that should trigger urgent, comprehensive investigation to determine if ventricular arrhythmia is present, and thus whether an implantable cardioverter defibrillator is needed. Even if the 12-lead ECG shows extensive conducting tissue disease (predisposing to high-grade AV block), the cause of brief, sudden-onset–sudden-offset syncope following MI is VT in about two-thirds of cases and bradyarrhythmia in only about one-third.

Disease of the left ventricle (LV). The worse the LV function, the more ominous the prognosis in syncope. Syncope in hypertrophic cardio-myopathy is an independent risk factor for early death.

Effort-induced syncope is worrying (see below). Conversely, syncope occurring after effort is often vasomotor in nature and is usually not dangerous.

Syncope in Wolff–Parkinson–White (WPW) syndrome, in which heart rates in atrial fibrillation (AF) can exceed ≥250 bpm.

Syncope resulting in injury. The more profound the injury, the more the chance that a 'dangerous' cause underlies these attacks.

Physical examination

Physical examination during a syncopal event is rarely possible but can be diagnostic. More commonly patients are only examined some time after the event. At that stage the key is to determine if there is any evidence of:

- cardiac disease, especially aortic stenosis or heart failure
- postural hypotension: the patient should be asked to stand upright from the sitting or lying position, and their BP measured every minute for 5 minutes

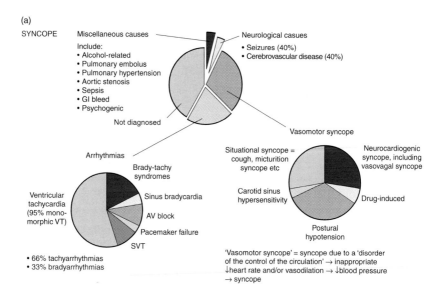

(a)

SYNCOPE

Miscellaneous causes

Include:
- Alcohol-related
- Pulmonary embolus
- Pulmonary hypertension
- Aortic stenosis
- Sepsis
- GI bleed
- Psychogenic

Not diagnosed

Neurological casues
- Seizures (40%)
- Cerebrovascular disease (40%)

Vasomotor syncope

Arrhythmias

Brady-tachy syndromes

Ventricular tachycardia (95% mono-morphic VT)

Sinus bradycardia

AV block

Pacemaker failure

SVT

- 66% tachyarrhythmias
- 33% bradyarrhythmias

Situational syncope = cough, micturition syncope etc

Carotid sinus hypersensitivity

Neurocardiogenic syncope, including vasovagal syncope

Drug-induced

Postural hypotension

'Vasomotor syncope' = syncope due to a 'disorder of the control of the circulation' → inappropriate ↓heart rate and/or vasodilation → ↓blood pressure → syncope

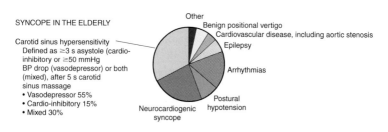

SYNCOPE IN THE ELDERLY

Carotid sinus hypersensitivity
Defined as ≥3 s asystole (cardio-inhibitory or ≥50 mmHg BP drop (vasodepressor) or both (mixed), after 5 s carotid sinus massage
- Vasodepressor 55%
- Cardio-inhibitory 15%
- Mixed 30%

Other
Benign positional vertigo
Cardiovascular disease, including aortic stenosis
Epilepsy

Arrhythmias

Postural hypotension

Neurocardiogenic syncope

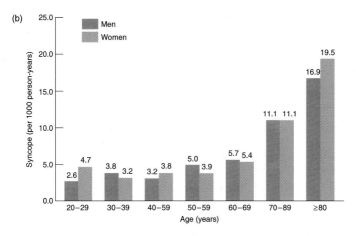

Figure 8.1
(a) Causes of syncope. GI, gastrointestinal; VT, ventricular tachycardia; AV, atrioventricular; SVT, supraventricular tachycardia; BP, blood pressure. Adapted with permission from Davey P. *Medicine at a Glance*. Oxford: Blackwell Science. (b) Incidence of syncope. Reprinted with permission from Soteriades ES, Evans JC, Larson MG *et al*. Incidence and prognosis of syncope. *N Engl J Med* 2002; **347**: 878–85.

- neurological disease, either suggestive of old stroke or of other intracranial pathology such as a tumour.

Investigation

The 'cardiological' approach to diagnosis in syncope is as follows.

First, determine if an arrhythmia is present during an attack. The resting ECG (Table 8.1) may indicate the risk of arrhythmias. These may include long QT interval or evidence of old MI, conducting tissue disease, or genetic causes of syncope such as hypertrophic cardiomyopathy, hereditary long QT syndrome types I to V (see Table 8.5) or Brugada syndrome. Obtaining an ECG during an attack is central to the diagnosis: if attacks are frequent then 24-hour ECG recordings or loop recorders may yield diagnostic information (see Chapter 12); if not then provocative or invasive studies may be required (see Chapter 13). The diagnostic yield of the various tests is shown in Table 8.2.

Second, determine if circulatory control is abnormal or not. A disruption in circulatory control is most commonly diagnosed on the basis of the clinical

Table 8.1 ECG findings in syncope

	Normal	Q waves	Long PR interval or RBBB + axis or LBBB	LVH	Long QT interval
Cardiac disease	• Sick sinus syndrome • Intermittent AV block	• VT • Intermittent CHB	• CHB • VT	• Aortic stenosis • VT	• Heart failure • Hereditary long QT syndrome
Vasomotor syncope	Yes	Yes	Yes	Yes	Unusual
Other diseases	Neurological disease	Less likely	Less likely	Seizures relating to CVA	Drug-induced QT interval prolongation

RBBB, right bundle branch block; LBBB, left bundle branch block; CHB, complete heart block; LVH, left ventricular hypertrophy; VT, ventricular tachycardia; AV, atrioventricular; CVA, cerebrovascular accident.

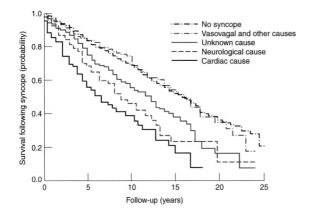

Figure 8.2
Prognosis in syncope. Vasomotor syncope has a benign prognosis, whereas all other forms of syncope are associated with an adverse prognosis. Adapted with permission from Soteriades ES, Evans JC, Larson MG *et al.* Incidence and prognosis of syncope. *N Engl J Med* 2002; **347**: 878–85.

Table 8.2 Diagnostic yield of various tests in syncope

Test	Diagnostic yield (%)
Holter monitor	2
EPS without SHD	6
External loop recorder	20
Tilt table test	11–87
EPS with SHD	41
Internal loop recorder	83–94

EPS, electrophysiological study; SHD, structural heart disease.

features (see Table 8.3); however, there are many investigations that may help. Carotid sinus massage (see p. 292; often conveniently carried out when a 24-hour ECG is being fitted) and tilt table testing (see p. 290) are commonly performed.

Third, in selected cases that have a neurological bent, investigate the electrical behaviour of the brain with an electroencephalogram (EEG), which will be abnormal between attacks in some 50% of patients with seizures (although also abnormal in some 1–2% of the normal population). Determine whether or not structural central nervous system abnormalities are present using computed tomography (CT) or magnetic resonance imaging (MRI) head scan.

Investigation results: 'alarm' signals

Investigation results that suggest a dangerous aetiology and that should provoke an urgent response include:

Q waves suggesting an old MI, raising the possibility of VT. Syncopal VTs have a very poor prognosis if not adequately treated.

Left ventricular hypertrophy (LVH), suggesting hypertensive heart disease or aortic stenosis. The latter is a particularly important diagnosis to make as early surgery can be life-saving.

Conducting tissue disease (especially a long PR interval, right bundle branch block with axis deviation or full left bundle branch block). This suggests that intermittent complete heart block may underlie symptoms. Some physicians would regard the finding of extensive conducting tissue disease together with a classic description of bradyarrhythmic symptoms (a 'Stokes–Adams' attack) as sufficient indication to implant a pacemaker, without attempting to conclusively prove that symptoms arise from intermittent high-grade AV block (provided that the patient is not post-MI, in which case invasive studies to investigate syncopal VT are often indicated).

Structural heart disease on cardiac ultrasound or from other investigations (eg coronary angiography).

Long QT interval (hereditary or acquired long QT syndrome), *inverted T waves in leads V1 to V3* (arrhythmogenic right ventricular dysplasia) and *ST elevation in leads V1 to V3* (Brugada syndrome, in which syncope relates to polymorphic VT) are all associated with ventricular arrhythmias, which can lead to premature death.

Management of syncope of unknown cause

The diagnosis of the cause of syncope rests on a characteristic history and (where possible) the results of diagnostic investigations. If a diagnosis cannot be achieved, what should be done?

The commonest and often best approach is to do nothing, provided there are no 'alarm' features (as above). If a dangerous cause of syncope is suspected then 'aggressive' cardiac investigations are justified [eg implanting a 'loop' recorder device and/or a full electrophysiological study, the latter particularly if ventricular arrhythmias are suspected (eg post-MI or where LV function is impaired for another reason)]. If symptoms are frequent and intrusive then tilt-table testing (with or without the addition of isoprenaline and/or glyceryl trinitrate) and carotid sinus massage are often appropriate to clarify if vasomotor syncope is present and its exact mechanism if so.

Prognosis in syncope

Prognosis in syncope depends on the cause and severity of any underlying heart disease (Figure 8.2). Vasomotor syncope has no adverse impact on prognosis, whereas undiagnosed syncope has some adverse impact, presumably as some of these patients have serious but difficult-to-diagnose pathology.

Causes of syncope

Unknown

The largest single group of causes of syncope is, frustratingly, 'unknown'. This is a valid diagnosis to make, provided appropriate investigations have been carried out to exclude serious pathology. The prognosis in these patients is worse than that of age-matched controls and worse than that of patients with vasomotor syncope. This implies that some of these patients have either a dangerous cause for syncope (which has been missed) or significant underlying heart or neurological disease (which itself has an adverse impact on prognosis).

Vasomotor syncope

This is the largest single group of identified causes of syncope (Table 8.3). There are many subclasses (see below) but they all have in common some intermittent disruption of circulatory control that causes the blood pressure to sink too low, provoking either syncope or near-syncope. Often symptoms are 'situation-dependent', ie they occur only in certain well-defined circumstances. For example, syncope may only occur in the shower just after morning rising – rising without showering does not provoke symptoms, nor does showering in the evening. Symptoms may be provoked by coughing, standing still or after exercise. However, syncope on effort is usually not vasomotor in origin – it is an 'alarm' signal (see below).

Most patients with vasomotor syncope are upright when symptoms occur. They often have a short prodromal period during which they experience

Table 8.3 Forms of vasomotor syncope

	Vasovagal syncope	Neurocardiogenic syncope	Carotid sinus hypersensitivity	Micturition syncope	Postural hypotension
Age	Usually young	Any age; more common in middle age	Usually elderly	Usually elderly; only occurs in men	More common in the elderly or diabetic
Position when syncope occurs	Upright	Almost always upright; usually does not occur immediately on standing (if so, think of postural hypotension), often occurs when standing still after walking, eg when out shopping	Usually when standing, can occur when sitting	Passing urine, usually in the middle of the night (vasodilated from a warm bed ± alcohol)	Standing – immediately
Preceding symptoms	Modest warning	Pre-syncope = 'near' syncope = 'as if about to black out', for up to 1 minute	Often none	Often none	Presyncope very common
Diagnostic test	Usually none required; if intrusive consider tilt-table test	Tilt-table test • Bradycardic: symptoms with ↓heart rate • Vasodepressor: symptoms with ↓SBP • Mixed • Cerebral (see text)	Bradycardia (≥ 3 s asystole) ± hypotension (≥ 50 mmHg fall) on CSM. CSM done while lying and on standing	History of syncopal event and of prostatism	Postural blood pressure
Utility of pacing	None	Complete response in pure bradycardic syncope only, otherwise no or partial response	Good response in bradycardic syncope	Not useful	Not useful

SBP, systolic blood pressure; CSM, carotid sinus massage.

some form of warning, often interpreted as being due to 'vagal' switch-on. They may feel nauseated, light-headed and/or rather nonspecifically unwell. After a minute or two (sometimes less) syncope occurs (during which patients fall to the ground). Syncope may be prevented by sitting or lying down during the prodromal warning period or sometimes by 'concentrating' very hard (which presumably activates the sympathetic nervous system). Although injury may occur with syncope, this is rather infrequent, which suggests that many of these patients still have some protective mechanisms left as they fall to the ground.

Syncope is brief, usually less than a few minutes, and the patient appears grey and pale but not usually 'as if dead'. After assuming the horizontal posture consciousness is rapidly restored, usually within 1–2 minutes, and during this phase patients may sweat profusely. Full faculties are immediately restored (unlike in epilepsy). If patients do not fall or lie down during an episode of vasomotor syncope, it is possible for a secondary hypoxic seizure to occur. The history is then complicated, as some features of a seizure disorder are present.

Treatment is in many cases difficult and not universally successful. Often the best advice is to avoid those situations known to provoke symptoms. If symptoms are frequent and treatment insisted on by the patient, it is often difficult to know exactly what to do. It is often, however, important to document the exact changes in heart rate and blood pressure before and during the syncopal episode, often by using a tilt-table test. If there is evidence of profound bradycardia during an event (ie ≥3–5 seconds of asystole) then pacemaker implantation may be tried, although this is often unpredictable in effect and may modify rather than remove attacks.

Prognosis in vasomotor syncope is for a normal life expectancy: pacemaker implantation does not improve outcome.

Specific forms of vasomotor syncope

Vasovagal attacks. See above.

Neurocardiogenic syncope. This is a complex syndrome wherein blood pressure falls due to inappropriate bradycardia and/or peripheral vasodilatation. The bradycardia is 'reflex', ie not due to sinus node or conducting tissue disease. The underlying pathophysiology is complex and only partially understood. There may be changes that are central in the function of serotonergic neurones, which partly explains the (partial) response to selective serotonin reuptake inhibitors (SSRIs). There may also be abnormalities in the reflex loop whereby the heart determines the amount of blood contained within it and the amount ejected in order to control the central blood pressure. This reflex loop may misinterpret haemodynamic data and inappropriately signal to the circulation to lower the blood pressure. Beta-receptors are involved, explaining why β-blockers may help in the treatment of neurocardiogenic syncope.

Neurocardiogenic syncope almost always occurs only in the standing position, sometimes only after patients have stood still for a while (eg while looking into a shop window). Standing still provokes symptoms because it reduces cardiac output. During exercise the gastrocnemius muscle pump improves venous return to the heart, so helping to maintain cardiac output, but this only occurs on effort; at rest (or when standing still) the pump ceases, venous return to the heart decreases and cardiac output falls, exacerbating any decrease in blood pressure due to bradycardia or vasodilatation.

The diagnosis of neurocardiogenic syncope depends on finding a characteristic history and on excluding more serious causes of syncope (where appropriate). Tilt-table testing (see Chapter 13) has some limited use (Figure 8.3).

Treatment of neurocardiogenic syncope is difficult: if possible, avoidance of provoking situations is the best advice. Pacemakers may be used if profound bradycardia occurs, although they do not treat any vasodilator component to the syndrome so some symptoms may persist despite pacing. SSRIs and β-blockers have also been tried with occasional success.

Carotid hypersensitivity syndrome. Here the carotid body baroreceptors are hypersensitive to external stimuli. Usual day-to-day pressures on the carotid, such as turning the neck, cause inappropriate carotid receptor discharge. The brain stem incorrectly believes that the blood pressure is too high and activates the vagus nerve, causing inappropriate bradycardia and/or peripheral vasodilatation, and syncope may occur. The diagnosis rests on a positive carotid sinus massage test (see Chapter 13, Figure 13.1). In this test first one then the other carotid artery is massaged firmly at the level of the cricoid cartilage for several seconds. If bradycardia leading to ≥3 seconds of asystole or a fall in systolic blood pressure ≥50 mmHg occurs, the test is said to be positive. If bradycardia is a marked

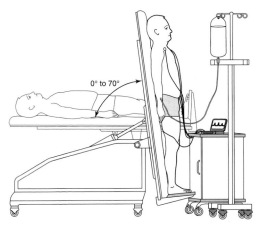

0° to 70°

Figure 8.3
Fasted patients are placed in a darkened quiet room, rested supine for 30 minutes, then strapped to the tilt table and placed in the 70° upright position. Blood pressure and heart rate are continuously monitored – see Chapter 13 for criteria for positive tests.

component of syncope then pacemaker implantation can relieve symptoms.

Situational syncope, including during cough and micturition. These are typical vasomotor syncopal episodes. Typically patients are older men, either with chronic obstructive pulmonary disease (COPD) in cough syncope or prostatic hypertrophy in micturition syncope. Prolonged coughing or nocturnal micturition leads to syncope. The diagnosis is made from the history. Investigations are not helpful except to exclude more serious disease. Treatment of the primary pathology may help.

Postural hypotension. Patients with postural hypotension usually have an autonomic neuropathy (often caused by diabetes) such that when they stand blood immediately pools in the legs, so the blood pressure falls on standing instead of rising. Symptoms then occur, usually of presyncope ('stars in the eyes'); syncope itself is unusual. The symptoms are exacerbated by standing still and relieved by moving around (activating the gastrocnemius pump and so improving venous return and cardiac output). The diagnosis is made by measuring the blood pressure on prolonged standing. There are no diagnostic ECG changes. Treatment is difficult, but support stockings or fludrocortisone may be helpful. Physical reconditioning may help unfit patients.

Arrhythmias

Syncopal tachyarrhythmias

In order for tachyarrhythmias to cause syncope either the heart must beat very fast or there must be substantial impairment to LV function. Ventricular arrhythmias are much more likely at any given heart rate to cause syncope than are supraventricular arrhythmias. This is because in ventricular arrhythmias the activation pathway across the ventricle is very abnormal so the coordination of cardiac mechanical activity is also quite abnormal, thus impairing cardiac performance. The tachyarrhythmias causing syncope include:

Table 8.4 Diagnostic criteria for the hereditary long QT syndrome

Findings		Points
ECG	Duration of QTc[†]	
	>480 ms$^{1/2}$	3
	460–470 ms$^{1/2}$	2
	450 ms (men)$^{1/2}$	1
	Torsades de pointes[‡]	2
	T wave alternans	1
	Notched T wave in three leads	1
	Low heart rate for age[§]	0.5
Clinical history	Syncope[‡]	
	with stress	2
	without stress	1
	Congenital deafness	0.5
Family history[¶]	Family members with definite long QT syndromes[**]	1
	Unexplained sudden cardiac death below 30 years among immediate family members	0.5
Scoring	<1 point: low probability of long QT syndrome	
	2–3 points: intermediate probability of long QT syndrome	
	>4 points: high probability of long QT syndrome	

*In the absence of medication or disorders known to affect these ECG features.
†Calculated by Bazett's formula, where QTc=QT interval/√(RR interval).
‡Mutually exclusive.
§Resting heart rate below the second percentile for age.
¶The same family member cannot be counted in both aspects of the family history.
**Definite long QT syndrome = a long QT syndrome score >4.
QTc, heart rate corrected QT interval.
Reprinted with permission from Schwartz PJ, Moss AJ, Vincent GM, Crampton RS. *Circulation* 1993; **88**: 782–4.

Ventricular tachycardia causes syncope partly because the heart rate can be quite high, often 180–220 bpm, and partly because many patients with VT have substantial impairment of LV function. Diseases predisposing to syncopal ventricular tachyarrhythmias include any structural disease affecting the LV; coronary artery disease; LVH, which makes VT much more likely during ischaemia (thus patients with hypertensive heart disease are much more likely to die of ventricular tachycardia or fibrillation during an MI); and adverse genes, especially hereditary long QT syndrome, Brugada syndrome and hypertrophic cardiomyopathy. Hereditary long QT syndrome can be a difficult diagnosis to make. Diagnostic criteria have been proposed (Table 8.4). The ECG usually, but not always, shows bizarre abnormalities to the T and/or U waves in addition to the long QT interval. There are several possible genetic defects (Table 8.5); prognosis does relate to sex (males are less likely to die), genotype and the degree of QT interval prolongation (Figure 8.4).

Table 8.5 Molecular genetics of long QT syndrome (LQTS)*.

LQTS type (year discovered)	Chromosomal locus	Mutant gene (alternative name)	Ion currents affected by the mutant gene
LQT1 (1991)	11p15.5	*KCNQ1(KVLQT1)*	Decreased slowly activating delayed rectifier K⁺ repolarization current (I_{Ks})
LQT2 (1994)	7q35–36	*HERG*	Decreased rapidly activating delayed rectifier K⁺ repolarization current (I_{Kr})
LQT3 (1994)	3p21–24	*SCN5A*	Increased Na⁺ current (I_{Na}) due to late reopening of the sodium channel
LQT4 (1995)	4q25–27	*Ankyrin B*	Possibly increased late Na⁺ current (I_{Na})
LQT5 (1997)	21q22.1–22.2	*KCNE1 (minK)*	Decreased slowly activating K⁺ repolarization current (I_{Ks})
LQT6 (1999)	21q22.1–22.2	*KCNE2 (MiRP1)*	Decreased rapidly activating K⁺ repolarization current (I_{Kr})
LQT7 (2001)†	17q23	*KCNJ2*	Decreased inwardly rectifying K⁺ current ($I_{Kir2.1}$)

* A single mutation (heterozygous state) in any one of the *LQT1* to *LQT7* genes results in an autosomal dominant form of LQTS (Romano-Ward syndrome). The presence of two mutations (homozygous state) in either the *LQT1* or the *LQT5* gene results in a severe autosomal recessive form of LQTS with associated deafness (Jervell and Lange–Nielsen syndrome).
† Mutations in *LQT7* are responsible for Andersen syndrome, a rare neurologic disorder characterized by periodic paralysis, skeletal developmental abnormalities and QT prolongation.

Pre-excited AF, ie AF in Wolff–Parkinson–White (WPW) syndrome, can cause syncope as the heart rate can be very high, often ≥250 bpm (Figure 8.5).

Atrial fibrillation can occasionally cause syncope in the absence of WPW syndrome if there is very severe impairment to LV function or if in those with sinus node disease there is a prolonged 'sinus' pause following termination of an episode of paroxysmal AF.

Other supraventricular tachycardias. These can cause syncope if another mechanism also comes into play, such as vasomotor syncope.

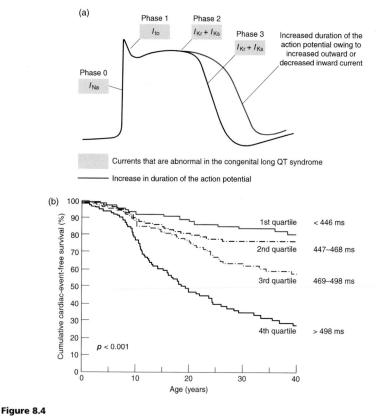

Figure 8.4
(a) Changes in the action potential in the hereditary long QT syndromes. (b) Although the exact genetic mechanism in any individual does influence prognosis, an important and relatively easily obtained estimate can be gained from the amount of QT interval prolongation, as shown here. Reprinted with permission from Priori SG, Schwartz PJ, Napolitano C *et al. N Engl J Med* 2003; **348**: 1866–74.

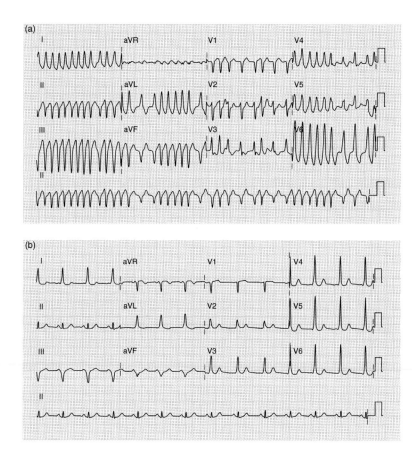

Figure 8.5
(a) Atrial fibrillation in a patient with WPW syndrome. The heart rate is high, irregular and there is a broad QRS complex. After restoration of sinus rhythm (b), a typical pattern of WPW syndrome is seen, with an obvious delta wave in the chest leads.

Syncopal bradyarrhythmias

Bradyarrhythmias must be fairly profound to cause syncope; pauses of at least 4 seconds are needed, which translates to heart rates of ≤ 5–20 bpm. The common causes of syncopal bradyarrhythmias are:

Complete heart block usually causes syncope as immediately after normal AV conduction ceases there is a period of asystole lasting around 10–30 seconds. After this asystolic episode a pacemaker below the disconnected

161

AV node 'takes over' from the sinoatrial node (SN), usually at a rate of 20–40 bpm. Typically patients who develop complete heart block therefore blackout without any warning and serious injury occurs (bone fractures, including bilateral 'black eyes' suggestive of a skull-base fracture). Full consciousness is rapidly restored once the lower-order pacemaker starts firing. This characteristic sequence of events at the start of an episode of complete heart block is known as a Stokes–Adams attack. Although complete heart block is by far the commonest cause of such a Stokes–Adams attack, occasionally this symptom can arise from syncopal ventricular tachycardia.

Sinus node disease can cause syncope in one of two ways. Either the SN rate spontaneously drops low enough to cause syncope or the SN is slow to start after a tachycardia (typically AF) stops. The diagnosis of SN disease is usually made from the 24-hour ECG. Two patterns are seen: inappropriate bradycardia only, or bradycardia alternating with tachycardia. The prognosis in intrinsic SN disease depends on whether or not there is heart disease present: in the absence of any structural heart disease SN disease has no impact on prognosis (so one can hold back from inserting a permanent pacemaker as it will not improve the outlook), whereas if heart disease is present, SN disease will worsen prognosis (so one should consider inserting a pacemaker).

Bradyarrhythmias associated with vasodilatation can also cause vasomotor syncope (see above).

Effort-related syncope

Effort-induced syncope is rare but important, as sometimes it indicates serious disease with a high chance of sudden cardiac death.

Aortic stenosis can cause effort-induced (pre)syncope, usually in association with effort-induced breathlessness and angina. This is an extremely worrying symptom that can easily and quickly escalate to cause sudden cardiac death. The diagnosis is usually easy to make from the physical examination and confirmed by a cardiac ultrasound. The ECG commonly (but not always) shows LVH. Urgent aortic valve replacement is indicated.

Effort-induced arrhythmias can cause syncope, either because they are very fast or because there is associated structural heart disease. The most common syncopal effort-induced arrhythmia is syncopal VT, either due to ischaemic heart disease or to right ventricular dysplasia (right ventricular outflow tract tachycardia). The diagnosis can often be relatively easily established from an exercise ECG.

Pulmonary hypertension can cause effort-induced syncope. The pulmonary artery pressure needs to be very high for the cardiac output to be reduced to such a critical level that exercise causes syncope. Severe pulmonary hypertension can be primary (a rare disease) or secondary (common, often due to COPD) in aetiology. Pulmonary artery hypertension can be suspected from the clinical examination [left parasternal heave, high jugular venous pressure (JVP)] and/or from the ECG (right axis deviation, dominant R wave in V1). The cardiac ultrasound usually (but not always) confirms the diagnosis, although not the cause of the pulmonary hypertension.

Post-effort syncope usually has a quite different mechanism from effort-induced syncope and often is due to excessive 'switch-on' of the vagus nerve. This can occur in anyone, but is most likely in the physically fit. The diagnosis is made from the history and from exclusion of more serious disease.

Seizures

A seizure disorder is an extremely rare cause of undiagnosed syncope, as the other stigmata of generalized seizures are usually so obvious that the right diagnosis is made immediately. However, some patients have unwitnessed seizures and can present to cardiology outpatient departments as 'unknown syncope'. The clues that the diagnosis is a seizure disorder come first from the associated incontinence and tongue biting, and second from the fact that full recovery after the episode takes many hours. Investigations in suspected seizures include the EEG (abnormal between attacks in 50% with a seizure disorder and in 1–2% of the normal population). If seizures are confirmed then neuroimaging (eg head CT or MRI scan) may be appropriate to exclude underlying structural brain disease.

Some cardiac diseases can present as apparent seizures – a consequence of cerebral anoxia from temporary loss of cardiac output. This can occur in vasomotor syncope if the patient is not allowed to lie flat; indeed some 'twitching' is very common in this disorder. Seizures may also occur with bradyarrhythmias (especially intermittent complete heart block). Tachyarrhythmias occasionally present as seizures. Acquired heart disease is the commonest cause of predisposition to syncopal ventricular tachycardias; however, the most striking cases (although exceptionally rare) are due to polymorphic VT caused by congenital long QT syndrome. Patients with this disorder can be treated for many years with anticonvulsant therapy before the right diagnosis is made (interestingly, some anticonvulsants have class 1 antiarrhythmic properties and some forms of congenital long QT syndrome respond to these drugs, perhaps explaining the positive response to this inappropriate therapy).

Other causes of syncope

There are a number of other conditions that can present as apparent syncope.

Hyperventilation

This is an extraordinarily common condition and usually causes light-headedness, dizziness and parasthaesia; however, occasionally patients can hyperventilate to such an extent that unconsciousness occurs. The exact mechanism is unclear. The diagnosis is essentially one of exclusion, although asking patients to hyperventilate in the clinic can, by reproducing exact symptoms, occasionally be diagnostic.

Narcolepsy

Narcolepsy has a strong genetic aetiology and is being increasingly clinically recognized. The key feature is sudden onset of sleep, often in situations containing unvaried external stimuli. Catalepsy is a related condition in which loss of postural tone with preservation of consciousness occurs, often in response to strong emotion (laughter or anger). Narcolepsy and catalepsy may occur together. The diagnosis of these conditions is often made from the history. Amphetamine derivatives may be useful in treatment.

Hypovolaemia

A quick reduction in circulating blood volume from acute haemorrhage can result in syncope. Trauma is an obvious cause; occasionally a concealed gastrointestinal haemorrhage is responsible.

Chapter 9

The ECG in arrhythmia

Arrhythmias can produce varying symptoms, including:

- none
- palpitations
- breathlessness, usually in those with pre-existing cardiac disease (see Chapter 6)
- angina, usually in those with pre-existing cardiac disease
- blackouts or near-blackouts (see Chapter 8)
- sudden cardiac death.

Arrhythmias are conveniently divided into bradyarrhythmias and tachy-arrhythmias.

Bradyarrhythmias

Bradyarrhythmias are arbitrarily defined as heart rates ≤40 bpm. The common causes are as follows:

Sinus bradycardia

It is unusual for a sinus bradycardia to cause symptoms, unless the heart rate is very low (≤30 bpm), it drops suddenly (eg by ≥20 bpm in a few seconds), or it fails to increase when needed (eg during exercise) if sinus node chronotropic incompetence is present. Symptoms, when they occur, may comprise tiredness, effort intolerance or (rarely) syncope or presyncope. However, most sinus bradycardias are asymptomatic.

ECG recognition

Sinus bradycardia is recognized when the heart rate is slow but each PQRST complex is normal (Figure 9.1). If chronotropic incompetence is present the 24-hour ECG monitor will show a low, almost 'fixed' heart rate unresponsive to activity, often staying ≤50 bpm (Figure 9.2).

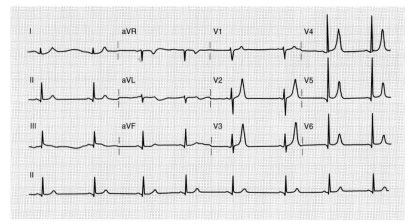

Figure 9.1
ECG showing a sinus node bradycardia. Prominent sinus arrhythmia (irregularity of the RR interval) suggests that the cause of the bradycardia may be a prominent vagal reflex.

Causes

Sinus bradycardia can be caused by drugs that slow the heart rate (eg β-blockers, some calcium channel blockers, digoxin, long-term amiodarone), intrinsic sinus node disease [usually benign fibrosis (age-associated) or due to coronary artery disease (CAD)] and hypothyroidism. A very common 'physiological' cause is physical fitness – indeed, a resting sinus bradycardia is a marker for physical fitness and can be used to measure the strength of any training effect.

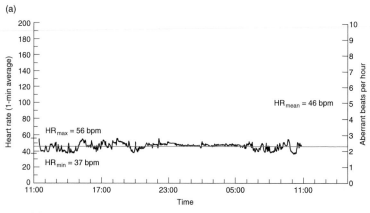

Figure 9.2(a)

(b)

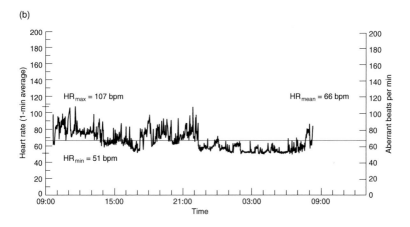

(c)

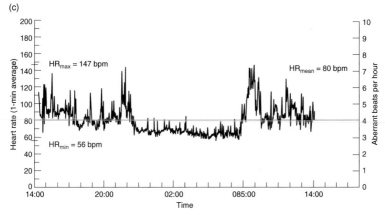

Figure 9.2

Tachograms obtained from 24 hour ECGs. (a) This tachogram (heart rate recorded over 24 hours) shows a prominent sinus bradycardia throughout the recording. Note that there is very little difference between the day- and night-time heart rates. This prominent example of sinus node disease was induced by amiodarone. Compare with (b) a normal but inactive individual and (c) a normal and active individual. HR_{max}, HR_{min}, HR_{mean}, maximum, minimum, mean heart rates respectively.

Prognosis

In health there is an inverse relationship between resting heart rate and longevity – ie within physiological limits, the lower the resting heart rate, the better the outlook.

Following myocardial infarction (MI), β-blockers improve prognosis in proportion to how much they slow the heart rate. Thus, in this situation a slow heart rate is undeniably a good thing. Therefore β-blockers should never be stopped or the dose reduced just because an asymptomatic sinus bradycardia has been found.

In patients with intrinsic sinus node disease there is no adverse impact on prognosis unless there is underlying myocardial or coronary artery disease, in which case sinus node disease worsens the outlook. Thus, in patients with sinus node disease and a structurally normal heart one can hold back from implanting a pacemaker, whereas in those with structural heart disease (eg following MI) one should consider a pacemaker more strongly.

Therefore, most sinus bradycardias have no adverse impact on prognosis and the outlook is that of any underlying heart disease.

Treatment

Treatment of bradycardia depends on the cause and the symptoms. Often no treatment is needed. If symptoms are present, stopping contributing drugs can help. If additional treatment is required an atrial pacemaker may be useful.

Atrioventricular block

This is a much more serious cause of a slow heart rate than sinus node bradycardias. The forms of atrioventricular (AV) block are as follows.

First-degree atrioventricular block

First degree AV block is seen on the ECG as a prolongation of the PR interval (Figure 9.3). The normal PR interval prolongs at low heart rates and in those with a high vagal tone (the latter usually being due to physical fitness) and this needs to be considered when deciding whether or not the PR interval is pathologically prolonged. In practice, however, it is often reasonable to regard a PR interval of longer than 200 ms as being pathological (ie ≥5 small squares on a standard-speed ECG recording); see Figure 9.4.

Causes of PR interval prolongation. These include:

- most heart diseases
- ischaemic heart disease, especially during an inferior wall MI
- idiopathic fibrosis of the conducting tissues, commonest in the elderly

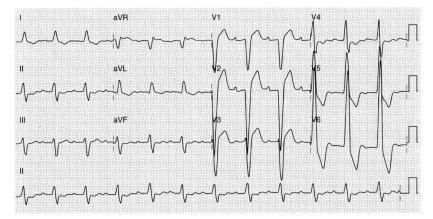

Figure 9.3
PR interval prolongation, in association with left bundle branch block. This combination of extensive conducting tissue disease suggests that the patient is at significant risk of high-grade atrioventricular (AV) block. A Stokes–Adams attack should be assumed to be due to the temporary asystole that accompanies the onset of high-grade AV block. In such symptomatic individuals one should therefore have a very low threshold for implanting a pacemaker.

- myocarditis, especially when due to acute rheumatic fever, diphtheria or (more commonly now) Lyme disease; sarcoidosis is a rare cause
- 'physiological' due to high vagal tone in the physically fit and in many normal individuals at night.

Prognosis. This depends on the cause, but the condition may not progress. Infra-Hissian block is rather more likely to progress than AV node disease – however, the level of block can only be determined invasively, which is rarely indicated. In some patients the conducting tissue disease progresses to higher forms of AV block, with a dramatic impact on life expectancy.

Treatment. Usually none is required. However, a long PR interval is a clue that the heart may be prone to higher grades of AV block, which may cause symptoms such as syncope or near-syncope. Thus, if blackouts are occurring and the patient is found to have a prolonged PR interval, consideration should be given to implanting a pacemaker (ventricular or dual chamber).

Second-degree atrioventricular block

In second-degree heart block some but not all of the impulses reach the ventricle, and so QRS complexes do not follow every P wave. Second-degree AV block is subdivided into Mobitz type I and II heart block (Figure 9.5). In

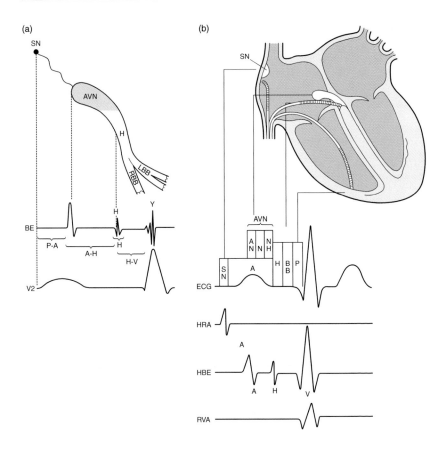

Figure 9.4

Different mechanisms may underlie PR interval prolongation. (a) PR interval prolongation may relate to disease in the atrioventricular (AV) node, the bundle of His or the bundle branches. Disease in any of these structures may be visible on the ECG as PR interval prolongation. Adapted with permission from Narula OS, Schlerlab BJ, Samet P et al. Atrioventricular block: localization and classification by His bundle recordings. *Am J Med* 1971; **50:** 228–37. (b) It is only possible to determine the exact mechanism of any PR interval prolongation from invasive studies in which electrodes are placed in the right atrium, along the bundle of His and in the right ventricle, and conduction times measured, so determining where the block lies. BE, bipolar intracardiac electrogram; S, sinoatrial node conduction; A, atrial conduction; V, ventricular conduction; AVN, atrioventricular node conduction; H, His bundle conduction; BB, bundle branch conduction; P, Purkinje fibre conduction; R, right; L, left; N, node; HRA, high right atrial intracardiac ECG; HBE, His bundle ECG; RVA, right ventricular apex ECG. Adapted with permission from Braunwald E, Zipes DB, Libby P. *Heart Disease: A Textbook of Cardiovascular Medicine*. Philadelphia: WB Saunders.

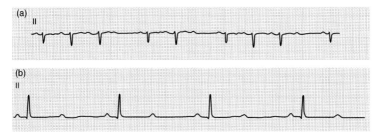

Figure 9.5
Types of second-degree heart block. (a) Wenkeback (or Mobitz type II) heart block: gradual prolongation of the PR interval leads to a dropped beat. (b) Mobitz type I heart block: a regular number of beats are conducted, here every second beat.

Mobitz type I (formerly called Wenkeback) the PR interval of each succeeding beat gradually prolongs until a P wave fails to be conducted to the ventricle and a 'dropped' beat occurs. In Mobitz type II, each conducted beat is followed by a fixed number of nonconducted beats – usually one but sometimes more. The ratio of total P waves to conducted beats is used in describing the pattern, eg two to one, three to one.

Symptoms. These depend on whether or not there are episodes of higher-grade (third-degree) AV block. If third-degree AV block does not occur patients often complain of breathlessness, fatigue and effort intolerance; if it does occur patients often experience syncope.

Causes. The common causes of second-degree AV block include idiopathic conducting tissue fibrosis, any form of structural heart disease [especially ischaemic heart disease (IHD)] and inflammatory conditions of the heart (eg myocarditis, especially due to sarcoidosis or Lyme disease).

Prognosis. The outlook without definitive treatment is very poor in Mobitz type II heart block, as most patients rapidly progress to complete heart block, then asystole and death. If syncope has occurred, it should be assumed that complete heart block is at least intermittently present, and the prognosis is much worse than that of second-degree heart block without syncope.

Treatment. Permanent pacing is indicated, and if there has been syncope or presyncope then a temporary pacing wire should be inserted immediately as a prelude to implanting a permanent system.

Third-degree atrioventricular block

Third-degree AV block is otherwise known as complete heart block

(Figure 9.6). There is no electrical connection between the atria and the ventricles, and so impulses cannot be propagated down the conducting tissue into the ventricle. In this situation the heart will stop unless tissue within the conducting system develops its own automaticity. This is usually but not always the case, and a subsidiary pacemaker forms below the level of the block. The lower the level of this pacemaker, the broader will be the QRS 'escape' complex. Unfortunately this subsidiary pacemaker is unreliable and prone to stopping, with consequent asystole. Third-degree AV block is recognized on the ECG by there being no relation between the P waves and the QRS complexes.

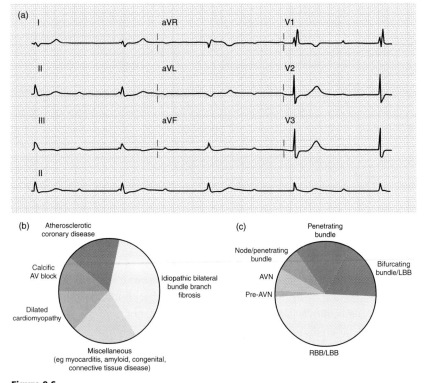

Figure 9.6
(a) Third-degree heart block (complete heart block). There is no relation between the P waves and the QRS complexes. (b) Causes of atrioventricular (AV) block. (c) Site of AV block. RBB, right bundle branch; LBB, left bundle branch; AVN, atrioventricular node. (b) and (c) adapted with permission from Davies MJ, Anderson RH, Becker AE et al. The Conduction System of the Heart. London: Butterworth, 1983.

Symptoms. When third-degree AV block starts the heart usually becomes temporarily asystolic. This often lasts for 10–30 seconds and the patient suffers a blackout. Sometimes the period of asystole is shorter and the patient nearly but not totally blacks out – ie presyncope. In the classic Stokes–Adams attack:

- sudden loss of consciousness occurs without any warning, resulting in loss of all postural tone
- patients fall to the floor with no intact protective reflexes so significant injury, particularly to the head, may occur
- patients appear 'dead' during the event, which only lasts a few seconds (occasionally up to a minute or so but never longer, unless secondary seizure activity has occurred)
- patients recover rapidly (ie within a few minutes) and completely following the episode, as a lower-order pacemaker takes over. Sweating or increased facial colouring may occur during recovery.

Thus syncope or near-syncope in this situation indicates a period of asystole, which has a high risk of recurrence, often prolonged and resulting in sudden cardiac death. It is an ominous symptom and indicates a need for immediate pacing.

Prognosis. The natural history of third-degree AV block is for the heart to beat slower and slower and then stop. Most patients with untreated, acquired, symptomatic complete heart block are dead within 6 weeks.

Treatment. This is by permanent pacemaker implantation, covered with immediate temporary pacemaker insertion if there has been any syncope or near-syncope or if the heart rate is exceptionally slow (arbitrarily, ≤30 bpm), or if the escape beats have a continually changing morphology. Permanent pacemaker implantation returns the patient's life expectancy to normal.

Infra-Hissian conducting tissue disease

Disease of the conducting tissue below the bundle of His is common.

Right bundle branch block

Right bundle branch block (RBBB) is recognized by a broadening of the QRS complex with a positive late deflection in lead V1 (Figure 9.7). It may be an isolated abnormality of one part of the conducting tissue or a more generalized process affecting all of the specialized conducting tissue, in which case a long PR interval and/or QRS axis deviation may be present (Figure 9.8). A long PR interval with RBBB and right or left QRS axis deviation is called 'trifascicular block', and indicates extensive conducting tissue disease with at least a moderately high risk of progressing to complete AV block. Indeed, if symptoms of syncope occur in the presence of trifascicular block, it is often wisest to assume that they relate to transient asystole consequent to intermittent complete heart block, and to implant a pacemaker. The exception to this rule is when the patient has underlying ischaemic heart disease and an old MI. Here, despite the presence of extensive conducting tissue disease, syncope may relate to a ventricular arrhythmia, especially ventricular tachycardia (VT). Accordingly, consideration should be given to performing a diagnostic ventricular stimulation study to assess whether an implantable cardioverter defibrillator (ICD) is appropriate therapy.

Causes of RBBB include:

- No apparent cardiac disease: this is true for many patients, particularly young people and those with 'partial' as opposed to 'complete' RBBB (Figure 9.9); this is reflected in the community incidence of RBBB versus left bundle branch block (LBBB) (Figure 9.10).
- Isolated conducting tissue disease.
- Generalized cardiac disease, which damages both the myocardium and the conducting system. This includes most heart disease, especially IHD, as well as the much rarer inflammatory heart diseases (such as myocarditis, especially that caused by Lyme disease).
- Right heart strain can cause RBBB; this may arise from acute or chronic thromboembolic lung disease, fibrotic lung disease or occasionally from an atrial septal defect (ASD).

Prognosis. This depends on the underlying heart disease. In itself RBBB has no impact on longevity.

Treatment. None is necessary, unless there are symptoms and ECG evidence of higher-grade AV block, in which case a pacemaker is justified.

Full left bundle branch block

LBBB is recognized by broadening of the QRS complex and a late positive deflection in the left-sided chest leads, especially V5 and V6 (Figure 9.7). Partial LBBB is associated with QRS axis deviation – rightwards for block of

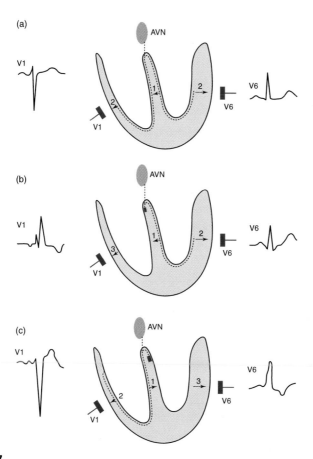

Figure 9.7

Mechanism of the ECG appearance of right bundle branch block (RBBB) and left bundle branch block (LBBB). (a) Normal intraventricular conduction: 1, septal activation from both bundle branches but primarily from the left; 2, free-wall activation occurring simultaneously in the two ventricles. (b) RBBB: 1, septal activation for the intact LBB; 2, free-wall activation in the left ventricle by normally timed propagation through the intact LBB; 3, late unopposed free-wall activation in the right ventricle by impulse propagation for the left ventricle. (c) LBBB: 1, septal activation from the intact RBB; 2, free-wall activation in the right ventricle by normally timed impulse propagation through the intact RBB; 3, late unopposed free-wall activation in the left ventricle by impulse propagation from the right ventricle. Adapted with permission from Sandøe E, Sigurd B. *Arrhythmia Diagnosis and Management: A Clinical Electrocardiographic Guide*. St Gallen: Fachmed.

the smaller anterior fascicle, leftwards for block of the larger posterior fascicle – often without any dramatic increase in QRS duration (Figure 9.8). If conducting tissue disease is extensive then there may be associated PR interval prolongation.

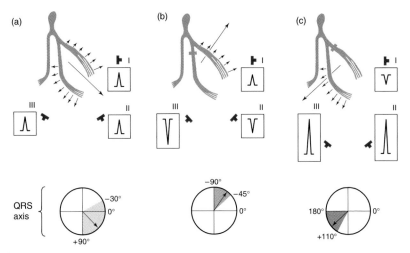

Figure 9.8
Mechanism of the ECG appearance of (a) normal function, and of partial block of the (b) left anterior fascicles and (c) left posterior fascicles. When partial block of the left bundle occurs there is no broadening of the QRS complex, as the left anterior and posterior fascicles connect via small branches over their entire length, so depolarization is not prolonged. Instead, a shift in the QRS axis occurs as shown, caused by the predominant early depolarization, which is determined by which fascicle remains viable.

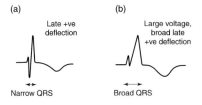

Figure 9.9
Appearance of (a) partial versus (b) complete right bundle branch block. +ve, positive.

Causes. It is considered that LBBB, unlike RBBB, is always pathological, indicative of some underlying heart disease. It is certainly almost always acquired (Figure 9.10). Common causes include:

- IHD
- aortic valve disease (especially calcific aortic stenosis, in which the calcium encrusting the valve 'burrows' down into the interventricular septum, interfering with the function of the conducting tissue contained within)

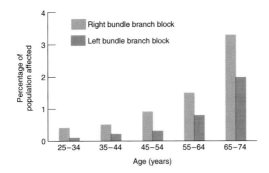

Figure 9.10
Community incidence of right and left bundle branch block.

- cardiomyopathy
- advanced left ventricular hypertrophy (LVH).

However, many patients with asymptomatic LBBB do not have severe, progressive heart disease.

Prognosis for LBBB is that of the underlying heart disease (except where AV block has occurred, in which case the prognosis is dramatically worse and a pacemaker is indicated).

Treatment. Usually none is given for the LBBB itself; however, any associated heart disease must be diagnosed and treated. If heart muscle disease is present and has caused advanced heart failure only poorly (or not at all) responsive to conventional therapy then 'resynchronization' therapy may be indicated.

Extrasystoles

Extra beats are classified according to which part of the heart they originate from.

Atrial extrasystoles

Atrial extrasystoles are recognized on the ECG by premature atrial beats, usually (but not always) with an unusual P wave morphology indicating an origin other than the sinoatrial node (SN) (Figure 9.11). The QRS complex is usually narrow as the normal conduction route through the AV node and onward remains intact.

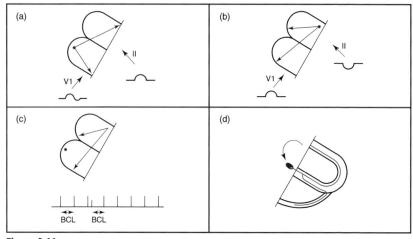

Figure 9.11
Mechanism and appearance of atrial extrasytoles. (a) Normal. (b) Ectopic atrial pacemaker, causing a different vector of depolarization and thus a different P wave shape. (c) Sinoatrial node invaded by a retrograde impulse and reset. This resetting of thesinus node means that after many atrial extrasystoles the next heart beat occurs after the basic cycle length (BCL). (d) All impulses still pass down the atrioventricular node and specialized conducting tissue, so the final QRS complex is narrow.

Causes

Atrial extrasystoles may be caused by any disease associated with stretching of the atria (eg hypertension, previous MI, valvular heart disease, cardiomyopathy) or by a toxic insult to the heart (eg alcohol, thyrotoxicosis, low K+ concentration). In many patients atrial extrasystoles are idiopathic. Most normal people have a few atrial extrasystoles every day.

Symptoms

Most people do not feel atrial extrasystoles; if they do, they sense an 'extra beat'. Occasionally, patients do not feel the extrasystole, but feel the stronger beat that follows it (Figure 9.12). Patients may feel that their heart 'stops, then restarts with a thud'.

Significance and prognosis

Atrial extrasystoles are usually of no great significance, and the prognosis is that of any underlying heart disease. However, in some patients they are associated with electrical instability of the atria, and thus with more sustained atrial arrhythmias such as atrial fibrillation (AF).

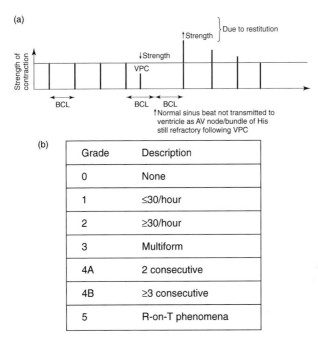

Figure 9.12

Mechanism of symptoms with ventricular premature contractions (VPCs). (a) 'Restitution' is a basic property of myocytes, which means that the greater the R–R interval, the stronger the strength of contraction. (b) Lown's grading of ventricular premature beats

Ventricular extrasystoles

Ventricular extrasystoles [sometimes termed ventricular premature contractions (VPCs)] are recognized on the ECG as premature beats (ie occurring before the normal sinus beat would occur) with a wide QRS morphology, without any preceding P wave (Figure 9.13). They are usually followed by a 'compensatory' pause, which comprises the remaining part of the RR interval of that cardiac cycle and the whole of the RR interval of the next cardiac cycle.

Pathophysiology

Although VPCs can occur in completely normal hearts, they are much more likely to occur in damaged hearts. Indeed, in some patients they may be a marker of cardiac damage. There are multiple mechanisms for VPCs, including increased automaticity of ventricular tissue [an electrical

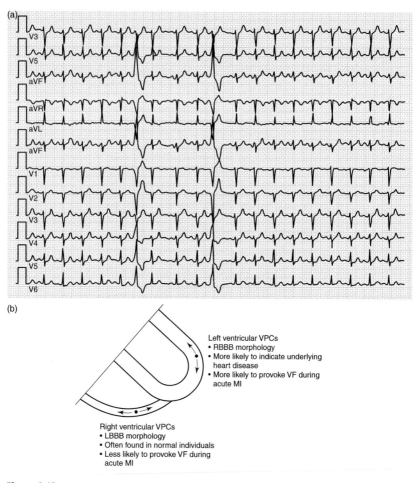

Figure 9.13

(a) ECG appearance of right ventricular premature contractions (VPCs) and (b) relevance of right and left VPCs. VPCs often originate outside specialized conduction tissue; they thus spread slowly and cause broad QRS complexes. RBBB, right bundle branch block; LBBB, left bundle branch block; VF, ventricular fibrillation; MI, myocardial infarction.

phenomenon due in some cases to 'triggered after-depolarizations' (Figure 9.14), recognized when the VPCs have a regular relationship between themselves and are unrelated to the preceding sinus beat] and reentry (indicated when multiple VPCs occur, each with the same coupling interval to the immediately preceding normal sinus beat).

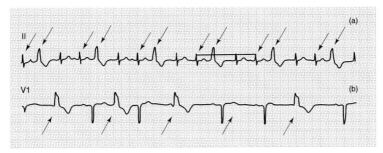

Figure 9.14
Mechanisms for ventricular premature contractions (VPCs). VPCs can be due to (a) reentry, in which case they have a constant relationship with the preceding sinus beat, or (b) enhanced automaticity, in which case they are separated from each other by a constant interval and are not related to the previous sinus beat. Adapted with permission from Wagner GS. *Marriot's Practical Electrocardiology*, 10th edn. Philadelphia: Lippincott, Williams and Wilkins.

VPCs are more likely to occur at low heart rates as bradycardia prolongs the QT interval and long QT intervals promote 'triggered activity' (ie repetitive action potentials occurring during the repolarization phase of the preceding action potential). Bradycardia (eg during rest) can thus promote VPCs and higher heart rates (eg during daytime activity) can suppress them. It is not just heart rate that influences VPC frequency – sympathetic tone does as well (by promoting 'triggered activity'). Thus when sympathetic tone is high the VPC frequency increases. Accordingly anxiety, which promotes sympathetic outflow, increases the chance of VPCs. Perhaps paradoxically, sympathetic tone can be quite high even when the heart rate is relatively low – thus a very powerful substrate for VPCs is night-time bradycardia combined with anxiety.

Causes

Although they can occur in normal hearts, VPCs are often a manifestation of cardiac damage. Thus they occur in:

- IHD
- hypertension
- cardiomyopathy
- valvular heart disease, especially if this has induced LV dysfunction
- toxic heart disease (alcohol, cytotoxic chemotherapy, hypereosinophilic syndromes)
- hypokalaemia in damaged hearts.

Significance

The significance of VPCs differs dramatically depending on whether or not there is any underlying heart disease. In structurally normal hearts VPCs have no adverse impact on prognosis.

In structural heart diseases, however, particularly post-MI, the more VPCs there are, the greater is the chance of a sustained ventricular arrhythmia occurring and resulting in sudden cardiac death (SCD) (Figure 9.15). Previously this led to unsuccessful attempts to suppress VPCs (and so SCD) pharmacologically with class I antiarrhythmic drugs in patients with frequent VPCs following an MI. Although VPCs were suppressed in these trials, the incidence of nonsustained VT and more sustained ventricular

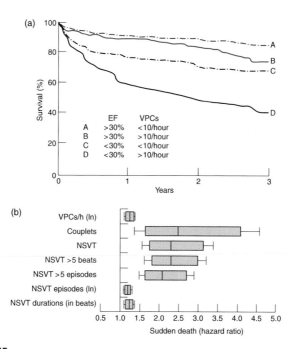

Figure 9.15

(a) Relationship between ventricular premature contractions (VPCs) and survival following myocardial infarction (MI). The graph shows post-MI patients (A, B, C and D) stratified according to ejection fraction (EF) and VPC frequency. In those with substantial LV systolic dysfunction excess VPCs are associated with a decreased survival. (b) The relationship between ventricular arrhythmias and sudden cardiac death in heart failure. NSVT, nonsustained ventricular tachycardia. Adapted with permission from Bigger JT. Relation between left ventricular dysfunction and ventricular arrhythmias after myocardial infarction. *Am J Cardiol* 1986; **57**: 8B–14B.

arrhythmias increased and SCD rates increased dramatically! In the modern era an excess of VPCs in association with moderate LV impairment (ejection fraction 30–40%) would indicate a low threshold for further invasive tests of cardiac electrical stability, to assess the need for an ICD.

Symptoms

Many patients have no symptoms. The thinner the patient, the greater the chance that they will feel the extrasystoles.

Symptoms can arise from the VPC itself, with patients complaining of 'extra beats' either as isolated phenomena or as repeated episodes. Patients usually experience slow, irregular palpitations. The differential diagnosis includes AF, although here the palpitations are usually felt to occur at a much higher rate.

Symptoms may also arise from the compensatory pause following the VPC (Figure 9.12). Patients may feel that their heart 'stops then restarts with a thud' (as the postextrasystolic beat is increased in strength for physiological reasons).

Whatever the symptoms are they often frighten the patient, which increases sympathetic outflow (and thus the chance of further VPCs), in an escalating pattern. As VPCs can be promoted by long QT intervals, some patients only experience symptoms at night (see above), others only when sitting down during the day or after exercise (ie when the heart rate is low and the QT interval long).

Grading of VPCs

When grading VPCs it has become conventional to use the Lown system (Figure 9.12) which is based on:

- the frequency of VPCs (0, grade 0; ≤30 per hour, grade I; >30 per hour, grade II)
- whether VPCs have different shapes (grade III), or occur 'back-to-back', ie in couplets (grade IVA) or triplets (grade IVB); or in higher runs, ie VT, nonsustained if lasting less than 30 seconds and terminating spontaneously
- the timing of VPCs, particularly whether or not they fall on the T wave of the previous beat (grade V).

The rationale for this grading system is that it is considered by some clinicians to predict the likelihood of sustained ventricular arrhythmias.

Investigations

Investigations in people with VPCs aim to ascertain whether or not there is any heart disease present, and if so its nature and severity. There is some use in determining VPC frequency and whether or not there is any evidence of any higher-grade ventricular arrhythmias (eg nonsustained ventricular tachycardia; see below). This can be done from a 24-hour ECG recording. If very frequent VPCs or higher-grade arrhythmias are seen in the presence of substantial LV dysfunction (ie ejection fraction ≤30–40%) then invasive electrophysiological studies to determine the benefit from an ICD may be indicated.

Treatment

VPC treatment focuses on the underlying heart disease. β-blockers can suppress many (but not all) VPCs (despite their heart-rate-slowing properties) and should be tried if the patient is symptomatic. It is difficult to know what drugs are appropriate for asthmatics, but occasionally calcium channel blockers with heart-rate-slowing properties are used (providing LV dysfunction is not present). Digoxin lessens sympathetic outflow and increases vagal outflow, and has a theoretically beneficial role. Class I antiarrhythmic drugs should not be used in the treatment of uncomplicated VPCs.

Sustained tachyarrhythmias

Clinical history and physical examination

The nature of a sustained tachyarrhythmia can often (but not always) be suspected from the clinical features:

- Demographics: previous cardiac history [young and no heart disease favours supraventricular tachycardia (SVT) whereas older and known heart disease favours VT].
- Symptoms: collapse favours VT, fast pre-excited AF or an SVT in the presence of substantial damage to LV function.
- Signs: in examining any patient with an arrhythmia it is important to determine the haemodynamic status (ie heart rate, blood pressure and evidence of poor tissue perfusion, eg cold skin, confusion or oliguria) and whether there is any evidence of heart failure. Haemodynamic collapse suggests VT or a supraventricular arrhythmia with significant structural heart disease.

Diagnosis

The diagnosis of sustained tachyarrhythmia can often be confirmed from the ECG alone.

If the arrhythmia is 'narrow complex' (ie the QRS complex is ≤120 ms), the arrhythmia is clearly of supraventricular origin. If it is irregular, it is likely to be AF, whereas if it is regular, it is likely to be atrioventricular nodal reentrant tachycardia (AVNRT; most commonly) or atrioventricular reentrant tachycardia (AVRT; rarer). AVN blocking drugs [adenosine, β-blockers or verapamil (note: never β-blockers and verapamil together)] will terminate AVNRT or AVRT and slow atrial tachycardia (AT) or AF.

If the arrhythmia is 'broad complex' (ie the QRS complex is broader than 120 ms), the diagnosis may not immediately be apparent. A broad complex tachycardia can be either a supraventricular tachyarrhythmia with bundle branch block (so-called 'SVT with aberrancy') or a ventricular tachyarrhythmia.

Management of broad complex tachyarrhythmias

If the patient is severely unwell (ie in a state of haemodynamic collapse), immediate treatment is needed – usually DC cardioversion. However, in a less 'sick' patient fuller and more leisurely assessment can take place, including a full history and physical examination.

Clinical history

A long history of paroxysmal arrhythmias (palpitations) terminated by 'vagal' manoeuvres strongly suggests that the arrhythmia is supraventricular – usually AVNRT or AVRT. However, underlying disease of the heart, especially IHD, increases the likelihood of either AF (usually easily determined from the ECG) or VT (see below).

Physical examination

There are a number of signs that may help differentiate a broad complex supraventricular arrhythmia from a ventricular arrhythmia (Table 9.1):

Is there any evidence of haemodynamic collapse? The greater the haemodynamic impairment the more likely an arrhythmia is to be ventricular in origin. However, be aware that many patients with VT have no

Table 9.1 Diagnosis of broad complex tachycardia

	Favours SVT	Favours VT
Known heart disease	Less usual	Common
Long history of palpitations	Common	Unusual
Haemodynamic collapse	Rare (pre-excited AF, SVTs with severe structural heart disease)	Commoner but still unusual
Heart rate	Unhelpful	Unhelpful
Pulse irregularity	Marked in AF, otherwise very regular	Occasionally mild
Blood pressure	Usually 'normal' (ie SBP ≥120–140 mmHg)	Often 'low' (ie SBP ≤120 mmHg)
JVP	Regular and bounding	Intermittent 'cannon' waves
First heart sound	Regular intensity	Fluctuating intensity
Response to vagal manoeuvres	Often	Very rarely
Response to adenosine	Arrhythmia usually breaks; may slow markedly but temporarily (atrial tachycardia, AF)	Very rarely

SVT, supraventricular tachycardia; VT, ventricular tachycardia; AF, atrial fibrillation; SBP, systolic blood pressure; JVP, jugular venous pressure.

haemodynamic disturbance at all, and equally patients with very fast supraventricular arrhythmias, or moderately fast supraventricular arrhythmias along with LV dysfunction (eg AF complicating an acute MI), may have haemodynamic compromise. Thus do not rely solely on haemodynamic status to differentiate SVT from VT.

Are intermittent 'cannon' waves seen in the jugular vein? These are found in ventricular arrhythmias but not in SVTs (in which a regular 'bounding' neck venous pulse occurs). The explanation for cannon waves in VT is that as the atria beat independently of the ventricles (in most cases), the atria occasionally contract onto a closed AV valve (tricuspid and mitral). No blood can pass from the atria to the ventricles, so blood pumps in a retrograde fashion either back into the lungs or up the great veins of the neck, where it causes intermittent pulsing. Thus 'cannon' waves are usually indicative of VT and a 'bounding' neck pulse (due to the atria contracting on a closed AV valve) is usually indicative of SVT. However, as some cases of VT have retrograde one-to-one VA conduction, which results in atrial systole occurring after ventricular systole (and thus the atria contracting on a closed AV valve), bounding neck venous pulses cannot be relied on to distinguish SVT from VT.

Does the first heart sound vary in intensity? If so VT is likely to be present. The first heart sound consists mainly of mitral valve closure, the intensity depends on how fully open the valve is when ventricular systole commences – the more open the valve, the louder the first heart sound. The position of the valve is in part determined by the timing of atrial systole in relation to ventricular systole, and as the atria (usually) beat independently of the ventricles in VT there is no consistency in the timing between atrial and ventricular systole, and accordingly there is no consistency in the intensity of the first heart sound.

Does the arrhythmia 'break' with 'vagotonic' manoeuvres? These are actions that increase vagal outflow to the heart, eg the Valsalva manoeuvre (bearing down, as if constipated), drinking ice-cold liquids, ocular massage, and immersing the face in a bowl of ice-cold water (the 'diving' reflex). Arrhythmias that use the AV node as an obligatory part of the circuit are terminated by such actions, whereas arrhythmias that do not are either transiently slowed (eg AF or automatic supraventricular arrhythmias such as AT) or not affected at all (eg ventricular arrhythmias).

Response to adenosine? Adenosine given as an intravenous bolus results in temporary and complete AV heart block, causing all arrhythmias using the AV node to be slowed (AF or AT) or terminated (AVNRT or AVRT). Ventricular arrhythmias are usually unaffected.

ECG diagnosis

The ECG gives clues to the origin of broad complex tachyarrhythmias. If the complexes are very irregular then the arrhythmia is likely to be AF. If the complexes look like RBBB or LBBB (Figure 9.16) then the arrhythmia is likely to be supraventricular. Otherwise the standard rules for the ECG diagnosis of VT apply (see p. 207).

If it is impossible to reliably and confidently differentiate whether a broad complex arrhythmia is SVT with aberrancy or VT then the arrhythmia must be treated as VT. This usually means that DC cardioversion to attempt to terminate the tachycardia is indicated.

Specific arrhythmias

Sustained supraventricular tachyarrhythmias

There are a number of sustained supraventricular arrhythmias. As a generalization, they all give rise to bursts of rapid palpitations (sudden onset

QRS contours favouring ventricular tachycardia

	Wellens[a]	Gulamhusein[b]
V1	15/15 (100%)	84/86 (98%)
V1 / V6	7/7 (100%)	177/187 (95%)
V6	27/31 (87%)	189/190 (100%)
V6	17/17 (100%)	38/40 (94%)

QRS contours favouring ventricular aberration

	Wellens[a]	Gulamhusein[b]
V1	38/41 (93%)	55/55 (100%)
V6	44/47 (94%)	27/27 (100%)

Figure 9.16

ECG features helpful in determining the origin of broad complex tachycardias. In each expression y/x here x is the number of times the contour was encountered and y is the number of times it was ventricular in origin. [a] Wellens HJJ. *Am J Cardiol* 1982; **49**: 186–93 and *Am J Med* 1978; **64**: 27–33. [b] Gulamhusain S. *J Electrocardiol* 1985; **18**: 41–50. Adapted with permission from Wagner S. *Marriot's Practical Electrocardiography*, 10th edn. Philadelphia: Lippincott, Williams and Wilkins, 2001.

and offset, defined duration, sometimes terminated by Valsalva manoeuvres) with an ECG showing a 'narrow-complex' tachycardia. Sometimes the atrial stretch that occurs during an SVT provokes the release of atrial natriuretic peptide and so a postevent polyuria.

Atrial tachycardia

Atrial tachycardia is a common rhythm disturbance. The causes are the same as for AF (see below) but the electrical mechanism is quite different (Figure 9.17); there is usually an anatomically fixed electrical focus in the atria that discharges impulses at a moderately high rate (usually 140–180 bpm). In between beats the atria are electrically silent. Thus the ECG (Figure 9.18) shows a high rate of P waves (morphologically abnormal as they originate from a site distant to the SN) separated by an isoelectric atrial line, with each P wave usually being followed by a QRS complex (although sometimes the AV node cannot transmit all the impulses bombarding it and a 'block'

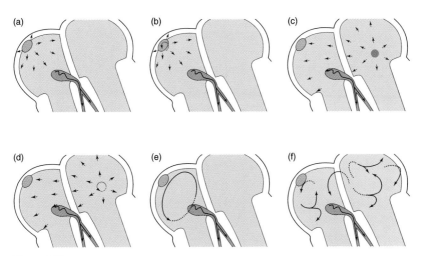

Figure 9.17
Mechanisms of atrial tachycardias. (a) Sinus tachycardia has the same P wave morphology as normal sinus rhythm. (b) The very rare sinus node reentrant tachycardia has the same P wave morphology as sinus rhythm. The clue to the diagnosis is that the heart rate is 'fixed' – best seen on a 24-hour ECG. Atrial tachycardia can also be due to (c) an automatic focus or (d) a micro-reentrant circuit. In either case the surface P wave morphology differs from normal sinus rhythm. (e) Atrial flutter is due to a macro-reentrant circuit in the right atrium and causes a characteristic continuous 'saw-tooth' baseline in the inferior leads. (f) Atrial fibrillation (AF) is often due to continuous reentry within the atria. The atria are continually electrically active and generate continuous, randomly changing 'fibrillation' waves. (For other mechanisms of AF see Figure 9.21). Reprinted with permission from Crawford MH, DiMarco JP. *Cardiology*. London: Mosby.

occurs, often with a two- or three-to-one ratio. The QRS complex is narrow unless there is a concomitant bundle branch block.

Symptoms are of sudden-onset, rapid, regular palpitations, not responding to 'vagal' manoeuvres (see below). Occasionally, if there is significant underlying heart disease, patients can become breathless during episodes. The tachycardia can induce chest pain in those with CAD. Syncope or presyncope can occur but are exceptionally rare, and are either confined to those with very severe underlying heart disease or indicative of SN disease (and a sinus pause following termination of the arrhythmia; see below). Very rarely the arrhythmia is not felt and therefore not treated for several months. The ventricular rate will thus be ≥150–170 bpm over this time period. This will cause ventricular function to deteriorate, and a so-called 'rate-related' cardiomyopathy will develop with breathlessness due to heart failure. This is usually reversible over several months provided the arrhythmia is terminated or the heart rate is controlled meticulously by drugs or AV node ablation.

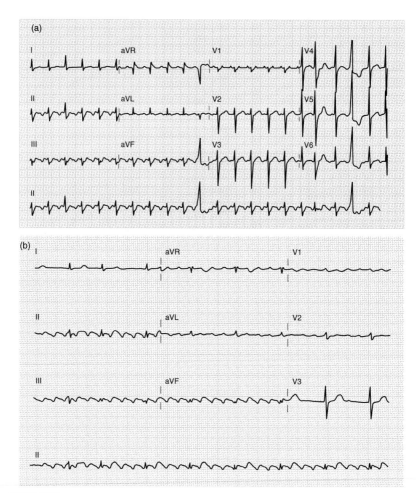

Figure 9.18
ECGs of atrial tachycardia. (a) The rhythm strip shows a tachycardia, the nature of which is not immediately apparent. However, inspection of lead V1 shows two atrial complexes for every QRS complex. The principle differential diagnosis in this situation is atrial flutter. However, lead V1 shows that the P wave returns to the isoelectric line between beats, and the inferior leads (lead II, III and aVF), which reveal atrial flutter best, do not show the typical 'saw tooth' pattern of atrial flutter. Compare with (b) typical atrial flutter, with a 'saw-tooth' baseline in the inferior leads.

Investigation is to exclude underlying heart disease (usually a cardiac ultrasound is sufficient). A 24-hour ECG recording is sometimes indicated.

Treatment is of the underlying heart disease. If the episode does not terminate spontaneously then DC cardioversion may be indicated, but usually this is not needed. Antiarrhythmic drugs, especially class III agents such as amiodarone, may prevent recurrent episodes. Due to the potential side-effects of amiodarone, a better strategy may be to accept that further episodes are likely to occur and aim for heart rate control during episodes via an AV node-blocking drug such as a β-blocker and/or digoxin.

Atrial flutter

Atrial flutter is a common rhythm disturbance, often (but not always) occurring in association with or followed by AF. It is due to a macro-reentrant circuit (Figure 9.19) in an enlarged right atrium and is therefore likely to be due to structural heart disease. This should be clarified via a cardiac ultrasound. Patients experience rapid, regular palpitations or present with complications of the underlying structural heart disease (eg heart failure). The risk of systemic emboli is significantly less than in AF. The ECG appearances are classic (Figure 9.18b): as there is continuous atrial activity, continuous activity is seen in the ECG, most commonly in the inferior leads. Almost invariably the atria beat at 300 bpm. The AV node cannot conduct impulses at this high rate, and accordingly some degree of 'block' occurs so that the ventricles beat once for every two, three, four or more atrial beats. Thus the ventricles beat at a slower rate than the atria. The commonest block is two-to-one, which results in a heart rate of exactly 150 bpm – this is so common that any tachyarrhythmia of 150 bpm should be considered to be atrial flutter until proven otherwise.

Treatment involves terminating the arrhythmia (DC cardioversion with anticoagulant cover) and/or slowing the heart rate response (digoxin, β-blockers, calcium channel blockers with AV node-blocking properties, such as diltiazem or verapamil, and occasionally amiodarone). If recurrent episodes occur (which is likely), these can either be accepted and the heart rate controlled, or be suppressed with antiarrhythmic drugs (eg amiodarone). There are two interventional approaches that are useful in the small number of patients who are resistant to, or experience unacceptable side-effects from, conventional drug treatment. First, the macro-reentrant circuit can be ablated (Figure 9.20). Second, the occasional patient may be sufficiently symptomatic (and drug-resistant or drug-intolerant) as to require AV node ablation and ventricular pacemaker insertion.

Atrial fibrillation

AF is probably the commonest serious disturbance of the heart rhythm. Although it can occur in the absence of any obvious form of heart disease (in

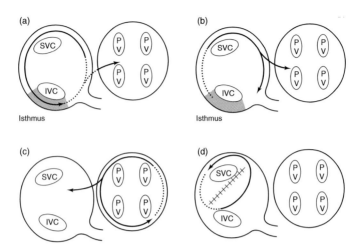

Figure 9.19
Mechanism of atrial flutter (the heart is observed from the front; thus the right atrium appears on the left and vice versa). (a) Typical atrial flutter, with an anticlockwise circuit in the right atrium. (b) Atypical atrial flutter, with a clockwise circuit in the right atrium. (c) Very atypical atrial flutter, with a macro-reentrant circuit in the left atrium. (d) Postsurgical atrial flutter, commonly related to scar tissue formation in patients with congenital heart disease. SVC, superior vena cava; IVC, inferior vena cava; PV, pulmonary vein. Reprinted with permission from Murgatroyd FD, Krahn AD, Klein GJ *et al*. *Handbook of Cardiac Electrophysiology*. London: Remedica, 2000.

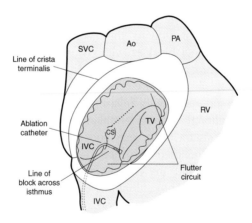

Figure 9.20
Ablation of macro-reentrant circuit in atrial flutter. SVC, superior vena cava; Ao, aorta; PA, pulmonary artery; IVC, inferior vena cava; CS, ostium of coronary sinus; TV, tricuspid valve; RV, right ventricle. Adapted with permission from Murgatroyd FD, Krahn AD, Klein GJ *et al*. *Handbook of Cardiac Electrophysiology*. London: Remedica, 2000.

which case it may relate to electrical instability in the left atrium around the origin of the pulmonary veins – so-called 'idiopathic' or 'lone' AF), it may also reflect heart disease or other processes, including:

- IHD, which can be complicated at any time by AF. In particular, AF can occur during the acute phase of an MI, in which case it is associated with more extensive coronary disease and worse LV function. Unsurprisingly, AF complicating an MI is therefore associated with a significantly decreased long-term prognosis. AF can also complicate the chronic postMI phase of IHD with an incidence proportional to the severity of the heart failure (Figure 9.21)
- sinus node disease can underlie AF; this can often be diagnosed from a 24-hour ECG, whether or not AF is present during the recording
- hypertension
- valvular heart disease, especially mitral stenosis
- congenital heart disease, especially ASD (in which case atrial arrhythmias are very common, whether or not the ASD has been closed)
- cardiomyopathy, particularly that due to alcohol
- excess alcohol, even in the absence of overt cardiomyopathy
- thyrotoxicosis
- pneumonia; AF indicates more severe infection and a higher early mortality
- pulmonary emboli
- chronic obstructive pulmonary disease (COPD) or other chronic lung disease
- idiopathic, or 'lone' AF (ie no cause found); this occurs in some 20–50% of cases. Some authorities have further classified this form of AF into 'vagal' (ie where episodes of AF start when the heart rate is low, eg night) and 'adrenergic' (ie relating to sympathetic outflow, eg with episodes occurring during or shortly after exercise).

Pathophysiology. There are three possible mechanisms. In the first, the atria are continually active, with multiple (at least seven) different waves continually moving across the atria (Figure 9.21). In the second mechanism there may be a rapidly firing focus near the pulmonary veins, from which waves of electricity flow along continually altering paths. In the third (rarer) form, a rapid reentry circuit may occur in one or other atria. All mechanisms are associated with the typical irregular ECG baseline containing fibrillatory waves. The key ECG clue to the diagnosis of AF, in addition to the irregular baseline, is that the QRS complexes occur irregularly. Whatever the exact

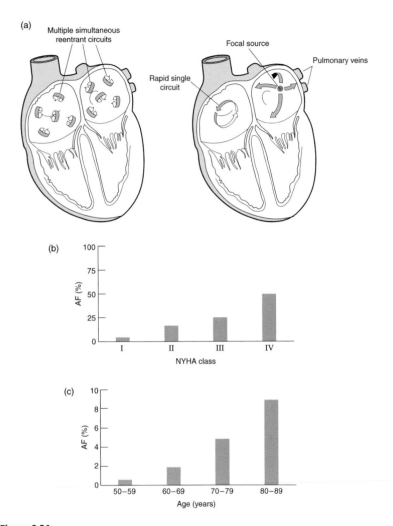

Figure 9.21

(a) The three mechanisms of atrial fibrillation (AF): multiple reentrant wavelets; a focal source, usually near the pulmonary veins, with the subsequent path varying continuously from beat to beat; and a micro-reentrant circuit, with the subsequent path varying continuously. Reprinted with permission from Crawford MH, DiMarco JP. *Cardiology*. Mosby, London. (b) Prevalence of AF in chronic heart failure relates to New York Heart Assocation (NYHA) grading. Reprinted with permission from Maisel WH, Stevenson LW. Atrial fibrillation in heart failure; epidemiology, pathophysiology and rationale for therapy. *Am J Cardiol* 2003; **91 (6A)**: 2D–8D. (c) Prevalence of AF in a US population. Reprinted with permission from Kannel WB, Wolf PA, Benjamin EJ, Levy D. Prevalence, incidence, prognosis and predisposing conditions for atrial fibrillation: population-based estimates. *Am J Cardiol* 1998; **82 (8A)**: 2N–9N.

mechanism, the AV node is continually bombarded with electrical impulses, accounting for the high heart rate. Effective mechanical activity of the atria ceases, accounting for stasis of blood in the left atrial appendage, thrombus formation and so systemic emboli.

Symptoms of AF include:

- None.
- Symptoms from tachycardia: fast, 'irregularly irregular' palpitations in those with normal hearts. Breathlessness (from heart failure) also occurs in those with significant impairment of LV function. Occasionally ischaemic chest pain occurs, in those with CAD. Syncope or near-syncope during tachycardia is very rare and is usually associated with severe underlying impairment of LV systolic and/or diastolic function. Tachycardia can occur at rest and/or during exercise, an important point when considering drug therapy.
- Symptoms from irregular heart rate: a very small number of patients develop marked symptoms due to heart rate irregularity, even when the absolute rate is well controlled.
- Symptoms from systemic thromboembolism: in AF the left atria tends to generate thrombi, which usually do not interfere with cardiac function but which can be expelled from the heart causing arterial occlusion elsewhere, commonly in the brain (stroke), limbs (ischaemic arm or leg) or gut (mesenteric ischaemia, causing an 'acute abdomen'). The risk of left atrial thrombi developing relates to the duration of AF (very low risk if ≤48 hours), patient's age (risk increases significantly if ≥65 years), presence of structural heart disease [especially acute MI, impaired LV function, mitral stenosis and hypertension (even if meticulously controlled)].
- Symptoms from any associated sinus node disease: these symptoms cause a sinus pause after the AF terminates, before the sinus node pace-maker takes over. This pause typically lasts 3–5 seconds and may result in syncope.

Terminology in atrial fibrillation is confusing (Figure 9.22). 'New-onset AF' refers to a new episode (within 48 hours), 'paroxysmal AF' refers to repeated attacks terminating spontaneously (usually within a few hours, almost always within a few days); 'persistent AF' refers to attacks lasting longer than 7 days, usually requiring specific therapy for termination. Both paroxysmal and persistent AF can recur. 'Permanent AF' is AF that is not self-terminating and for which cadioverting therapy is not planned.

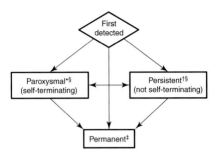

Figure 9.22

Forms of atrial fibrillation (AF): *episodes that generally last <7days (most last less than 24 hours); †episodes usually lasting >7 days; ‡cardioversion failed or not attempted; §either paroxysmal or persistent AF may recur. Reprinted with permission from ACC/AHA Task Force on Practice Guidelines and ESC Committee for Practice Guidelines and Policy Conference in collaboration with North American Society of Pacing and Electrophysiology. ACC/AHA/ESC guidelines for the management of patients with atrial fibrillation. *Eur Heart J* 2001; **22**: 1852–923.

Investigations aim to confirm that the diagnosis is AF (from an ECG obtained during an attack) and exclude any underlying heart disease (cardiac ultrasound scan is mandatory) and thyrotoxicosis. A 24-hour ECG recording may be indicated to assess whether or not atypical symptoms are due to AF and whether occult paroxysms of AF continue despite treatment, and to observe the heart rate response over 24 hours.

Treatment. During an acute attack the aim is to slow the heart down (using digoxin and β-blockers), to terminate the arrhythmia (DC cardioversion or a class I agent such as flecainide or propafenone – provided AF has been present ≤48 hours, otherwise cardioversion can result in systemic emboli) and to anticoagulate to prevent systemic emboli. Many attacks terminate spontaneously, usually within 24 hours.

In persistent AF there are two possible approaches. First, there is the 'rate-control' strategy: accept AF and aim for heart rate control and anticoagulation. This is a highly effective strategy in many, although it has the disadvantage that long-term therapy with heart-rate-slowing and anticoagulant drugs is required. Second, there is the 'rhythm-control' strategy: attempt to restore and then maintain sinus rhythm. This can be an effective strategy. Success depends on the chance of initially restoring sinus rhythm (decreased in the presence of AF ≥18 months or significant structural heart disease) and the drive to recurrent episodes of AF (background rate ±25% per year, increased by high alcohol intake, thyrotoxicosis and structural heart disease). The rate of spontaneous relapse is felt to be so high that antiarrhythmic drug therapy is usually justified (which exposes patients to possible side-effects). Unfortunately, this policy is not 100% effective and although it may reduce further episodes of AF it cannot prevent all of them – something that some patients find quite upsetting. There is increasing consensus that the first strategy is the best treatment policy in persistent AF (Figure 9.23).

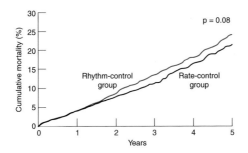

Figure 9.23
Prognosis in 'rate' versus 'rhythm' control strategies for atrial fibrillation (AF). The data presented here come from the AFFIRM trial – a large randomized study comparing a strategy of accepting AF, anticoagulating and controlling the heart rate ('rate-control' group), versus a strategy of attempting to establish and maintain sinus rhythm using electrical and pharmacological therapy ('rhythm-control' group). These data are consistent with data from other trials. Adapted from The Atrial Fibrillation Follow-up Investigation of Rhythm Management (AFFRM) investigators. A comparison of rate control and rhythm control in patients with atrial fibrillation. *N Engl J Med* 2002; **347**: 1825–33.

There are two methods of restoring sinus rhythm in AF: synchronized DC cardioversion (which requires heavy sedation or a short-acting general anaesthetic) or chemical cardioversion (usually with a class I agent, eg flecainide or propafenone). For 'elective' DC cardioversion a general anaesthetic is generally used, whereas for emergency DC cardioversion in 'sick' patients (especially if there is significant hypotension) heavy sedation can be used, particularly using amnesic drugs such as the benzodiazepines.

AF increases the heart rate (indeed, if it does not do so, one should question whether or not there is any associated conducting tissue disease). This high heart rate occurs at rest and can usually be fairly readily controlled with digoxin. Exercise also leads to excessive rises in the heart rate; this can often be readily controlled by a β-blocker but not by digoxin alone. Thus most patients with AF need both digoxin and a β-blocker for heart rate control. A very small number of patients cannot tolerate these AV nodal-blocking drugs or find their action ineffective, and amiodarone may be useful. If this is unsuccessful, then AV node ablation with permanent ventricular VVI-R pacing can be effective.

Atrial pacing can have a role in preventing episodes of AF. This is especially true in sick sinus syndrome, in which sinus bradycardia (which increases the dispersion of atrial repolarization and thus promotes atrial 'reentry') predisposes to AF. Atrial extrasystoles, which also promote AF, can be suppressed by pacing. Thus pacing the sinus node at a fairly high heart rate (eg ≥60–70 bpm) can suppress the tendency to AF. More sophisticated pacing algorithms are being developed to enable suppression of AF by complex electrophysiological means. An automatic, implantable atrial defibrillator has been developed but is still experimental.

Antiplatelet drugs and warfarin both have a role in AF. The stronger the tendency towards left atrial thrombi, and hence systemic emboli, the better is warfarin (compared with aspirin) in preventing systemic thromboemboli. Left atrial thrombi are more likely with increasing age (≥65 years) in those with hypertension, structural heart disease and for the month following DC cardioversion (due to temporary 'stunning' of the atria impairing contractile function, so promoting stasis of blood, thrombosis and consequent thromboembolism).

In practice it is reasonable to use aspirin in patients with all of the following:

- age ≤65 years
- no structural heart disease (eg IHD, valvular heart disease, echocardiographic increase in LA or LV dimensions)
- no treated hypertension (as hypertension emerges from most of the trials as being a strong predictor of stroke in nonwarfarinized AF)
- not scheduled for cardioversion.

Warfarin [International Normalized Ratio (INR) 2.5–3.0] should be used for everyone else, assuming there is no comorbid disease (eg falls, dementia or excess alcohol intake) and that there are no issues over compliance. There remain uncertainties about the best anticoagulation regime in the very elderly (≥80 years).

Atrioventricular nodal reentrant tachycardia

AVNRT is the commonest form of regular SVT. It is caused by an accessory conduction path within or near to the AV node (Figure 9.24). This pathway is felt to be present life-long but only comes into play very occasionally. During episodes of tachycardia a 'circus' movement develops within the AV node tissue and the accessory pathway (Figure 9.24). Each time the electrical current passes around the circuit an impulse is sent down to the ventricle. As the circuit is small, it does not take long to be completed, and thus tachycardia results.

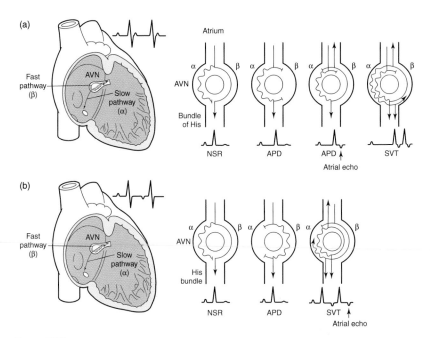

Figure 9.24

Mechanism of atrioventricular nodal reentrant tachycardia (AVNRT). In typical AVNRT (a) the atrioventricular node (AVN) possesses two parallel pathways, one capable of conducting slowly (α) but with a short refractory period, the other capable of conducting quickly (β) but with a long refractory period. An atrial premature depolarization 'hits' the node when the fast pathway is still refractory. It passes down the slow pathway. By the time it reaches the distal end of the AVN, the fast pathway is no longer refractory, and the impulse can pass in a retrograde fashion up the fast pathway, then down the slow pathway again, setting up a self-sustaining reentrant circuit. As the ventricle is activated only shortly before the atria, the (abnormally shaped) P wave is either 'hidden' in the QRS complex (in two-thirds of cases), or appears just afterwards (in about one-third of cases). In the rare atypical form of AVNRT (4% of cases) (b) the fast pathway is the anterograde one and the slow pathway the retrograde one. Atrial activation occurs some time after ventricular activation, so the P wave follows the QRS complex by such a long time period that it appears as if the P wave just precedes the next QRS complex – so-called 'long RP tachycardia'. The other long RP tachycardias include sinus tachycardia and sinus node reentrant tachycardia. NSR, normal sinus rhythm; APD, atrial premature depolarization; SVT, supraventricular tachycardia. Reprinted with permission from Braunwald E, Zipes DP, Libby P. *Heart Disease: A Textbook of Cardiovascular Medicine*. Philadelphia: WB Saunders, 2001.

Symptoms of AVNRT:

- sudden-onset, fast, regular palpitations
- well-defined duration of palpitations (ie a clear-cut number of seconds or minutes, unlike 'appreciation of sinus tachycardia' symptoms, for which the patient often finds it difficult to establish a duration)
- 'vagal' manoeuvres (see above) may terminate, by increasing the vagal outflow to the AVN, slowing conduction through it and thus 'breaking' the arrhythmia and restoring sinus rhythm
- 'post-event' polyuria occasionally follows (see below)
- chest tightness can occur during tachycardias, due either to very fast tachycardia (usually over 220 bpm) or to coexistent CAD
- 'bounding' neck pulse (see above), occasionally commented on by patients.

Syncope is very unusual and is not regarded as a classic symptom of AVNRT.

Demographics. Patients may have a long history of palpitations starting as a teenager, although (perhaps surprisingly given that the substrate is present life-long) often do not develop attacks until later life.

Diagnosis. Between attacks the ECG is normal. During an attack it shows a narrow complex tachycardia and is usually diagnostic (Figure 9.25).

Prognosis is for a normal life expectancy.

Treatment to terminate an acute attack of AVNRT aims to slow conduction through the AV node, thus 'breaking' the arrhythmia. This can be done using physiological 'vagotonic' manoeuvres that increase vagal outflow to the AV node (see above) or via pharmacological measures [intravenous adenosine, or another AV node-blocking drug (a β-blocker or verapamil, but never the two together)].

No prophylaxis may be required if symptoms are infrequent (other than teaching the valsalva manoeuvre). If symptoms are more frequent then drugs that slow conduction through the AV node (digoxin, β-blockers and some Ca^{2+} channel blockers) may be useful. If symptoms are intrusive despite this, or if there is drug intolerance, then it is possible to ablate the extra pathway percutaneously (however, as the extra pathway runs close to the normal AV node, there is an approximately 1% chance of permanently damaging the normal conduction pathway, making a permanent pacemaker essential (Figure 9.26).

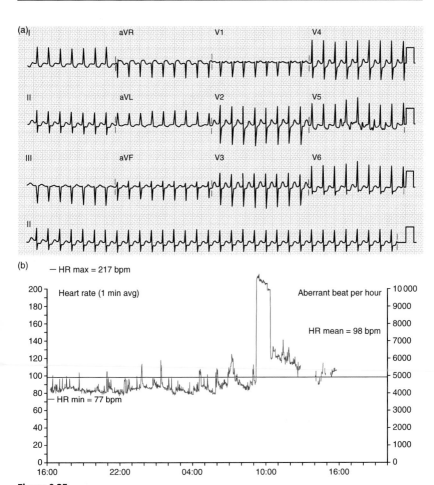

Figure 9.25

(a) ECG showing atrioventricular nodal reentrant tachycardia (AVNRT). The ECG shows a narrow complex tachycardia without a well-defined P wave. (b) The tachogram from a 24-hour tape shows a sudden increase in heart rate at the onset of a SVT and a sudden decrease when it terminates.

Atrioventricular reentrant tachycardias

AVRTs are due to accessory conduction pathways between the atria and the ventricles. These may be seen on the ECG between attacks as a 'delta' wave with a short PR interval and a 'slurred' QRS upstroke. This pattern of ECG is indicative of Wolff–Parkinson–White (WPW) syndrome. The size of the delta wave can vary dramatically (Figure 9.27). In concealed WPW syndrome no changes are visible on the resting ECG between attacks.

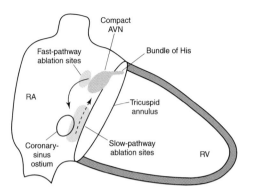

Figure 9.26

Ablation of the pathway supporting the atrioventricular nodal reentrant tachycardia (AVNRT) circuit. 'Slow pathway modification' has a success rate of 98–100%, a recurrence rate of 0–2% and a 0–1.3% chance of inducing high-grade AV block. 'Fast pathway' ablation has a success rate of 82–96%, a recurrence rate of 5–14% and a 0–10% chance of inducing high-grade AV block. Thus slow pathway ablation is the preferred treatment for AVNRT. RA, right atrium; RV, right ventricle. Reprinted with permission from Morady F. Drug therapy: radio-frequency ablation as treatment for cardiac arrhythmias. *N Engl J Med* 1999; **340**: 534–44.

The delta wave in WPW syndrome originates from the fact that normal physiological impulses passing down the AV node are delayed (this is part of the normal function of the node), whereas impulses passing down the abnormal accessory conduction pathway are not and so arrive at the ventricle earlier than the normal impulse (the ventricle is said to be 'pre-excited', ie depolarized earlier than normal). Thus the PR interval is shortened. The impulse from the accessory pathway starts to depolarize the ventricle via cell-to-cell depolarization rather than via the specialized conducting tissue of the heart, so QRS complexes have a broad 'slur', the delta wave.

Mechanisms for tachycardia in WPW syndrome. These fall into three categories. First, in orthodromic tachycardia impulses pass down the AV node, into the ventricle, up the accessory pathway back into the atria, then back down the AV nodal pathway, etc (Figure 9.28a); the ECG usually shows a narrow complex tachycardia. Second, in antidromic tachycardia (much rarer) impulses pass down the accessory pathway into the ventricle, 'short-circuit' up the AV node back into the atria, pass back down the accessory pathway, etc; the ECG may show a broad complex tachycardia (Figure 9.28b). Third, there is AF: ventricular ectopic beats generate electrical

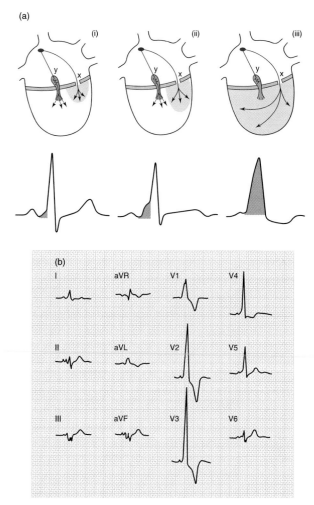

Figure 9.27
(a) The size of the delta wave in Wolff–Parkinson–White (WPW) syndrome depends on how far ahead of the normal atrioventricular (AV) conduction (y) the electrical impulse passing down the accessory pathway (x) arrives at the ventricle. If the accessory wavefront arrives only marginally ahead of the normal AV wave (i) then there is a small delta wave. Quicker accessory path transmission (ii) increases the size of the delta wave, and in the very quickest pathways (iii) the delta wave can be very large indeed. Reprinted with permission from Sandøe E, Sigurd B. *Arrhythmia Diagnosis and Management: A Clinical Electrocardiographic Guide*. St Gallen: Fachmed. (b) In this example of WPW syndrome the delta wave is very well developed.

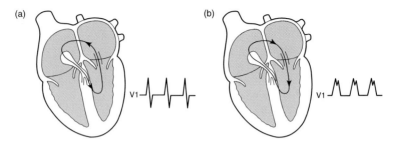

Figure 9.28
Mechanism of tachycardia in AVRT. Most tachycardias are orthodromic (a). The QRS will be narrow, as activation is via the specialized conducting tissue of the heart. Occasionally antidromic tachycardias (b) occur. As activation here is via the accessory pathway, ventricular depolarization will not occur via the specialized conducting tissue and so the QRS complexes will be broad. Reprinted with permission from Braunwald E, Zipes DP, Libby P. *Heart Disease: A Textbook of Cardiovascular Medicine*. Philadelphia: WB Saunders, 2001.

impulses, which pass in a retrograde fashion up the accessory pathway into the atria, where they meet the normal sinus beat and interfere with propagation of current flow across the atria, ie the atrial circuits 'break up', reentry occurs and AF ensues.

AF occurs in some 20% of patients with WPW syndrome. In normal patients with atrial fibrillation the AV node, although continually bombarded with electrical impulses, only allows a maximum of 160–180 impulses per minute to reach the ventricle, so the maximum heart rate is around 160–180 bpm (which is at the upper limit of the normal physiological range). In 'pre-excited' AF impulses can (in some patients) be transmitted down the accessory pathway to the ventricle at a much higher rate – so fast that there is inadequate time for the heart to fill, thus decreasing cardiac output and blood pressure. In these circumstances coronary perfusion becomes reduced and myocardial ischaemia occurs, provoking ventricular fibrillation (VF) and sudden cardiac death. The ECG of 'pre-excited' AF shows a broad, slurred QRS complex as most of the ventricular activation occurs from electricity spread down the accessory pathway (Figure 9.29).

Symptoms of AVRT:

- none
- recurrent episodes of sudden-onset, fast, regular palpitations, terminated by 'vagal' manoeuvres
- AF, and so 'irregularly irregular' palpitations; as the heart rate may be very

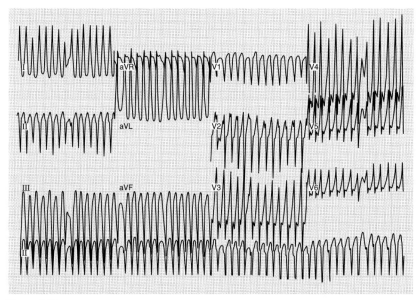

Figure 9.29
'Pre-excited' atrial fibrillation (AF). The rhythm is AF, although this is not easy to determine as the heart rate is so high (the higher the heart rate in AF, the more regular AF appears). However, there is significant irregularity, indicative of AF, and occasionally the atrial beat passes through the atrioventricular node to 'capture' the ventricle. The most characteristic feature is the 'slurred' upstroke due to the 'delta' wave, especially visible in the lateral chest leads. This pattern is pathognomonic of pre-excited AF.

high, patients with 'pre-excited' AF may feel faint or even die suddenly (in AVRT the incidence of AF is about 20% and the incidence of sudden cardiac death is 1–3%)

• sudden death.

Treatment (Figure 9.30). The acute attack of AVRT can be terminated by drugs that slow conduction through the AV node. Adenosine is probably the best, causing a very brief period (less than a few seconds) of complete heart block. Alternatives include β-blockers or certain Ca^{2+} channel blockers (but never combine verapamil with a β-blocker as lethal bradyarrhythmias can occur). Prophylaxis may be achieved with AV node-blocking drugs such as β-blockers, verapamil, diltiazem and digoxin. Definitive treatment is percutaneous ablation of the AV accessory pathway. In the treatment of pre-excited AF both adenosine and amiodarone (as well as verapamil and

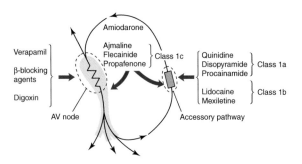

Figure 9.30
Drug treatment of atrioventricular reentrant tachycardia (AVRT) in Wolff–Parkinson–White syndrome. Drugs that slow AV conduction are good treatments for AVRT, but unless they also slow conduction through the accessory pathway they are very bad in 'pre-excited' atrial fibrillation (AF) as they can then lead to more conduction down the pathway and a speeding up in the ventricular response to the AF, provoking dangerously high rates. Drugs that only slow conduction through the accessory pathway are, however, safe in AF. Adapted with permission from Sandøe E, Sigurd B. *Arrhythmia Diagnosis and Management: A Clinical Electrocardiographic Guide*. St Gallen: Fachmed.

digoxin) should be avoided as they block conduction down the normal AV node but not the accessory pathway, thus increasing conduction down the accessory pathway and increasing the heart rate (sometimes dangerously). In the treatment of pre-excited AF drugs are best avoided and the preferred treatment is cardioversion, followed by elective pathway ablation.

Risk stratification is vital for all patients with AVRT, (probably) even in the absence of symptoms, as some patients have accessory pathways that can conduct very quickly, allowing for very high heart rates in AF. AF occurs in about 20% of WPW patients. Pre-excited AF can be dangerous and may cause sudden cardiac death (as above). The ability of the accessory pathway to conduct AF at dangerously high rates can be ascertained from invasive electrophysiological studies. If great, the patient is at risk of sudden cardiac death; the risk of ablating the pathway is much less than the risk of conservative treatment and should thus be performed.

Ventricular tachyarrhythmias

There are three forms of ventricular tachyarrhythmias: ventricular premature contractions (VPCs) (see p. 179), ventricular tachycardia (VT) and ventricular fibrillation (VF).

Ventricular tachycardia

VT is classified as:

- Nonsustained monomorphic VT: episodes of VT lasting less than 30 seconds and terminating spontaneously. There can be many such episodes in a day (Figure 9.31).
- Sustained monomorphic VT: episodes of VT lasting longer than 30 seconds that may terminate spontaneously or may need therapy (see below) to terminate. Monomorphic VT often (but not always; see fascicular tachycardia, below) occurs in the setting of LV damage, often from a remote MI (scar tissue is needed to provide the substrate for the abnormal reentrant circuit) or other structural damage to the left ventricle.
- Polymorphic VT (see below).
- Ventricular fibrillation (see below).

The rhythm disturbance in VT originates within the ventricle. The arrhythmia can travel round the ventricle continuously due to a 'circus' movement or originate from a single focus that discharges continuously at a high rate (a so-called 'automatic focus') (Box 9.1). An arrhythmia that travels continuously around the same ventricular pathway results in monomorphic VT (ie each VT beat has the same shape), whereas if the circuit changes continuously then polymorphic VT results (ie each successive VT beat has a different shape). Although both forms of VT can degenerate into VF, the risk is usually considered higher with acquired polymorphic VT than with monomorphic VT.

ECG features of monomorphic VT. There is a tachycardia (heart rate usually 120–220 bpm). The QRS complexes are broad. P waves may not be visible, but if they are there is usually (but not always) no association between the P waves and the QRS complexes. The diagnosis is usually obvious, but on occasions it can be difficult to differentiate VT from supraventricular arrhythmia with a 'bundle branch block' (so-called 'SVT with aberrant conduction' or 'SVT with aberrancy'). If one is in doubt, the patient should always be initially treated as if they have VT. Helpful ECG features suggestive of VT include:

- independent P wave activity. Occasionally 'capture' beats may be seen, when the P wave fortuitously passes through the AV node and captures the ventricle, causing a normal PQRST beat in the middle of a run of VT. Sometimes the ventricle is partially captured, and a 'fusion' beat occurs, midway in shape between a normal sinus beat and a VT complex

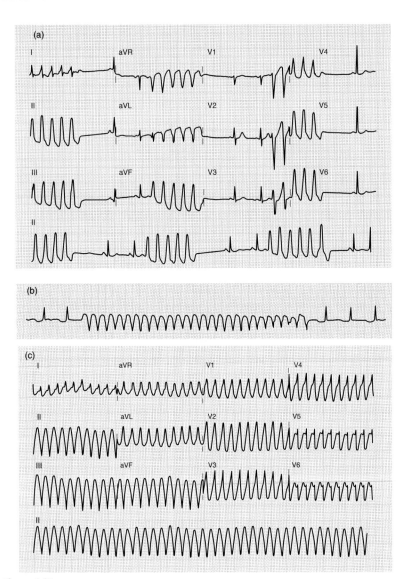

Figure 9.31
(a) Multiple episode of nonsustained ventricular tachycardia (VT). (b) A typical 'run' of VT seen during intensive care monitoring. Although quite a long run, it is less than 30 seconds and terminates spontaneously and so is classified as nonsustained monomorphic VT. (c) Sustained monomorphic VT. This ECG shows a broad complex tachycardia, identified as VT by broad QRS complexes and (on careful inspection of the rhythm strip) P waves occasionally independent of ventricular activity (ie AV dissociation, pathognomonic of VT). (Unusually, the second ear of the V1 complex is larger than the first – in most VT the first ear is larger.)

Box 9.1 Mechanisms of different forms of ventricular tachycardia (VT)

Abnormal automaticity

- May relate to 'late' after-depolarizations
- Good examples in animal models, human role less certain
- Suppressed by verapamil
- May underlie verapamil-responsive VT
- May be relevant in digoxin-toxicity-related VT and some ischaemia-related VT
- Not inducible, ie VT stimulation studies not useful for management

'Triggered' activity → polymorphic VT

- May relate to 'early' after-depolarizations (EADs)
- Often related to ↑ QT interval, which is commonly due to:
  - Drugs (eg antipsychotics, antihistamines, antiarrhythmics)
  - Medical conditions (eg critical myocardial ischaemia, heart failure, alcoholic liver disease, diabetes)
  - Rarely due to genetic disease: hereditary long QT prolongation
- Promoted by ↓ heart rate → further ↑ QT interval (so may occur in complete heart block, at night or when resting)
- Enhanced by ↑ sympathetic outflow (which ↑ tendency to EADs), eg anxiety, exercise, sudden sounds
- Promoted by ↓ [K⁺] and ischaemia
- Suppressed by:
  - pacing to ↑ heart rate → ↓ QT interval
  - β-blockers
  - optimal [K⁺]
- Treatment also involves removing the underlying cause

'Reentry' → monomorphic VT

- Suggested when:
  - VT can be induced/terminated by VPCs
  - Continuous electrical activity occurs during VT
  - Pacing can 'capture' ventricle and/or reset VT
  - Slow conduction during normal sinus rhythm, often seen as 'late' potentials, ie a scar is often present
  - excising or ablating a critical part of the pathway prevents the arrhythmia
- Common in IHD
- Possible in normal heart VT (eg bundle branch reentry)
- Promoted by catecholamines, ↓ [K⁺], ischaemia
- Electrophysiological studies useful to:
  - demonstrate presence, significance and need for ICD
  - ablate substrate (sometimes)

VT, ventricular tachycardia; EAD, early after-depolarizations; VPC, ventricular premature contraction; IHD, ischaemic heart disease; ICD, implantable cardioverter defibrillator.

- very broad QRS complexes
- QRS morphology is unlike RBBB or LBBB
- precordial lead concordance: ie all the chest leads have either a dominant R wave or a negative R wave (see Figure 9.16).

ECG features of VT of right and left ventricular origin.

- Right ventricular origin: LBBB pattern. Associated right axis deviation suggests that the VT originates in the RV outflow tract, and this may be due to RV dysplasia.
- Left ventricular origin: suggested by a RBBB pattern. Associated left axis deviation suggests that the VT originates in the fascicle of the conducting tissue (so-called 'fascicular tachycardia').

Clinical features. Symptoms experienced in VT can vary greatly, and depend to a certain extent on the severity of the underlying heart disease, arrhythmia speed and various other factors (including 'cardiovascular fitness', ie how well an individual can tolerate a low blood pressure). Common symptoms in VT include (Figure 9.32):

- sudden-onset, fast, regular palpitations
- presyncope or syncope, with or without palpitations
- haemodynamic collapse, with near unconsciousness and cardiogenic shock
- sudden cardiac death.

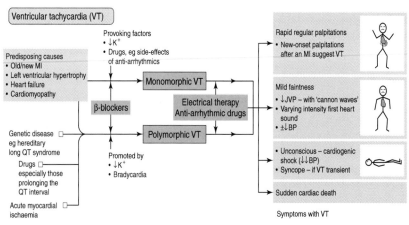

Figure 9.32
Summary of the causes, consequences and treatment of monomorphic and polymorphic VT.

Predisposing cardiac disease. Most (but not all) patients with monomorphic VT have underlying structural heart disease. Ischaemic heart disease is common, particularly an old MI. Patients with an ejection fraction ≤40% and nonsustained VT on a 24-hour ECG are at increased risk of sudden cardiac death, mainly from ventricular arrhythmias; those with inducible VT on electrophysiological testing are at particularly high risk. Cardiomyopathy may also underlie monomorphic VT, especially the form known as 'RV dysplasia', which can cause RV outflow tract VT. RV dysplasia can be diagnosed echocardiographically but the appearances may be subtle; if this diagnosis is under serious consideration and the ultrasound has not been diagnostic, magnetic resonance imaging of the heart should be undertaken; the resting ECG often shows partial RBBB or T wave changes in leads V1 to V3 but can be disturbingly unremarkable. Any other disease process affecting the ventricles (especially the LV but also the RV) may predispose to monomorphic VT. LVH is a potent factor predisposing to VT – patients with LVH who suffer an MI are much more likely to die from an acute phase ventricular arrhythmia than those without LVH.

Provoking factors. There are several factors that can promote an episode of VT in the presence of structural heart disease:

- Drugs: eg those with class I antiarrhythmic properties, and especially those prolonging the QT interval (eg macrolide antibiotics, nonsedating antihistamines; these drugs can also provoke polymorphic VT in structurally normal hearts (see below).
- Hypokalaemia: a powerful provoker of VT in the presence of heart disease but very rarely a cause of ventricular arrhythmia in its absence.
- Bradycardia: in some subjects, sometimes for both monomorphic and polymorphic VT; probably via prolongation of the QT interval, which promotes early after-depolarization.

Treatment of an episode of sustained monomorphic VT. This depends on the situation. For haemodynamically well-tolerated VT some authorities recommend trying antiarrhythmic drugs (eg lignocaine or sotolol) with continuous ECG monitoring. Other approaches include inserting a temporary pacing wire and terminating the arrhythmia by 'overdrive' pacing (pacing at a rate 10–30 bpm higher than that of the VT, then either slowly turning the rate down or stopping the pacing suddenly, so allowing normal sinus rhythm to take over) or 'underdrive' pacing (same principle, pacing rate just below that of the VT). If the VT is not well tolerated or if the above treatment has failed then DC cardioversion should be used, under heavy sedation or general anaesthesia. This is likely to be effective. If not, high-dose amiodarone should be given intravenously, if possible with a low dose of a β-blocker. Over- or under-drive ventricular pacing can then be retried. If this fails, cardioversion should be repeated once the patient is fully loaded with amiodarone.

Following an episode of monomorphic VT a full cardiac 'workup' should take place: LV function should be ascertained; the nature of any coronary disease should be determined by coronary angiography; and invasive electrophysiological studies may be indicated.

If VT has been well tolerated then pharmacological treatment (β-blockers, amiodarone) may be tried in the long term. However, if there has been any suggestion of haemodynamic instability, if VT is very easily induced during electrophysiological tests, or if LV function is poor, the patient should probably have an ICD inserted.

There are two rare forms of VT that respond to specific and unusual therapies. The correct diagnosis is therefore important, and is usually suspected from the following.

Fascicular tachycardia. If the QRS complex shows a RBBB pattern with left axis deviation (Figure 9.33), then the VT may be due to fascicular tachycardia, a rare form of VT unrelated to structural heart disease (although this must always be formally excluded). It is relatively benign (unless class I antiarrhythmic agents are given, in which case the prognosis worsens dramatically) and responds to β-blockers or verapamil.

RV outflow tract VT. If the QRS complex shows an LBBB pattern with right axis deviation then the VT may be due to RV outflow tract tachycardia, which may relate to a RV cardiomyopathy or dysplasia. This tachycardia is more malignant than fascicular tachycardia, especially if treated with class I antiarrhythmic agents. Thus, although this form of VT may respond to some drugs (including β-blockers), the threshold for implanting a ICD should be low.

Polymorphic ventricular tachycardia

Polymorphic ventricular tachycardia is recognized by continually changing VT morphology. One form of polymorphic VT involves a continually shifting

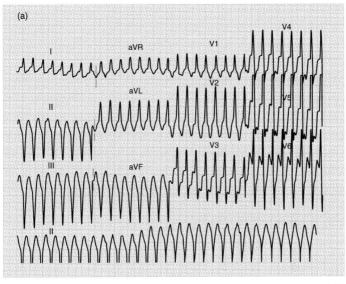

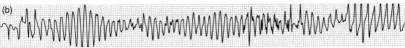

Figure 9.33
ECG appearance of ventricular tachycardia (VT). (a) Monomorphic VT, of right bundle branch block morphology. There is clear atrioventricular dissociation, shown in lead V1. (b) A short run of polymorphic VT occurring during an exercise test and terminating spontaneously.

axis, termed 'torsade de pointes'. Various factors can underlie polymorphic VT:

- drugs alone: nonsedating antihistamines (particularly in association with grapefruit juice), antipsychotics, antidepressants and macrolide antibiotics such as erythromycin can all provoke potentially life-threatening polymorphic VT, often via prolonging the QT interval
- drugs in conjunction with LV dysfunction
- structural heart disease, especially if severe
- 'metabolic' disturbance: particularly low K^+ and/or Mg^{2+} concentrations, usually in the presence of at least mild structural heart disease
- primary electrical abnormalities of the heart: particularly QT interval prolongation, inherited (very rare) or acquired (most commonly due to heart failure). Episodes of VT are particularly likely to occur at rest (when the heart

rate is low and thus the QT interval long) or with sympathetic activation – thus a characteristic time is in bed in the morning (low heart rate, long QT interval) when the alarm clock goes off (sympathetic stimulation)

- low heart rate: by prolonging the QT interval.

Symptoms in polymorphic VT depend, like those in monomorphic VT, on the speed of the arrhythmia (collapse and syncope are more likely with fast VT, palpitations with slow VT), the severity of any underlying heart disease (the more severe the damage to ventricular function, the greater the chance of collapse) and the duration of the arrhythmias (the longer the VT, the less well it is tolerated).

Thus characteristic symptoms of polymorphic VT include:

- palpitations alone (relatively rare)
- palpitations with 'presyncope' (relatively rare)
- syncope, usually without preceding palpitations (common, and can easily degenerate into VF)
- sudden cardiac death (common).

Polymorphic VT is promoted by:

- drugs: all should be assessed and any relevant drugs stopped
- hypoakalaemia: must be treated
- bradycardia: often due to sinus node disease or to heart-rate-slowing drugs that do not block the adrenergic system (eg calcium channel blockers).

Treatment of polymorphic VT. Acute episodes can be terminated by DC cardioversion. Further episodes in the acute phase can then be prevented by: pacing at moderately high heart rates (usually ≥90 bpm); maintaining an ideal K^+ concentration; and if possible giving β-blockers.

Following an acute episode the underlying mechanism should be determined. If a drug is responsible, it should be withdrawn. If the mechanism involves structural heart disease then this should if possible be treated (especially revascularization for CAD). Permanent pacing at a high heart rate may well prove effective, if possible combined with β-blocker therapy. Not infrequently an ICD may be required.

Ventricular fibrillation

Ventricular fibrillation is due to completely chaotic electrical activity of the ventricle, with continually changing reentrant circuits. There is no effective cardiac mechanical activity and so no cardiac output. The patient blacks out and will die unless prompt effective treatment is given immediately. Basic life support (external cardiac massage and artificial ventilation) may maintain life until external defibrillation can be applied to restore sinus rhythm.

Causes of VF include the following:

Acute phase of an MI. Most deaths during acute MI are due to ventricular arrhythmias. The incidence of acute phase VF is largely unrelated to the size of the MI. For this reason patients with an acute MI should be positioned right next to a defibrillator along with a nurse who can use it! Provided 'acute phase' VF is promptly treated by defibrillation there is little impact on long-term prognosis, quite unlike acute phase AF, which is associated with a significantly worse medium-term outlook.

Following MI. The risk of VF is significant, being worst in those with the greatest impairment of LV ejection fraction (EF). The risk can be lessened by long-term β-blocker therapy and by implanting a prophylactic ICD. This should be reserved for those patients at the very highest risk of developing VT or VF in the medium term following an MI. These patients can be identified on the basis of the EF (the lower the EF the higher the risk – EF ≤30% conveys substantial risk), by the presence of nonsustained ventricular arrhythmias on 24-hour ambulatory ECG recordings, and from ventricular stimulation studies (showing easily provoked, sustained, haemodynamically unstable VT).

Critical coronary disease. All patients with unexplained VF should have coronary angiography, as critical proximal multivessel coronary disease underlies some (indeed many) episodes of VF. If severe CAD is found then revascularization is usually appropriate. Postrevascularization VT stimulation studies are indicated to ascertain whether the heart has a persisting 'scar' capable of sustaining a VT circuit. If it does then an ICD may also be required.

Any structural heart disease. This is true both for acquired heart disease and for genetic heart disease (such as hypertrophic cardiomyopathy, Duchenne muscular dystrophy and Freidrich's ataxia).

Cardiac hypertrophy.

Wolff–Parkinson–White syndrome. Occasionally VF is the consequence of WPW syndrome, with pre-excited AF degenerating into VF. Accessory pathway ablation can be totally preventive.

Genetic disease. This includes hypertrophic cardiomyopathy, long QT syndrome and Brugada syndrome.

ECG diagnosis. The ECG in VF is totally chaotic. Initially the complexes are of large amplitude, but in the absence of successful treatment the amplitude declines markedly after the first minute or two (Figure 9.34).

Investigation. Full investigation of VF, including coronary angiography and sometimes full electrophysiological studies, is indicated to define the underlying mechanism, and so determine the best preventive therapy.

Treatment of VF involves immediate DC cardioversion, and, once clinical stability is re-established, antiarrhythmics (β-blockers, amiodarone), drugs to improve LV function (angiotensin-converting enzyme inhibitors), revascularization if appropriate, and in some (probably most) ICD implantation (age and general fitness allowing).

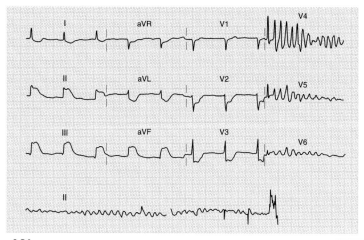

Figure 9.34
Inferior wall myocardial infarction, with VF occurring in the latter stages of the recording. The rhythm strip, on this rather old ECG machine, is recorded after the main ECG, not contemporaneously. This shows that VF continues and the amplitude declines rapidly.

Chapter 10
The ECG in ischaemic heart disease

The ECG is most helpful in the management of ischaemic heart disease (IHD). Its use varies according to which clinical syndrome is being evaluated.

Classification of ischaemic heart disease

There are many different classifications of ischaemic heart disease; the following, based on the stability of symptoms, ECG findings and troponin levels, is commonly used:

- asymptomatic coronary disease
- stable angina
- crescendo angina
- acute coronary syndromes:
  - troponin-negative acute coronary syndromes
  - non-ST segment elevation myocardial infarction (non-STEMI)
  - ST segment elevation myocardial infarction (STEMI)
- complications of IHD include arrhythmias and heart failure and can occur in any of the above phases of IHD.

One of the key differences between stable angina and the acute coronary syndromes (ACS) is that in the former the symptoms arise from a stenosis due to a stable plaque in the coronary circulation, whereas in the latter they arise from an 'unstable' plaque (atheroma with superimposed thrombus) in the coronary circulation. As a consequence of the thrombus on the plaque the coronaries often partially occlude (giving rise to pain at rest – one of the key clinical pointers to the presence of ACS) and can also occlude completely, producing an MI and various consequences, including death. Although death can occur in those with stable plaques, it is much more common in those with unstable 'hot' lesions, and this explains why it is so crucial to separate stable angina from ACS. The most helpful clinical clue to enable this is the presence or absence of rest pain.

Asymptomatic coronary artery disease

Most if not all adults have coronary artery disease (CAD) – it is endemic in Western societies. In many people only relatively minor plaques are found, but in some asymptomatic individuals the disease can be surprisingly severe. The prognosis in asymptomatic CAD is much better than in 'anatomically' similar, symptomatic individuals. Most authorities do not recommend that asymptomatic individuals be screened for the presence of high-grade lesions, even if at high risk of CAD. This is partly because there is no highly reliable method (exercise testing has high false-positive and false-negative rates, and isotope imaging exposes patients to unacceptable risks, as do more invasive approaches) and partly because the data are not clear about what should be done to individuals with CAD and no symptoms [other than treat CAD risk factors (which should be aggressively treated anyway) and add aspirin (which likewise should be taken by all high-risk individuals)].

The resting ECG in most asymptomatic people is normal. However, as up to one-third of MIs are 'silent' (especially in the elderly and those with diabetes) it is possible that the ECG of apparently asymptomatic patients can show old MIs (see below). Exercise tests carried out on those with asymptomatic CAD can be normal, even if the disease is severe, or can show any form of ST segment depression, at any workload. Statistically, however, the more severe the CAD the more likely there is to be substantial ST segment depression occurring at a low workload during exercise stress testing.

Stable angina

Stable angina is recognized as being present when patients present with 'long-standing' symptoms (pragmatically, for three or more months) typical of effort angina [ie retrosternal chest ache rapidly (≤2 min) relieved by rest], occurring reproducibly at the same intensity of exercise. The key feature in stable effort angina is that the amount of effort required to provoke symptoms is stable from day to day. Symptoms do not occur at rest.

The role of the ECG in stable angina is firstly to confirm the diagnosis and secondly to evaluate prognosis, and so the need for invasive assessment and revascularization. The resting ECG in stable effort angina that has not yet been complicated by an MI is usually normal, regardless of the severity of the underlying CAD, but may show evidence of:

- previous myocardial damage – either pathological Q waves, loss of R wave height, or persistent T wave flattening or inversion. Previous MI suggests impairment of left ventricular (LV) function and, as LV function is a prime determinant of outcome, a worsened prognosis
- left ventricular hypertrophy (LVH) if long-standing hypertension has been present. LVH is associated with more severe CAD and an increased risk of ventricular arrhythmias during an MI. It is therefore a marker for adverse prognosis, and in addition to mandating vigorous blood pressure control should lower the threshold for angiography. LVH interferes with the interpretation of the exercise test
- conducting tissue disease, especially left bundle branch block (LBBB).

To confirm the diagnosis of stable effort angina, one ideally wishes to see an exercise test induce typical anginal symptoms, preferably with effort-induced ST segment depression (although this is not necessary for diagnosis; see Chapter 11).

Bear in mind that the ST segment response during exercise in those with CAD may be entirely normal, ie no ST depression may occur, even in those with severe CAD who are exercising at a high workload.

Crescendo angina

Crescendo angina is defined as a rapid deterioration in previously stable angina. Symptoms of chest pain occur at a much lower workload than usual. Symptoms do not occur at rest – if they do, the syndrome is an ACS (see below). Causes for crescendo angina include:

- an increase in the severity of the underlying stenosis, often due to thrombus forming on a pre-existing coronary atheromatous plaque and partially occluding blood flow
- anaemia
- atrial fibrillation.

Crescendo angina and new-onset effort angina (ie angina developing within 6–8 weeks) are both at least moderately high-risk clinical situations, in which the probability of an adverse event in the near future, particularly an acute MI, is significantly increased. As in stable angina, the resting ECG is usually normal; urgent exercise testing is indicated to assess prognosis, although some cardiologists would regard crescendo angina as being sufficiently high-risk to justify an immediate coronary angiogram without an exercise test (provided there are no uncertainties about the diagnosis of the angina). This is particularly so if patients are otherwise at high risk of having multivessel coronary disease [ie have a long history of stable effort angina, are ≥65 years, have multiple risk factors for CAD (especially diabetes), and are already optimally treated (especially if already taking aspirin)].

Acute coronary syndromes

In ACS symptoms due to myocardial ischaemia occur at rest:

- Angina at rest results in typical ischaemic chest pain: 'tight' retrosternal ache or heaviness lasting up to 20–30 minutes, not associated with any features suggestive of MI. The patient may be uncomfortable but is not usually in severe pain.
- In an MI the pain is usually but not always much more severe: 'the worst pain ever', 'an elephant on my chest', and additional symptoms of sweating, nausea and vomiting may occur. The patient appears grey or 'ashen'. Complications (including arrhythmias and/or heart failure) may be present.
- Arrhythmias, which may complicate an 'obvious' ACS [eg atrial fibrillation (AF) complicating the inpatient stay during an MI]. However, not infrequently the first presentation of an ACS is unheralded ventricular fibrillation (VF).
- Heart failure is occasionally the presenting feature of an ACS.

Classification

The classification of ACS is rapidly evolving. Previously, patients with unstable coronary plaques were classified according to their ECG and how much myocardial necrosis had occurred (as measured by conventional cardiac enzymes such as creatine kinase or aspartate aminotransferase) into one of the following categories:

- Unstable angina is angina with symptoms occurring at rest. The ECG can vary from normal to widespread changes (but, by definition, no ST segment elevation). Myocardial necrosis is minor, and less than the World Health Organization definition of an MI (a twofold or greater rise in conventional enzymes, ie not troponin).

- Non-STEMI is diagnosed when infarction-quality chest pain occurs, with an abnormal ECG (not ST segment elevation) and a rise in conventional cardiac enzymes ≥ two times the upper limit of normal.
- STEMI is diagnosed when infarction-quality pain occurs with ST segment elevation.

The modern classification of ACS uses three key features:

- symptoms
- ECG changes: divided into STEMI, and all others
- troponin levels. The higher the troponin level the greater the chance of an adverse event in the short and medium term (see below). It is crucial to realize that troponin level is not the only determinant of risk; although there is a broad correlation between increased troponin level and increased risk, there are some patients who can have a normal troponin level and still be at very high risk, and others who can have a raised troponin level and be at very low risk (see p. 234 for other determinants of risk).

Using this approach ACS are classified into:

- STEMIs: all patients with ST segment elevation due to myocardial ischaemia
- non-STEMIs: all ACS with elevated troponin levels but no ST segment elevation. These patients' ECGs are usually abnormal in other ways. They can be subdivided into low, medium and high risk (see below)
- troponin-negative ACS, likewise subdivided into low, medium and high risk.

Approach to managing suspected acute coronary syndrome

There are several steps to the management of a patient with a suspected ACS.

First, it is important to be certain that the patient's symptoms relate to myocardial ischaemia (see below).

Second, it is important to assess any comorbid disease as this influences both treatment and the decision threshold for coronary angiography. For example, coexistent diabetes increases the risk of ACS and so lowers the threshold for angiography. Chronic lung disease (eg chronic obstructive pulmonary disease) may preclude the use of β-blockers. Anaemia may exacerbate any anginal symptoms and increase the risk of bleeding from anticoagulants if the cause is gastrointestinal pathology. Dementias, frailty and disseminated cancer all raise the threshold for angiography.

Third, it is important to determine the risk of early and late complications from the ACS. LV function is a key determinant of risk, amongst other factors (see below). It should be ascertained clinically (history of MI or heart failure, or evidence of heart failure), from the ECG (Q waves or poor R wave height) and by cardiac ultrasound. Extent of CAD should be ascertained clinically (a long history of symptomatic CAD suggests multivessel involvement), from the resting ECG (ACS in a post-MI patient with ECG changes remote from the territory of the infarct suggests multivessel involvement) and from the exercise ECG (widespread ST segment depression at a low workload increase the chance of multivessel disease). Clearly, definite diagnosis of the extent of the CAD requires a coronary angiogram.

Fourth, the right medical and interventional therapy should then be administered.

Are symptoms due to myocardial ischaemia?

It can be astonishingly easy, or conversely really quite difficult, to determine if symptoms are due to myocardial ischaemia or an alternative disease process. Although typical symptoms of ischaemia often relate to genuine myocardial ischaemia, and vice versa, unfortunately many patients with ACS have atypical symptoms, and many patients with typical symptoms of 'myocardial ischaemia' turn out to have alternative pathology (eg gastro-oesophageal reflux or oesophageal spasm). Thus, although the exact nature of the symptoms can be highly useful, they can on occasions mislead.

Furthermore, the ECG can do the same! Although as a generalization abnormal ECGs are associated with ACS and normal ECGs with other diagnoses, this is very far from being a universal truth. Many patients with ACS have normal ECGs and many patients with chest pain not due to ACS have abnormal ECGs. Thus the ECG cannot often be relied on to establish or exclude the diagnosis.

Given these facts, how does one in practice reach a diagnosis? Different clinicians use different approaches. However, many use the presence of a number of 'trumping' features to establish the diagnosis, including:

- Current symptoms being identical to those during a previous episode of unequivocal myocardial ischaemia. For example, the patient may have experienced an MI in the distant past, and current symptoms, although of a lesser intensity, are of the same quality.

- Background history of undiagnosed but still unambiguous, deteriorating effort angina, now occurring at rest.
- In the absence of the above, appropriate risk factors (especially age, diabetes, smoking and high cholesterol) and pains quite typical of myocardial ischaemia (retrosternal chest tightness or heaviness, occurring in episodes of ≤30 minutes).
- 'Trumping' ECG, eg ST segment elevation entirely typical of MI. Some ECG changes, although not 'trumping', are nonetheless highly suggestive, eg deep pan-anterior T wave inversion (a 'proximal LAD' pattern; Figure 10.1).
- Troponin level significantly raised (ie five to ten times the upper detect limit), with no other explanation (eg renal failure, pulmonary emboli, myocarditis). This is now one of the commonest ways to diagnose the atypical ACSs.
- Exercise/stress test carried out once symptoms have settled (ie ≥48 hours from last pain), showing characteristic symptoms with ECG changes and/or myocardial perfusion isotope defects or, on stress echo, induced regional wall motion abnormalities.

If doubt remains, one can proceed in several different directions. First, it may be appropriate to do no further investigations if one considers that even if the diagnosis is ACS the risk is low, eg in the patient who can achieve a high workload on exercise stress testing. Second, conversely, in many patients in this situation it is often appropriate to carry out coronary angiography both to clarify the diagnosis and for 'risk stratification'. Which approach is best depends on the clinical situation.

Myocardial infarction

By far the commonest cause of acute MI is occlusive thrombus occurring on an atheromatous plaque in the coronary circulation. However, there are a number of other possible causes:

- Cocaine-induced vasospasm, resulting in myocardial ischaemia sufficient to cause infarction.
- Patients with an aortic dissection backtracking to involve the right coronary artery (resulting in an inferior wall MI) can survive to reach hospital, whereas a dissection backtracking to involve the left main

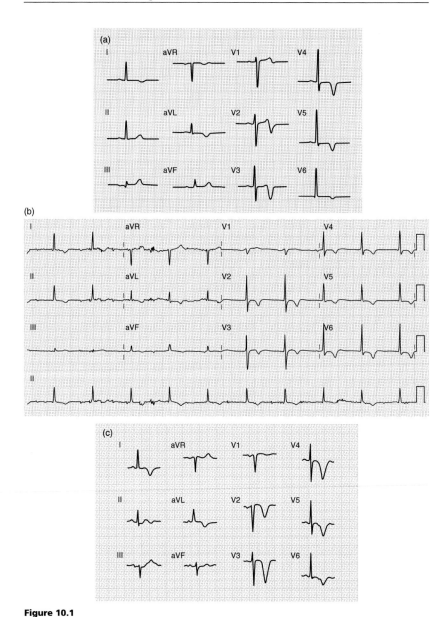

Figure 10.1

ECG patterns associated with a proximal left anterior descending coronary artery (LAD) lesion. (a) There are widespread T wave abnormalities, with the T waves in leads V2 and V3 being biphasic, whereas those more laterally are inverted. (b) Here there is T wave inversion affecting all the anterior leads (ie 'pan-anterior'), although the T waves are not particularly deep. (c) This is a worrying ECG and shows the classic T wave changes along with a dramatically prolonged QT interval.

coronary stem is almost invariably promptly lethal. Thus inferior MIs may very rarely be due to aortic dissection, whereas anterior infarcts are not.

- Spontaneous coronary artery dissection: rare, most commonly found in young women.
- Embolism down a coronary artery, either from thrombus arising in the left atrium during AF or (exceptionally rarely) from an endocarditic valve lesion or (even more rarely) a left atrial myxoma.

ECG in acute ST segment elevation myocardial infarction

The ECG in an acute STEMI goes through a variety of changes (see Figure 4.7).

Initially it may be normal! This accounts for 2% of MIs at presentation and for some of the 3–5% of patients who present with an MI to the A&E department and are sent home inappropriately [highly unfortunate as the incidence of acute phase high-grade ventricular arrhythmias in this group is around 30% (typical for most MIs); such arrhythmias are lethal in the community but readily treatable in hospital]. Thus if a patient presents to the emergency room with typical ischaemic chest pain then, almost regardless of the presenting ECG, they merit a period of inpatient observation.

Subsequently in the course of the STEMI 'hyperacute' T wave changes develop. Classic ST segment elevation then occurs, with the affected leads reflecting which artery is occluded (see p. 44). However, it is quite wrong to rely upon ST segment elevation to make the diagnosis of MI as only about 40–60% of patients with an MI have ST segment elevation on admission. Rather one should rely on the clinical findings and use the ECG to support these (see below).

If reperfusion therapy has been successful the ST segment elevation resolves, with preservation of R waves and without the development of pathological Q waves; occasionally this occurs spontaneously. After such temporary ST segment elevation substantial T wave changes may occur.

The less successful reperfusion therapy has been, the slower is the resolution of ST segment elevation and the more likely Q waves are to develop in the hours and days following the MI. As ST segment elevation resolves much more slowly in unsuccessful than in successful reperfusion, the speed of ST segment resolution is a reasonable measure of the efficacy of reperfusion therapy. What should be done if reperfusion therapy is unsuccessful is unfortunately quite unclear.

In the days and weeks following the MI most patients show T wave inversion and then normalization.

It is vital to understand that patients with substantial MIs may present without ST segment elevation. There are several reasons for this: a posterior MI (seen as ST segment depression in leads V1 to V3) may be misdiagnosed as angina [due to left anterior descending coronary artery (LAD) territory ischaemia] usually because the commonly associated inferior wall MI is absent; alternatively the MI may also involve extensive subepicardial rather than endocardial necrosis, resulting in ST segment depression rather than elevation (see Figure 4.3). It is thus best to make a diagnosis of MI on clinical grounds (ie ischaemic chest pain lasting longer than 20 minutes, with or without sweating) confirmed by any significant abnormality on the ECG, rather than relying solely on the 'classic' findings of ST segment elevation.

Determination of infarct-related artery

Inferior wall MI (ie ST elevation in leads II, III and aVF): caused by right coronary artery (RCA) occlusion in 80% of cases; circumflex coronary artery occlusion accounts for most of the remaining 20%. ST segment elevation greater in lead II than in lead III suggests RCA occlusion (if there is evidence of right ventricular infarction (ie ST elevation in the right-sided chest leads) then the occlusion is likely to be in the very proximal part of the RCA). ST elevation greater in lead III than in lead II suggests circumflex artery occlusion (especially if there is also evidence of lateral infarction, shown as ST elevation in leads I, aVL, V5 and V6, and evidence of posterior wall infarction, seen as ST depression in leads V1 to V3).

Anterior wall MI (ie ST elevation in leads V1 to V3): occlusion of the proximal segment of the LAD is suggested by substantial ST elevation in lead V1 (≥2.5 mm) or by ST depression in the inferior wall leads (II, III and aVF). Occlusion of the distal segment of the LAD is suggested by minor inferior lead ST depression or inferior lead ST elevation.

Posterior wall MI (ie ST depression in leads V1 to V3, proceeding to a dominant R wave in lead V1; see Figures 3.9 and 3.15): isolated posterior wall MI is likely to be due to circumflex coronary disease. If there is associated inferior wall MI, circumflex occlusion is suggested by greater ST elevation in lead III than in lead II; the reverse suggests RCA occlusion.

ECG diagnosis of full thickness MI

Difficulties in the diagnosis of full thickness MIs can arise if the ECG is already very abnormal due to previous myocardial damage. This is especially the case if previous MIs have left persisting ST elevation, for example in the anterior leads. It can be very difficult to determine whether or not these changes reflect old or new MI if patients present again with chest pain. There is no clear way past this problem; one approach, not always available, is to compare the current ECG with a remote one performed when the patient was well. If the ST elevation is greater, a presumptive diagnosis of further MI is made. Another approach is to essentially make the diagnosis of MI on the clinical features (severe prolonged chest pain, with sweating, vomiting, etc) and use the ECG to confirm the diagnosis. If the patient has extensive coronary disease, they will often know what an MI feels like. This can be used to determine whether or not current symptoms are likely to be due to MI. In practice, one should have a very low threshold for undertaking 'hot' angiography in all such patients.

LBBB may also obscure diagnosis of MI. It has been held that LBBB precludes the diagnosis of MI. This is not entirely true, but it certainly makes it more difficult. Often it is best to go back to clinical criteria – MI is diagnosed by the presence of typically ischaemic and prolonged severe chest pain. In this setting if one finds LBBB one should administer a thrombolytic. Some authorities suggest that LBBB does not completely preclude accurately diagnosing an MI, and that if some or all of the following are present, an MI is likely: ST elevation ≥1 mm concordant to the QRS complex; ST depression occurring in leads V1 to V3; ST elevation ≥5 mm discordant to the QRS complex; and ST elevation in leads V5 or V6. These are rather complex criteria and are not yet of proven clinical usefulness.

ECG changes in acute coronary syndromes presenting without ST segment elevation

Patients presenting with an ACS without ST segment elevation on the initial ECG are collectively referred to as non-ST segment elevation ACS; if the troponin level is raised they are classified as non-STEMIs. These conditions are associated with many different ECG patterns. However, be aware that the ECG in ACS can vary greatly between patients and over time, and for this reason it is very important to frequently repeat the ECG during an admission with an ACS. Possible findings include:

Normal resting ECG: certainly possible, but unlikely if symptoms are genuinely due to myocardial ischaemia (ie multiple episodes of chest pain, each lasting ≥20 minutes). If a normal ECG is found in someone with a presumed diagnosis of unstable angina then two possibilities arise: the diagnosis of an ACS is wrong; or the patient has circumflex territory ischaemia [this can often result in very subtle ECG signs, of which the commonest is a dominant T wave in lead V1 (in health the T wave in this ECG lead is negative) – the best way to differentiate these two possibilities is often by coronary angiography].

T wave flattening in the territory of the affected coronary artery: this is unfortunately not a reliable sign, as many elderly patients have mild regional T wave changes not necessarily relating to an ACS.

T wave inversion in the territory of the affected coronary artery: although this can affect any territory, deep anterior T wave inversion is a particularly characteristic syndrome and is strongly associated with an active lesion in the proximal LAD (producing a 'proximal LAD pattern' ECG). Unstable angina with an active lesion in the proximal LAD is a high-risk clinical situation and usually benefits from aggressive medical and interventional therapy (see Figure 4.11).

ST segment depression (often, but not always, fluctuating): this is a marker of high risk and usually mandates coronary angiography (Figure 10.2).

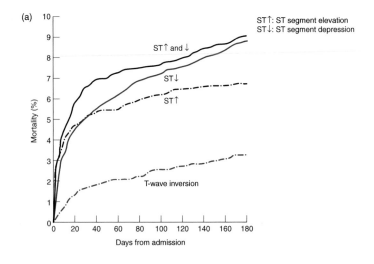

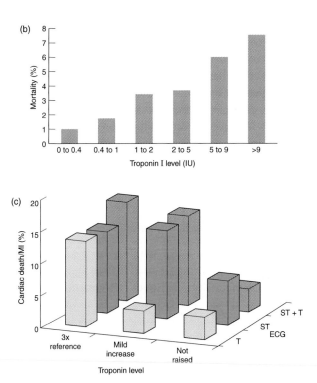

Figure 10.2

(a) Relationship between ST segment changes and outcome in acute coronary syndromes. Adapted with permission from Savonitto S, Ardissino D, Granger CB *et al*. *JAMA* 1999; **281**: 707–13. (b) Use of troponin levels to predict adverse outcome in acute coronary syndromes (graph shows 42-day mortality). Reprinted with permission from Morrow DA, Cannon CP, Rifai N *et al*. *JAMA* 2001; **286**: 2405–12. (c) Interaction between troponin level, ECG changes and adverse outcome. ST, ST segment changes (depression and/or elevation); T, T wave inversion. Reprinted with permission from Lindahl B, Venge P, Wallentin L, for the FRISC study group. *Circulation* 1996; **93**: 1651–7.

Intermittent ST segment elevation: this is an extraordinarily high-risk clinical situation, and one commonly associated with a high-grade, active lesion, with much thrombus formation and a great likelihood of proceeding to MI. Immediate angiography (with intensive medical therapy) is indicated. One diagnosis not to make in this situation is so-called Prinzmetal or 'variant' angina; this term has probably been responsible for more deaths than any other ECG term. This is because physicians make this diagnosis incorrectly, deny the patient angiography and thus allow the IHD-related ACS to proceed to a full thickness MI. In its pure form, Prinzmetal angina refers to chest pain with ST segment elevation occurring as a consequence of coronary artery spasm in arteries that are completely free of both atheromatous coronary disease and *in situ* coronary artery thrombus. Thus a correct diagnosis of Prinzmetal or 'variant' angina can only be made once coronary angiography has been undertaken. The role of 'provocative' agents (ie drugs given at the time of coronary angiography to determine the sensitivity of the coronary arteries to vasoconstrictors) is hotly debated. Most cardiologists feel that in practice these provocative drugs have no role in diagnosis, and indeed are dangerous as they may provoke an MI.

Mixed ST segment elevation and depression ACS: this is the very highest risk situation and mandates very urgent angiography.

Prognosis in acute coronary syndromes

Although the use of the ECG in risk-stratification has been discussed in the paragraphs above, it is vitally important to realize that a patient's overall risk is an amalgam of many factors and does not depend on the ECG features alone (see below).

Prognosis in ST segment elevation myocardial infarction

Short-term outcome (Figure 10.3) depends on:

- Age: the older the patient, the worse the outlook.
- Killip class (Figure 10.4): this reflects haemodynamic upset and the presence or absence of heart failure. The higher the Killip class, the worse the outlook.
- Size of MI: as determined by location (anterior ≥ inferior ≥ posterior), amount of ST segment elevation, and efficacy of thrombolysis (as reflected by speed of ST segment resolution, often estimated by determining whether or not the ST segment elevation in the lead with the most elevation resolves ≥50% within 2 hours), how much R wave height has been lost (and whether Q waves have developed), and cardiac enzyme rise.
- Diabetes: associated with a dramatically worse short- and long-term outlook.

These data have been incorporated into a risk prediction scoring system: the TIMI STEMI risk score. [Thrombolysis In Myocardial Infarction (TIMI) is a group of trialists based in the USA]. One point is given for each adverse factor and the predicted mortality can be read from a graph (Figure 10.5).

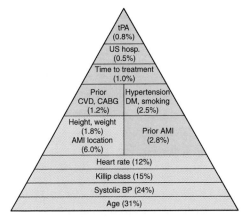

Figure 10.3
Factors determining outcome in acute ST segment elevation myocardial infarction. This pyramid demonstrates the relative proportion of the early mortality ascribed to each factor. It was determined by analysing patient data from the GUSTO IV trial. It can be seen that easily determinable clinical variables are strongly associated with much of the risk.

Class	Finding
I	No S3 (third ventricular heart sound) or rales
II	Rales in less than half the lung fields
III	Rales in more than half the lung field
IV	Cardiogenic shock

Figure 10.4
Killip class classification.

Long-term outcome depends on:
- age
- LV function, which can be estimated from the cardiac ultrasound and improved with angiotensin-converting enzyme (ACE) inhibitors and β-blockers
- extent of coronary disease, which can be estimated from an exercise test conventionally undertaken 4–6 weeks following a Q wave MI. If the exercise test is not reassuring, coronary angiography should be undertaken. Although this is the time-honoured approach, unfortunately the usefulness of exercise-induced ST segment depression in predicting future events, in the thrombolytic era, is rather low. There is no clear way past this problem

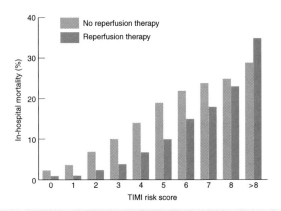

TIMI ST elevation myocardial infarction scoring system

Clinical risk indicator	Points
Historical	
Age (years)	
≥ 75	3
65–74	2
History of diabetes, hypertension or angina	1
Examination	
Systolic BP <100 mmHg	3
Heart rate >100 beats/minute	2
Killip class II–IV	2
Weight <67 kg	1
Presentation	
Anterior ST elevation or left bundle branch block	1
Time to reperfusion therapy >4 hours	1
Total possible points	14

Figure 10.5
TIMI ST elevation myocardial infarction risk prediction chart. Reproduced with permission from Morrow DA, Antman EM, Parsons L et al. JAMA 2001; **286**: 1356–9.

- presence of heart failure, which has some relation to LV function
- electrical instability – an important risk factor. Patients with severe LV dysfunction and frequent low-grade repetitive ventricular arrhythmias are at high risk of out-of-hospital cardiac arrest due to a ventricular tachycardia (VT), as are patients with low heart rate variability (see p. 283) or inducible VT on electrophysiological study (see p. 293). It is unclear which tests are routinely indicated post MI to determine electrical stability, as there is currently no clear strategy (in the UK) for the prediction and management of post-MI electrical instability
- control of risk factors for CAD.

Prognosis in non-ST segment elevation ACS

Acute coronary syndrome comprises a range of conditions, some of which can rapidly proceed to fatal MI. Equally there are many patients who are at low risk of further adverse events. In these latter patients angiography and/or other intervention is costly, confers no benefit and exposes the patient to risk. Provided that such low-risk patients can be reliably identified, they can then avoid the risks of these treatments and be managed with a less invasive therapy.

Conversely, if high-risk patients can be accurately identified then targeted intervention to minimize the risk of adverse events can be instituted, eg intensive anticoagulation (with platelet receptor IIb/IIIa receptor antagonists), percutaneous coronary intervention or coronary surgery.

Thus to accurately guide therapy in non-ST segment elevation ACS, it is vital to be able to identify low-, medium- and high-risk patients: this can be done on the basis of the clinical features along with ECG findings and troponin measurements (ie calculate total TIMI risk score from Box 10.1 and read prognosis from Figure 10.6).

The TIMI study group has found that patients at high risk of adverse complications are those who have the following features:

- multiple risk factors for coronary disease, ie a combination of at least two of the following: smoking, hypertension or hyperlipidaemia
- diabetes mellitus, especially long-standing type I or type II (non-insulin-dependent, NIDDM) at any time. Twenty percent of patients with NIDDM have an overt macrovascular complication at presentation, ie old 'silent' MI, stroke or peripheral vascular disease; however, in type I diabetes overt macrovascular disease is rare before 20 years of diabetes have elapsed
- old age: the older the patient, the higher the risk of an adverse complication from their unstable angina
- unstable angina developing while taking aspirin, ie 'aspirin failure'
- abnormal ECG. The highest risk marker is ST segment depression. Persisting T wave inversion, especially if affecting the anterior leads ('proximal LAD syndrome' pattern ECG) is also associated with an adverse outcome
- raised troponin levels. The higher the troponin, the more adverse the outcome. The interaction of the ECG and troponin is important. Abnormalities in either alone increase the risk; abnormalities in both substantially increase the risk (see Figure 10.2c and Box 10.1)

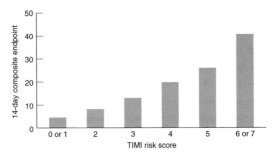

Figure 10.6
TIMI acute coronary syndrome risk score predication chart. The relationship between TIMI ACS risk score and the 14-day composite endpoint (death, MI, severe recurrent ischaemia requiring urgent revascularization). Reprinted with permission from Antman EM, Cohen M, Bernink PJLM *et al*. The TIMI risk score for unstable angina/non-ST elevation MI. *JAMA* 2000; **284**: 835–42

Box 10.1 TIMI non-ST segment elevation myocardial infarction scoring system

Score 1 point for each of the following:

- Age ≥65 years[†]
- ≥ Three risk factors for coronary disease*
- Significant coronary stenosis
- ST deviation
- Severe anginal symptoms (≥ two episodes/24 hour)
- Use of aspirin in last seven days
- Elevated serum cardiac markers[†].

*Family history, hypertension, hypercholesterolaemia, diabetes, current smoker

[†]Creatine kinase MB or cardiac-specific troponins.

Reprinted with permission from Morrow DA, Antman EM, Parsons L *et al*. Application of the TIMI risk score for ST-elevation MI in the National Registry of Myocardial Infarction. *JAMA* 2001; **286**: 1356–9

- recurrent episodes of symptomatic angina (ie recurrent episodes of anginal chest pain) despite appropriate therapy.

The more of the above risk factors present, the greater the risk. To estimate risk, one point is given for each of the seven categories above; the risk is then read from a chart. What level of risk is sufficiently high to justify angiography is debatable, and will reflect prevailing practice, access to facilities, remuneration (personal and institutional), amongst others factors. High risk is slightly arbitrarily defined, although a composite endpoint of more than 15% would be regarded as high risk by many cardiologists. Any patients who are high-risk should have coronary angiography in addition to aggressive medical therapy.

Risk stratification in medium- and low-risk non-ST segment elevation acute coronary syndromes: use of the exercise ECG

High-risk ACS is further risk-stratified by means of coronary angiography. Medium- and low-risk populations clearly contain some individuals who will go on to experience an adverse event. If it is possible to identify such patients, they can then be aggressively and intensively investigated and treated, leaving an even lower-risk population to be investigated and treated in a gentler manner. The key question therefore is how should medium- and low-risk ACS be further risk-stratified?

There are a number of approaches to this.

First, coronary angiography for all: a very aggressive approach with some support from the literature. However, most healthcare economies cannot support this.

Second, coronary angiography for all those with diabetes (this group is at very high risk of adverse complications) and 'targeted' for the rest. This is a very reasonable approach, given that the prognosis of diabetics with coronary disease is so poor.

Third, 'targeted' coronary angiography: patients (either all low-/medium-risk, or those without diabetes, as above) are selected for angiography on the basis of inducible ischaemia, with the threshold being lowest in those whose ischaemia is easiest to provoke. Thus, provided symptoms at rest have resolved (if not, angiography is indicated), an exercise test is undertaken. If symptoms or ECG changes (typically ST segment depression) occur then angiography is considered. In the UK it is usual to perform angiography if the exercise test is 'early-positive', that is chest pain or ≥2 mm of ST segment depression occur before stage III of the Bruce protocol. Other healthcare systems perform angiography at different thresholds.

Thus it is often easier to define those who do not need coronary angiography rather than those who do. In practice, those patients who do not need angiography have all of the following features:

- a clear-cut diagnosis of ACS
- symptoms have totally settled
- are not diabetic

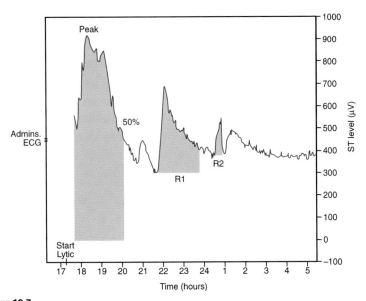

Figure 10.7
Example of continuous ST-segment monitoring during ST segment elevation MI.
Admis ECG, electrocardiography on admission; peak, peak ST level; 50%, moment of 50% ST reduction from preceding peak ST level; R1 and R2 are 2 recurrent ischemic episodes; grey zones reflect estimated area under the ST trends.
Reprinted with permission from Continuous ST-Segment Monitoring Associated With Infarct Size and Left Ventricular Function in the GUSTO-I Trial. *Am Heart J* 1999; **138(3)**: 525–32.

- no heart failure, either during the acute episode (when it may reflect critical multivessel coronary disease) or at any other time (when it may reflect impaired LV function)
- ejection fraction ≥40%
- ability to achieve a high level of exercise (end-stage II Bruce protocol or greater) without symptoms or substantial ST segment depression, defined arbitrarily as ≥2 mm depression.

Overall probably around 50–70% of patients with non-ST segment elevation ACSs should undergo angiography.

Ischaemic heart disease-related arrhythmias

Acute phase

Complete heart block

This arrhythmia most commonly occurs as a complication of an acute inferior wall MI, when it is often (but not always) haemodynamically well tolerated – if not, a temporary pacing wire is indicated. Usually complete heart block (CHB) complicating an inferior wall MI resolves after a few days – it is worth waiting up to 7–10 days before deciding whether or not permanent pacing is needed. CHB complicating an anterior wall MI is an ominous sign and indicates a large MI, usually with haemodynamic instability, associated with a very high mortality rate. Immediate temporary pacing is indicated, preferably with a dual chamber system.

Atrial fibrillation

An acute MI can be complicated by AF, which is associated with a larger MI and worse short- and long-term prognoses. Treatment is immediate cardioversion if there is significant haemodynamic instability, otherwise heart-rate control (digoxin, β-blockers, amiodarone) and anticoagulation.

Ventricular premature contractions

Ventricular premature contractions (VPCs) are not infrequent during the acute phase of an MI. They are (loosely) associated with a higher risk of acute phase VF; years ago this led to patients being given class I antiarrhythmic agents such as lignocaine to prevent VF. This was moderately successful, but unfortunately led to an increased rate of death from low-output heart failure. Probably the only treatment that both suppresses acute phase VPCs and lowers death rates is the use of β-blockers.

Nonsustained ventricular tachycardia

This may herald the onset of VF. Nonsustained VT sometimes reflects an arrhythmic substrate, eg LVH or a previous MI with an arrhythmogenic scar.

Sustained monomorphic ventricular tachycardia

This is an unusual rhythm disturbance during an acute MI, suggesting that a patient already possesses an arrhythmogenic scar, with the arrhythmia possibly being promoted by the acute MI interacting with this scar. These patients have a higher long-term risk of developing further VT. Treatment is as for any VT – cardioversion if not tolerated, over/underdrive pacing if tolerated. If sustained monomorphic VT complicates an acute MI then angiography with a view to revascularization is usually indicated. Many patients will need postrevascularization ventricular stimulation studies to determine the long-term risk of VT. If VT is inducible (especially if this occurs at a low level of the protocol) then an implantable cardioverter defibrillator (ICD) is usually indicated.

Polymorphic ventricular tachycardia

This is not rare, and often degenerates to VF. It does not particularly reflect a future arrhythmic tendency.

Ventricular fibrillation

VF can either occur *de novo* or follow an episode of VT. VF complicates an acute MI in about 30% of cases prior to hospitalization, accounting for the 30% or so of patients who die from an MI before admission to hospital. Once patients reach hospital, VF occurs in about another 5% – this explains why acute MI patients should be nursed in a coronary care unit, close to a defibrillator. Patients who have multiple episodes of VF complicating their MI should undergo immediate angioplasty to the artery where the infarct has occurred.

Chronic phase

Complete heart block

CHB can occur with chronic IHD, when it is due to fibrosis of the conducting tissue. This requires permanent ventricular pacing, with immediate insertion of a temporary wire if there has been syncope or near-syncope.

Atrial fibrillation

AF is common in those with impaired LV function, and this commonly occurs post MI, especially following an anterior wall MI. The chance of a long-term reversion back to sinus rhythm is low. Thromboembolic risk is high in this situation.

Ventricular premature contractions

These are very common following an MI. The higher the VPC frequency, and the higher the grade of VPC, the greater the chance of the patient developing sudden cardiac death (Figure 10.8). Studies have shown that most sudden cardiac death is due to ventricular arrhythmias (some 70–90%) and only 10–15% is due to a primary bradyarrhythmia (most commonly CHB) (Figure 10.9). These findings led to the hypothesis that if VPCs could be suppressed

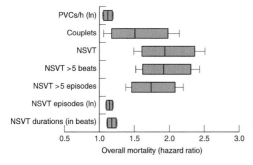

Figure 10.8

Relationship between ventricular arrhythmias and total mortality. Higher-grade ventricular arrhythmias are associated with an increased risk of death in those with heart failure. Reproduced with permission from Teerlink JR *et al*, on behalf of the PROMISE investigators. *Circulation* 2000; **101**: 40–6.

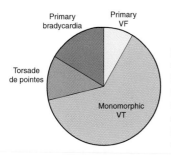

Figure 10.9

Causes of sudden cardiac death. This data comes from 24-hour ECG monitors being worn when the subjects died. VF, ventricular fibrillation; VT, ventricular tachycardia. Reprinted with permission from Bayes de Luna A, Coumel P, Leclerq JF. Ambulatory sudden cardiac death; mechanisms of production of fatal arrhythmia on the basis of data from 157 cases. *Am Heart J* 1989; **117**: 151–9

post MI then sudden cardiac death would likewise be reduced. This was tested by giving post-MI patients the class I antiarrhythmic flecainide (other class I agents were used as well). Unfortunately, although flecainide (and other class I drugs) suppressed VPCs, the incidences of nonsustained VT and sudden cardiac death were both increased. One reason for this may be that post-MI VPCs merely reflect the underlying arrhythmic mechanism, rather than being causally related to the induction of ventricular arrhythmias.

Ventricular tachycardia

This can complicate any phase of IHD but is most likely following an MI, especially if the MI has been large and associated with failure of reperfusion therapy (ie no acute ST segment resolution with thrombolysis). Patients with fast VT or VT associated with any haemodynamic instability should undergo invasive assessment of electrical stability (VT stimulation studies) and many will need an ICD.

Ventricular fibrillation

VF can develop in chronic IHD either *de novo* (less likely) or following a period of sustained VT (more likely). Treatment is immediate cardioversion (unlikely, as this arrhythmia usually occurs out of hospital), evaluation of the ischaemic burden (ie how much healthy heart is supplied by stenosed arteries), revascularization as appropriate, and often an ICD (especially if revascularization is not required, ie the VF relates to a 'scar'). Drug therapy (with β-blockers, amiodarone, ACE inhibitors, etc) is also usually needed. Patients at high risk of serious ventricular arrhythmias can be partly identified on the basis of MI size (ejection fraction ≤30% conveys high risk), VPC rate, and the results of a ventricular stimulation study, in which easy inducibility conveys a high risk. If patients are judged to be at high risk then an ICD should be implanted prophylactically.

Ischaemic heart disease-related heart failure

Pre-myocardial infarction related heart failure

Papillary muscle dysfunction

Papillary muscle dysfuntion is an unusual but not rare cause of heart failure. A critical stenosis occurs in the coronary artery supplying the papillary muscle. If myocardial oxygen demand increases (anxiety, exercise, etc) then ischaemia occurs in the papillary muscle; the mitral valve does not close properly during systole and mitral regurgitation develops. Mild heart failure can occur, resulting in breathlessness, anxiety, increased oxygen demand and more ischaemia, so increasing the severity of the mitral regurgitation and leading to even more severe heart failure, etc. This can rapidly progress to life-threatening pulmonary oedema, the signs being extreme breathlessness, cold and clammy skin, tachycardia and tachypnoea, and lungs filled with crepitations. The murmur of mitral regurgitation may not be heard during the acute episode (too much lung noise) and, as relieving the pulmonary oedema relieves the papillary muscle ischaemia, which lessens the severity of mitral regurgitation, the murmur later on may be so quiet as to be inaudible. During the episode of pulmonary oedema the ECG shows a sinus tachycardia and may show posterior wall ischaemia (ST/T wave changes in leads V1 to V3, especially ST segment depression). Once the heart failure has been successfully treated the ECG can become surprisingly normal, although there may be a dominant T wave in lead V1. Cardiac ultrasound after the episode has settled may be completely or nearly normal. The diagnosis is suspected when a patient at risk of coronary disease presents with acute left heart failure for which no other explanation can be found, and coronary angiography shows circumflex artery disease. Revascularizing the circumflex artery is appropriate treatment.

Heart failure relating to critical multivessel coronary disease

Proximal multivessel CAD can underlie life-threatening pulmonary oedema in the absence of MI. The usual presentation is surprising: one might expect these patients to have a long history of symptomatic coronary disease but this is rare. Most patients have a short (or even no) history of preceding angina, then present acutely with life-threatening pulmonary oedema, during which they may have ischaemic chest pain, although this is not invariable. The heart failure responds to standard medical therapy. The ECG during the episode shows a sinus tachycardia, and often non-specific ST changes, sometimes rather profound ST depression. The postepisode ECG may show any of the changes of an ACS, ie no changes, nonspecific ST changes, or deep T wave inversion in the distribution of any coronary artery (although not infrequently in the anterior chest leads). The troponin level is often raised, but as this is also the case with most nonischaemically mediated causes of pulmonary oedema, the finding does not discriminate from other diagnoses. The real clue that critical CAD underlies the acute heart failure is that no alternative cause can be found, the patient has risk factors for CAD, and the cardiac ultrasound may be normal or may show mild regional wall motion abnormalities. This means that patients with unexplained pulmonary oedema with risk factors for CAD should undergo diagnostic coronary angiography.

Heart failure due to hibernation

Critical coronary disease can lead to myocytes being so starved of oxygen that, to survive, they must 'switch-off' all nonessential activities. Contractile function is energy-expensive and therefore ceases; all remaining energies are dedicated to keeping the cells viable, so the cells start to 'hibernate'. If the number of hibernating cells is large, patients develop symptoms and signs of heart failure. The cardiac ultrasound shows poor contractile function, often with normal LV wall thickness. The ECG often shows well-preserved R waves; there may be substantial ST/T wave changes. Bundle branch block may occur. Hibernation should be suspected when patients present with heart failure and are found to have impaired LV function in the

241

absence of previous MIs. Alternatively, impaired contractile function is found in the territory of a critically stenosed artery. How can one predict whether revascularization will improve contractile function? In particular, can the ECG be used to answer the key question 'will cell contractile function return if revascularization occurs?' The short answer is 'no', but it can give some clues: successful revascularization is more likely if R waves are well preserved, or at least if there are 'volts' on the ECG (eg deep rather than very small Q waves). Pharmacological 'stress' cardiac ultrasounds may be predictive of revascularization success. The basis of this is that even hibernating cells can be encouraged to contract if stimulated with enough catecholamine; thus if contractile function picks up during dobutamine infusion then revascularization may improve pump function. Complex positron emission tomographic scans, which allow for an assessment of regional cell metabolism, may also be predictive but are not widely available. The same applies to functional magnetic resonance imaging.

Myocardial infarction-related heart failure

The commonest cause of heart failure during an MI is infarct-related myocyte death causing inadequate contractile force, a decreased ejection fraction, and so heart failure. The larger the infarct the higher the chance of heart failure. Accordingly, the prognosis is worse in patients with heart failure complicating their MI (Table 10.1). The ECG can show any of the changes of MI, although as the LAD is usually the largest coronary artery, heart failure is more likely with an anterior wall MI than with MI in another territory. Some cells in the peri-infarct zone can be reversibly damaged for a few days after an MI. Until recovery occurs, usually after a few days, they are alive but have no contractile function; they are 'stunned'. This means that even if heart failure is severe around the time of an MI, it is often worth instigating aggressive medical therapy for at least a few days, until these 'stunned' cells 'pick-up' their contractile function (which will help to lessen the severity of the heart failure), before making a decision about the utility or futility of therapy.

Papillary muscle infarction causes acute mitral regurgitation (MR) and extraordinarily severe pulmonary oedema. The diagnosis is suspected when a patient with a circumflex territory MI (shown on the ECG as ST segment depression in leads V1 to V3) develops severe pulmonary oedema. Patients are often critically unwell and extraordinarily breathless, with extreme tachypnoea. They sit bolt upright, trying to get relief. The signs are dominated by pulmonary oedema; the mitral murmur is usually not heard (too many

Table 10.1 Severity of pump failure and hospital mortality in acute myocardial infarction

Clinical category of heart failure	Pathophysiological basis	Equivalent clinical subsets		
		Killip	Cedars–Sinai	Equivalent haemodynamic subsets
Subclinical	Minimal or compensated LV dysfunction	I (1–3%)	I (1%)	I (CI >2.2, PCW <18) (3%)
Pulmonary congestion	Systolic and/or diastolic LV dysfunction and/or MR or VSD	II (3–5%)	II (3–5%)	II (CI >2.2, PCW >18) (9%)
Pulmonary oedema	As above but more severe	III (0–25%)	II (5–25%)	II (CI >2.2, PCW <18) (9%)
Low-output state/shock	As above	IV (30–60%)	IV (50–60%)	IV (CI >2.2, PCW >18) (51%)
– with pulmonary congestion/ oedema	Hypovolaemia	None	III (18%)	III (CI >2.2, PCW <18) (23%)
– without pulmonary congestion	Predominant RV infarction Brady-tachyarrythmias Cardiac rupture/ tamponade			

LV, left ventricle; CI, cardiac index (l/min/m^2); PCW, pulmonary capillary wedge pressure (mmHg); MR, mitral regurgitation; VSD, ventricular septal defect, RV, right ventricle. Reprinted with permission from Crawford MH, DiMarco JP. *Cardiology*. London: Mosby, 2001.

lung sounds; the MR is also often so severe that the MR jet is broad, nonturbulent and does not generate any murmur). Standard medical therapy often does not help – mechanical ventilation is needed. Transthoracic echocardiography is often unhelpful, 'missing' the MR, and only showing 'good' LV function (due to the offloading effect of the MR on the left ventricle). Occasionally a 'flail' papillary muscle is demonstrated. The diagnosis is made by having a high level of suspicion from the clinical situation, and confirmed by transoesophageal echocardiography LV cineangiography (the latter being carried out at the same time as coronary arteriography). The treatment is immediate mitral valve replacement surgery, with concomitant coronary artery bypass graft surgery if appropriate.

Ventricular septal defect causes predominant right-sided heart failure, ie peripheral oedema, and sometimes a poor cardiac output (which can be manifest as peripheral coolness or progressive renal failure). Patients are quite happy to lie flat (unlike in acute MR). The diagnosis is obvious from the loud murmur and is easily confirmed by cardiac ultrasound. Surgery is high-risk but may be life-saving. The ECG shows the acute infarct – it must be one that affects the septum, so is usually either in the LAD territory or affects the posterior descending coronary artery, which in 95% of patients is a branch of the RCA and in 5% a branch of the circumflex coronary artery.

Chronic phase IHD related heart failure

Adverse cardiac remodelling

This is a phrase used to describe the phenomena of the heart enlarging in the years following an MI, the most common cause of long-term post-MI heart failure. It can be recognized by the clinical features: a remote but usually quite large MI (thus often an anterior MI), an interval of no symptoms for several or many years, then symptoms typical for heart failure, without any angina. The ECG shows the old MI – usually a Q wave one, but little else of note. Cardiac ultrasound shows akinesis in the area of the MI, and more distant territories are often severely hypokinetic. Treatment is medical, with ACE inhibitors, β-blockers, diuretics and sometimes digoxin.

Hibernation

Long-term myocyte hibernation may not infrequently follow an MI. It is often a very difficult but important post-MI clinical problem to determine how much tissue is irreversibly damaged and how much is hibernating. Clues might be that a patient is known to have an MI in one territory but cardiac ultrasound shows that another territory is not working normally, and angiography shows a high-grade stenosis in the artery supplying this part of the heart. Nuclear/PET/MRI studies may be required to confirm viability. Revascularization has a role in selected patients.

Chapter 11

The exercise stress ECG

The exercise stress ECG is used to answer the following questions:

- Is coronary artery disease (CAD) present?
- If CAD is present, how severe is it?
- What is the prognosis?

The exercise test can rarely answer these questions unambiguously. What it can do is give some information about the probability of CAD being present, of it being extensive and of the prognosis being poor on medical therapy.

Principles underlying the exercise ECG

The principle of the exercise stress ECG is as follows: exercise increases cardiac workload and so myocardial oxygen demand. In the presence of flow-limiting CAD this increased demand for oxygen cannot be met and the myocardium becomes ischaemic. Myocardial ischaemia alters the electrophysiology of the myocytes, and this can be detected as ST depression.

The amount of cardiac work required to induce myocardial ischaemia will depend on how extensive and severe the CAD is: if several arteries are severely narrowed, myocardial ischaemia can be easily induced at a low level of exercise. Conversely, if there is only mild CAD then a high cardiac workload is required to induce ischaemia.

The amount of exercise required to induce myocardial ischaemia will thus correlate with the extent and severity of the underlying CAD. The more extensive the CAD is, the more likely is plaque rupture and so MI. For this reason, extent of coronary disease is one factor correlated with outcome in ischaemic heart disease (IHD). This means that the amount of exercise required to induce myocardial ischaemia will have some correlation with longevity. Thus the exercise test is useful not only in the detection of CAD but also in the prediction of prognosis. Large databases have been used to incorporate exercise test results into prognosis charts, a typical one being the Duke nomogram (Figure 11.1).

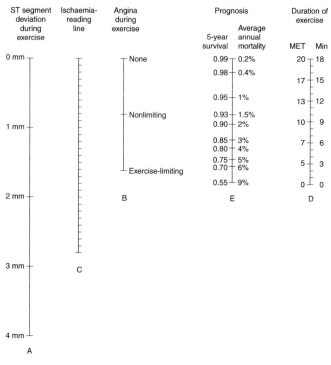

Figure 11.1
Duke nomogram. To use: mark on line A the maximum ST segment deviation seen during exercise; mark on line B the degree of angina during exercise; join the marks on lines A and B with a straight line; mark the point where this line crosses line C (the 'ischaemia-reading line'; mark on line D the duration of exercise (Bruce protocol) or metabolic equivalent levels (METs) achieved; join the marks on lines C and D with a straight line; where this line crosses line E, read off the patient's predicted mortality. Adapted with permission from Mark DB *et al.* Prognostic value of a treadmill score in outpatients with suspected coronary artery disease. *N Engl J Med* 1996; **325**: 849–53.

Safety

Exercise testing, in appropriately selected patients, is fairly but not completely safe. The risk of death is of the order of one in 10 000 for most patients, rising to three in 10 000 in the weeks following a myocardial infarct (MI). The risk of inducing a nonfatal MI is higher than this, as is the risk of inducing arrhythmias, which may or may not be well tolerated. For these reasons, exercise testing should only be carried out:

- in appropriate facilities: the room must be large, full resuscitation equipment should be present (including a defibrillator) and the facility must possess a full crash-team

- by personnel trained in advanced life support, including cardiopulmonary resuscitation and the use of an external defibrillator
- after informed consent.

Technique

The patient exercises according to a set protocol (see below), wired-up to a 12-lead ECG machine (Figure 11.2) that is set to automatically record an ECG every minute or so, although ECGs can be printed out at any time the operator wishes. The ECG machine usually has 'signal averaging' software that removes artefactual skeletal muscle 'noise'. The test is continued until:

- an ECG criteria has been passed (eg ≥2 mm of ST depression) *or*
- unacceptable symptoms have occurred (a 'symptom-limited' exercise test) *or*
- prespecified increases in heart rate have been achieved *or*
- the end of the protocol is reached.

It is usual to use symptom-limited tests for the majority of cases.

Protocols

The basic principle is that the patient exercises to increase cardiac workload (as above). How this is done does not really matter provided it is carried out in a standardized fashion. It has become traditional to use one of two forms of exercise.

The most frequently used form of exercise is a treadmill. There are many different protocols, but the Bruce protocol is standard, wherein the treadmill speed and slope are increased every three minutes (Figure 11.3). A reasonable workload in healthy late middle-aged subjects is attainment of the end of stage III of the protocol. In the modified Bruce protocol, often used in the early post-MI patient or in unstable angina, an extra three stages are added at the start.

The less frequently used form of exercise is a bicycle ergometer, used when patients have difficulty walking, for example due to balance problems or arthritis. It has the advantage that patients do not have to support their own weight. However, for this same reason it may be difficult to achieve a high cardiac workload. Frequently the resistance setting of the bicycle is adjusted

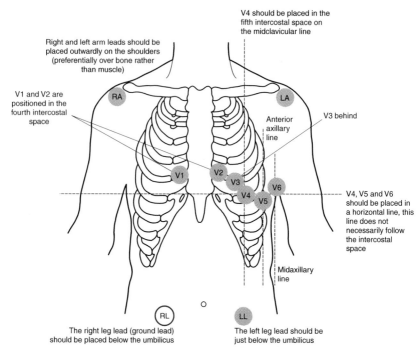

Figure 11.2
ECG lead placement for exercise testing. Reprinted with permission from ACC/AHA guidelines for exercise testing. *Circulation* 1997; **96**: 345–54.

so that the workload is increased by 25 watts every 3–4 minutes. A 'reasonable' workload is one ≥100 watts.

Monitoring during the exercise test

The most important monitoring is clinical: what does the patient feel and look like during the test? Severe symptoms (if patients become distressed, look ashen or otherwise appear unwell) should lead to the test being terminated, regardless of what other data shows. Likewise, falls in blood pressure or profound ECG changes are indications for terminating the test.

During exercise in healthy subjects the systolic blood pressure (SBP) increases progressively as exercise intensity increases, reflecting increased cardiac output, and the diastolic blood pressure falls progressively, reflecting peripheral vasodilatation. The SBP should be measured frequently during the stress test.

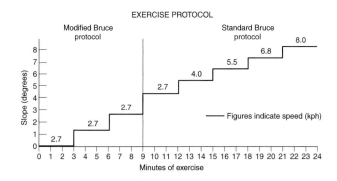

Figure 11.3
The Bruce protocol. Reproduced with permission from Houghton AR, Gray D. *Making Sense of the ECG*, 2nd edn. London: Arnold, 2003.

Blood pressure indications for terminating the exercise test

If a fall in SBP occurs with symptoms (eg light-headedness) then the test should be terminated, as this may mean that the patient has:

- critical multivessel CAD – an exercise-induced fall in blood pressure associated with symptoms consistent with hypotension ('dizziness', etc) is thus a relatively strong indication for angiography. This pattern is only infrequently seen
- poor left ventricular (LV) function
- left ventricular outflow tract (LVOT) obstruction, usually due to aortic stenosis, occasionally to hypertrophic cardiomyopathy. Heavy exercise with severe LVOT obstruction can occasionally result in death, so great caution should be used in deciding whether an exercise test is appropriate in this situation.

However, most often the blood pressure fall is artefactual and relates to the pre-test SBP being raised by anxiety. In this situation, the blood pressure falls as anxiety is dissipated by exercise. Thus the apparent fall in blood pressure on exercise is an artefact. The patient remains well during the test, free from dizziness and related symptoms. It is usually safe to continue the test despite the apparent fall in SBP.

ECG indications for terminating the exercise test

The ECG criteria for terminating the exercise test are as follows:

- Extensive ST segment depression (ie ≥2 mm) or elevation are usually held to be highly clinically relevant.
- Sustained arrhythmias [eg atrial fibrillation (AF), supraventricular tachycardias (SVTs) or sustained ventricular arrhythmias].
- Very frequent ventricular premature contractions (VPCs) and nonsustained ventricular tachycardia (NSVT), eg runs of four to five beats. Most ventricular extrasystoles are suppressed by exercise; however, VPCs and NSVT can be promoted by exercise in those with severe CAD, severe LV dysfunction, or if the heart has a tendency towards electrical instability. Very frequent VPCs and especially NSVT can degenerate into sustained ventricular tachycardia (VT) or ventricular fibrillation. Thus, VPCs and especially NSVT occurring during exercise should be observed closely; if VPCs are very frequent (eg ≥10–20/minute) or high-grade (eg recurring couplets, triplets or NSVT), or if these occur at a high cardiac workload, then consideration should be given to discontinuing the test to prevent a more sustained ventricular arrhythmia developing. Coronary angiography and tests for cardiac electrical stability (eg electrophysiological studies) are often indicated in this situation. Less frequent and isolated VPCs (ie not couplets, triplets, or NSVT) occur in those with more severe heart disease, although they are not independently associated with an adverse outcome (Figure 11.4).

Contraindications to exercise testing

Some situations increase the risk of an exercise test. Clearly, at some stage this increase in risk becomes such that exercise testing is too dangerous to carry out. However, perhaps surprisingly, this is only rarely the case, and as such there are a few absolute contraindications to exercise testing. The reasons for most contraindications are obvious. The most important ones are:

Acute MI. Obviously exercise during the acute throes of an MI is dangerous, but it is a little difficult to know at what point following an MI it becomes safe to use exercise testing to risk-stratify the patient. In practice the longer one

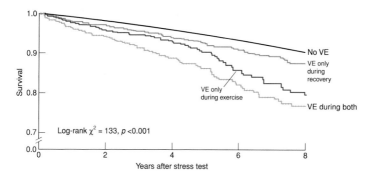

Figure 11.4

The significance of exercise-induced ventricular arrhythmias. Analysis of exercise tests from 29 244 patients showed an association between survival and exercise-induced ventricular ectopy, and ventricular ectopy during the recovery period (ectopy defined as ≥7 ectopics/min). Adjusting for baseline variables showed that only ectopy in recovery was independently associated with death (risk ratio 1.6, CI 1.3–1.9) whereas exercise-induced ectopy was not (risk ratio 1.2, CI 1–1.4). For ectopy occurring in the recovery period, higher Lown grade ectopy was independently associated with higher risk. Adapted with permission from Frolkis JP, Pothier CE, Blackstone EH, Lauer MS. Frequent ventricular ectopy after exercise as a predictor of death. *N Engl J Med* 2003; **348**: 781–90.

waits and the smaller the size of the MI, the lower the risk. Thus it is common practice to exercise patients with full thickness Q wave MIs at 4–6 weeks, whereas patients with smaller non-Q wave events are often exercised during the index admission, after being pain-free for 48 hours or so.

Unstable angina with ongoing chest pain is a relatively strong contraindication to exercise testing. Angiography is a better approach to risk stratification (and treatment). However, patients with acute coronary syndromes (ACS) who have been pain-free for ≥48 hours and who are free of high-risk features [ie the ECG has returned (virtually) to normal, LV function is good and troponin level has not been substantially raised] can be exercised with reasonable safety.

LVOT is an important although relative contraindication to a symptom-limited exercise test, as effort may provoke syncope and sudden death. Thus patients with significant aortic stenosis should not be exercised unless there are unusual circumstances. For example, it has become common practice to assess whether equivocal aortic valve gradients are significant by assessing the haemodynamic response to stress – by definition these patients do not have 'critical' aortic stenosis.

Arrhythmias that are not haemodynamically tolerated (eg VT, fast AF, complete heart block) are obvious contraindications. However, well-tolerated AF or complete heart block (especially if congenital) are not contraindications to exercise testing.

Severe comorbid illness (eg pneumonia, severe chronic obstructive pulmonary disease). What comorbid illness constitutes a significant contraindication is usually a matter for common sense.

Substantial pre-existing ST segment changes, especially if due to left ventricular hypertrophy (LVH), as inevitably ST segment depression will occur during exercise, regardless of whether or not CAD is present.

Full left bundle branch block (LBBB) 'conceals' any ST changes, thus making it impossible to obtain any ECG data from the test. However, as exercise capacity is the most important data obtained from the test (rather than ECG changes) a valid exercise test may still be obtained in the presence of LBBB.

Significant mitral stenosis is a relative contraindication, not because the test is dangerous (it probably is not) but because patients can have profound ST segment depression in the absence of CAD, thus rendering the test meaningless.

When the results of an exercise test would not alter future management. Curiosity is not usually a sufficient reason to undertake an exercise test.

Inability to exercise.

Interpretation of the exercise test

Correct interpretation of the exercise test depends on successfully amalgamating a wide range of data. The most important data for a correct interpretation include:

How much exercise can the patient do? This is a very powerful independent determinant of prognosis. Indeed, a patient who does not have CAD but is very exercise-limited (eg can only walk with a Zimmer frame) has a very poor prognosis, whereas if a patient has severe CAD (eg proximal three-vessel CAD) but can still achieve a high level of exercise (eg reach the end of stage V of the Bruce protocol) then, despite the severity of their heart disease, the outlook on medical therapy is excellent, hardly differing from healthy age-matched controls. Thus exercise capacity is in itself probably the most important information to be gained from the test – certainly more important than most ECG changes.

Nature of symptoms occurring during the test: the more typical symptoms are for CAD, the more likely coronary disease is to be present and 'vice-versa.

Rate–pressure product (= systolic blood pressure × heart rate) reflects cardiac workload (only an approximation, as exercise-induced changes in stroke volume are not taken into account). Symptoms and ECG changes occurring at a low cardiac workload are of greater prognostic significance than those occurring at a higher cardiac workload, regardless of the level of exercise actually achieved.

Chronotropic response to exercise: exercise increases heart rate in normal subjects, perhaps on average by about 20–25 bpm/Bruce stage. The heart rate increases more quickly in those who are physically unfit, and conversely may increase very slowly in those who are fit, have chronotropic incompetence due to sinus node disease, or are on β-blockers. The exercise test can be used to diagnose the rare patient whose effort intolerance relates to such chronotropic incompetence. If this is due to sinus node disease, the treatment is a rate-responsive AAI pacemaker.

Nature of any ECG changes: see below.

Complications: such as MI, arrhythmias, etc.

Normal ECG changes during exercise

The normal response of the ECG to exercise is tachycardia (see above) and shortened QT interval (see p. 18). However, some normal subjects can show ST segment depression during exercise, especially so-called 'up-sloping' depression, but also 'planar' and occasionally 'down-sloping' depression.

This raises the important point as to how one might suspect that ST segment depression during exercise reflects a normal heart rather than epicardial CAD. The clues are:

- Chest pain is atypical for myocardial ischaemia.
- The demographics (age, sex, smoking status, etc) make coronary disease unlikely.
- There are pre-existing ST segment changes in the resting ECG. Exercise usually makes any pre-existing ST segment changes worse, regardless of the aetiology of such changes (eg whether caused by hyperventilation, anxiety or old pericardial disease).

- The ST depression is up-sloping rather than planar (down-sloping ST depression is most likely to be associated with underlying CAD).
- ST depression quickly returns to the baseline once exercise ceases.
- There are no post-exercise ST changes (see below).

ECG changes during exercise in coronary artery disease

There are several responses of the ECG to exercise in coronary disease:

- no change from normal (not uncommon, even in those with severe CAD! This appreciable false negative rate is one of the great limitations of this test)
- ST depression (see below)
- ST elevation (see below)
- arrhythmias, especially VT.

Exercise-induced ST depression

The characteristic response of the ST segment to myocardial ischaemia is ST depression (see Chapter 4). This is because in angina due to coronary artery disease the subepicardium is more ischaemic than the subendocardium, and so following depolarization current continues to flow from the 'healthier' endocardium to the 'sicker' epicardium, so depressing the ST segment. However and (rather unfortunately) ischaemia is not the only cause of ST segment depression on the ECG. There are in fact so many other causes that it can sometimes be very difficult to know whether ST segment depression relates to atheromatous CAD or to another more benign process. How can this problem be resolved? The extent and pattern of ST segment depression during and after exercise can be helpful. As a generalization (although there are many exceptions), the more profound and widespread the ST depression, the more likely CAD is to be present and the more likely it is to be severe. Why this is so is unclear.

The various patterns of ST depression (see Chapter 4, Figure 4.8) seen during exercise are:

- Up-sloping ST segment depression. This pattern is least likely to be due to myocardial ischaemia (ie unlikely but not impossible). On occasions this pattern can be associated with critical CAD, usually (but not always) in the presence of multiple risk factors for CAD.

- Planar ST segment depression. This has a higher probability of being due to myocardial ischaemia.
- Down-sloping ST segment depression. This has the highest chance of reflecting genuine myocardial ischaemia. However, this pattern does not invariably mean CAD is present, and is one that can be seen with angiographically normal coronary arteries (eg in young women with no risk factors for atheromatous coronary disease).

Thus the pattern of the ST segment response can lessen or increase the chance of CAD being present, but cannot unequivocally diagnose the presence or absence of CAD. In particular, it is critically important to realize that patients with CAD, even if severe, may show no ST segment depression at all during exercise. Thus, as in any other aspect of the ECG, false-negative results are possible. Again and again in interpreting the ECG data one comes back to the basic fact that one should be strongly guided by the clinical features in deciding whether it is reasonable to limit investigations to an exercise test or whether further, possibly more invasive, tests are required.

Exercise-induced ST segment elevation

This has several possible explanations:

New-onset MI provoked by the exercise test (see above). This is usually associated with the typical features of MI (severe retrosternal chest pain radiating to the jaw or left arm, ashen appearance, sweating, vomiting). The ST segment elevation usually does not resolve with resting and treatment is immediate pharmacological and/or mechanical revascularization. The provocation of MI is one of the main serious complications of exercise testing. The rate of MI in those with IHD is lowest in patients who have stable angina and highest in those who have unstable angina following an acute MI. The risk is intermediate in unstable angina.

Critical stenosis of the supplying artery. Chest pain occurs, but not of infarction quality (ie no sweating, no vomiting, patient not ashen), and both ST segment elevation and the chest pain usually resolve promptly with rest. Urgent angiography is indicated.

Pre-existing occlusion of the supplying blood vessel, often with stenosis of the collateral blood supply. This is most commonly seen in patients with a chronically occluded right coronary artery, who have developed a collateral supply from the left anterior descending artery, which in turn has developed a stenosis. During the exercise test inferior lead ST segment elevation occurs, which resolved rapidly on resting. There has often been a partial or full thickness inferior wall MI in the past (seen electrocardiographically as inferior lead Q waves). Chest pain, perhaps surprisingly, may not occur during the exercise test. Angiography is indicated.

Pre-existing full thickness MI. The meaning of (painless) ST segment elevation occurring during exercise in the territory of a previous full thickness ('Q' wave) MI is variable, but this pattern commonly reflects no more than the old myocardial damage. It does not necessarily imply ongoing myocardial ischaemia and thus by itself is not an indication for angiography.

In summary, ST segment elevation during exercise, unless painless and in the territory of a previous full thickness Q wave MI, usually indicates inducible ischaemia in viable muscle and as such is held to be an indication for angiography.

ST segment changes following exercise

The ST segment response following exercise can be helpful in working out whether symptomatic atherosclerotic CAD is present. This is particularly true when trying to decide whether ST segment depression is 'normal' or relates to CAD. The different patterns seen include:

Immediate return of the ST segment depression to the isoelectric baseline, followed by no further ECG changes. This pattern, especially if the depression is upward-sloping, is one that is least likely to be due to CAD, although (as above) it does not exclude it.

T wave inversion following exercise. This usually (but not always) occurs only in those who have demonstrated ST segment depression during exercise. The earlier T wave inversion occurs, and the more profound it is, the more likely CAD is to be present. Thus T wave inversion occurring in the first minute after exercise is most likely to reflect CAD, whereas if T wave inversion does not occur until, say, the fourth or fifth minute after exercise then CAD is less likely. This response can also be seen in those without epicardial CAD but with another disease process, eg LVH.

Significance of ST segment changes

It is very important to realize that although the pattern of ST segment changes can certainly increase or decrease the probability of CAD, no pattern is unambiguously associated with the presence or absence of CAD. [In other words, although some patterns are more or less likely to be associated with CAD, any pattern of ST segment depression (or indeed, no depression at all!) can be found in those with significant CAD.]

How can this confusing picture be clarified? Factoring in the pretest probability of CAD can help. In patients with a very low pretest probability of CAD (such as young women) even gross ST segment changes are unlikely to be due to 'fixed' atheromatous CAD, whereas in those with very high pretest probabilities even rather mild or atypical changes are often associated with (severe) CAD. Age (Figure 11.5), typicality or otherwise of chest pain, and extent of ST segment depression are critical factors in determining whether or

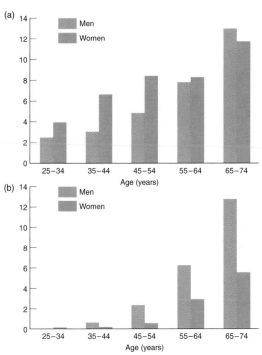

Figure 11.5
History of (a) angina and (b) myocardial infarction (MI) in men and women, plotted out according to age. Clearly, both angina and MI rates rise with age. Perhaps of greater interest is that despite the angina rates in women being higher than in men, the MI rate (a 'hard' outcome requiring the fulfilment of clear-cut diagnostic criteria) is much higher in men than in women. This emphasizes the fact that anginal symptoms in women are often not due to epicardial coronary artery disease. Adapted from Braunwald E, Zipes DB, Libby P. *Heart Disease: A Textbook of Cardiovascular Medicine*. Philadelphia: WB Saunders.

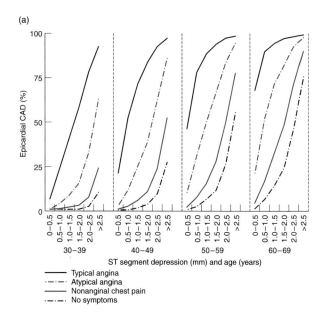

(a)

Typical angina
— · — Atypical angina
——— Nonanginal chest pain
— ·· — No symptoms

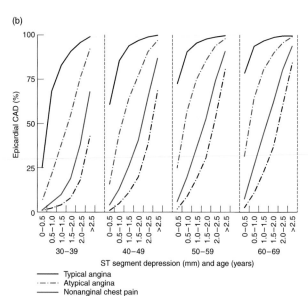

(b)

Typical angina
— · — Atypical angina
——— Nonanginal chest pain
— ·· — No symptoms

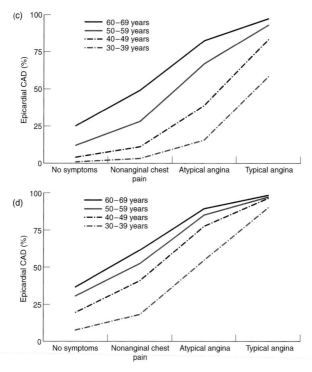

Figure 11.6
Prediction of the presence of epicardial coronary artery disease (CAD), related to typicality of symptoms, age and gender. (a) Data for women, stratified according to nature of chest pain, age of patient and amount of ST segment depression. (b) Similar data for men. In (a) and (b) the older the patient, the higher the probability of epicardial CAD, despite identical ST segment depression and nature of chest pain. Graphs (c) (for women) and (d) (for men) show that the probability of coronary artery disease depends strongly on age – subjects with 1.5–2.0 mm ST segment depression on an exercise test are compared at various ages. The older the patient, the higher the probability of coronary disease, despite identical ST segment changes and symptoms. Adapted with permission from Diamond GA, Forrester JS. Analysis of probability as an aid in the clinical diagnosis of coronary artery disease. *N Engl J Med* 1979; **300**: 1350–8.

not epicardial CAD is present (Figure 11.6). This again, therefore, emphasizes the value of clinical data in the interpretation of the ECG.

Diagnostic role of the exercise ECG

Perhaps the least useful aspect of the exercise test is in diagnosing the presence or absence of CAD. The usefulness of the exercise test in predicting prognosis is much greater (see later). To diagnose the presence of CAD, one classically wishes to see an exercise test provoke typical anginal symptoms and typical ECG changes (planar or downward-sloping ST segment depression, with postexercise deterioration along with T wave inversion). The more atypical the symptoms and ECG changes, the less likely CAD is to be present.

The diagnostic function of the exercise test rests on it significantly increasing or decreasing the post-test probability of CAD being present compared with the pre-test probability. If the pretest probability of CAD being present is in absolute terms very low then, even if an exercise test increases this chance substantially in relative terms, the absolute increase in chance is still low. (In other words, when the pretest probability is very low, false positives dominate the test results.) For example, young women with atypical chest pain have an extremely low probability of having epicardial CAD but a relatively high chance of having exercise-induced ST segment changes unrelated to any serious organic pathology. Indeed, most exercise-induced ST segment changes seen in this age group are not related to any serious disease process. Thus a 'positive' test will not substantially increase in absolute terms the post-test probability of CAD.

Furthermore, if the absolute probability of CAD being present is very high then even a negative test will not lower that probability sufficiently to rule out CAD. (In other words, in a very high-risk population, false-negative tests are common.) Thus the exercise test cannot in this situation be used to reliably exclude CAD, and another investigation (often coronary angiography) is more appropriate. Thus typical angina, limiting in nature, occurring in an elderly man is best investigated by coronary angiography rather than by exercise stress testing, as the overwhelming likelihood is that this patient has severe CAD that is likely to benefit from an intervention.

Thus the exercise test is not very useful in the diagnosis of CAD when the pretest probability of CAD being present is very high or very low. It is most useful when the pretest probability is intermediate. How does one determine the risk of coronary disease? Conventionally one determines the number of CAD risk factors present, and whether or not the chest pain is typical for the condition.

Obviously, the more risk factors present, the greater the risk of developing CAD. The most important risk factors are age, followed by smoking status, diabetic status, cholesterol level, history of treated hypertension and gender if middle-aged. Age is the dominant risk factor and can overwhelm virtually all the other risk factors. Thus a 20-year-old has an extraordinarily low risk of CAD (even if a male smoker with type 1 diabetes), whereas an 80-year-old, even with no other 'conventional' risk factors present, has a high chance of CAD (see Figure 11.7).

The more typical the symptoms are for angina, the more likely CAD is to be present. Typical angina is defined as a brief retrosternal chest heaviness or tightness (possibly radiating to the throat or left arm), reliably provoked by effort, not having been present prior to exercise, and relieved rapidly (<2 minutes) and totally by rest. Atypical pains are felt in an unusual site, have unusual characteristics (eg sharp, burning), are present other than when exercising (despite a good exercise capacity), are prolonged (may last for hours) and if exacerbated by effort take a long time to disperse afterwards (ie many hours). The less typical the pain, the less likely CAD is to be present, regardless of what ST segment changes are present. This is particularly true for all young patients ≤40 years and for women ≤55 years.

The more risk factors present, and the more typical the chest pain, the more likely there is to be CAD (Figure 11.6).

In clinical practice the exercise ECG is least helpful in the diagnosis of CAD in young men (≤35 years) and in slightly older women (≤45 years) unless very extensive risk factors are present (eg smoking + diabetes, or renal failure + hypertension), in which case the test may be useful at a younger age, say

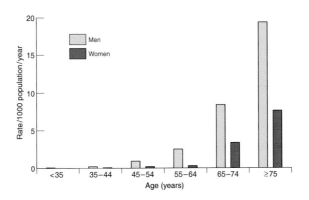

Figure 11.7
The relationship between age and death rates due to coronary artery disease in the UK. Increasing age is the dominant risk factor determining the probability of death.

30 years onwards for men and 35 years onwards for women. It has significant usefulness in older subjects, up to about 75 years for men and possibly 80 years for women, then again becomes less useful as age increases further, especially if symptoms are 'classic'.

Summary of the diagnostic role of the exercise ECG

An unambiguous diagnosis of CAD is not always easy to make from the exercise test, but it is possible to gain some idea of the likelihood of CAD being present. The following features increase this likelihood:

- Chest pain is 'typical' rather than 'atypical' (see above).
- Multiple risk factors are present, of which the most important are increasing age and, in younger patients (35–65 years), male gender.
- Exercise is limited by symptoms typical for myocardial ischaemia. This is usually typical angina, although in diabetics breathlessness can be readily accepted as an 'angina equivalent'.
- The resting ECG is normal.
- ST segment depression occurs at a low workload.
- ST segment depression is downward-sloping.
- T wave inversion occurs early on in the recovery period, ie within the first minute.
- ST segment elevation occurs (see above).

Role of the exercise test in estimating prognosis

Perhaps the most useful aspect of the exercise ECG is its role in estimating prognosis. Indeed this aspect is probably more useful than its diagnostic role. The reasons why the amount of effort that an individual can undertake relates to prognosis have been examined above, but in essence many diseases impair effort capacity in proportion to the severity of the disease, and disease severity usually relates to outcome.

Furthermore, physical fitness (which is reflected in exercise capacity) has a potent role in prolonging or shortening life, and this is true in disease as well as in health. Thus there are good reasons for believing that exercise capacity should reflect prognosis, and this hypothesis has been well borne out by the data in CAD. If exercise is limited by a disease process (eg cardiac, respiratory or neurological) then the prognosis is worsened by the complications of that disease process (eg cardiac, respiratory and neurological complications). Thus, the symptom that limits exercise dictates which organ system should be investigated and treated.

Prognosis in coronary disease depends on various factors, which are, in descending order of importance:

Age: probably the most potent determinant, regardless of other factors.

Exercise capacity (as measured by peak exercise capacity): a key parameter in predicting outcome. In assessing exercise capacity from the exercise test one needs to be certain that if low work capacity is found, this is not due to poor motivation during the test, as this will falsely skew the data. Submaximal effort endurance (which relates to peak exercise capacity, although not strongly) also has a prognostic role. Unfortunately, most exercise tests do not measure exercise endurance.

Extent of CAD is a key determinant of prognosis, and exercise capacity, along with the ST response to exercise, can indicate this (as above).

Ejection fraction also relates to outcome. Poor LV function has a rather dramatic adverse effect on outcome. An indication of ejection fraction can be obtained from the history (previous MI and/or symptoms suggestive of heart failure), the resting ECG (Q waves and loss of R wave height both suggest impaired LV function: an anterior MI usually results in more LV dysfunction than an inferior MI, which in turn is usually larger than a posterior MI) and if possible, although not always easily available, from the cardiac ultrasound scan.

Plaque stability is an important predictor of outcome. Patients with the least stable plaques (ie those most likely to ulcerate and thrombose) are clearly the most likely to develop an MI. Propensity to develop thrombosis on such plaques is very difficult to predict. However, once plaques have shown some instability (ie once the patient has had an admission with an ACS), one can get a better indication of this by using the peak troponin release measured during the index admission. Those patients with the most unstable plaques (as measured by microinfarcts caused by embolization of clot from the 'hot' lesion) are, unsurprisingly, the ones with the worst subsequent outcome, in part related to future plaque instability.

Other important factors impacting on prognosis include the following:

Extent of comorbid disease: the severity of any comorbid disease is relevant to prognosis, and this can be measured in a variety of ways. In respiratory disease spirometric findings, particularly vital capacity, and FEV$_1$ (forced expiratory volume at one second), as well as arterial blood gases, relate to outcome. In renal disease glomerular filtration rate, as measured by creatinine level, is often the key parameter, and in liver disease liver synthetic function as reflected in the plasma albumin or INR.

Clinical course: a much-underused measure of prognosis. In any disease, regardless of objective measures of severity, there are some patients who do well and others who do not. This is usually due to important but as yet unidentified aspects of their disease. It may well be that these factors can be measured (or at least estimated) clinically by observing the clinical course of the patient. Thus the patient who has a rapid decline in health is likely to continue to deteriorate, whereas the patient who has been stable for a prolonged period of time is more likely to remain well. One should not underestimate the 'feel' gained from observing the progress of a patient over time in estimating their prognosis.

Thus, to get a good indication of prognosis, one needs the data from the exercise test as well as data obtained from the clinical situation.

Summary of how to read an exercise ECG undertaken in suspected coronary disease

First, check the patients' name, demographics and test indication.

Second, look at the work capacity, and the symptoms that occurred during exercise. Were these symptoms responsible for the patient stopping exercise? Were they 'typical' for myocardial ischaemia? Crucially, did the patient attain a high level of exercise? This is important, as some patients fail to exercise much for noncardiac reasons, eg stopping in early stage II of the Bruce protocol, when there are no cardiac symptoms or significant ECG changes, whereas if they had managed to get further, substantial cardiac symptoms and/or ECG changes might have occurred. Thus one can only say that an exercise test is negative for symptoms and ECG changes if a high workload has been achieved. It is best to be quite explicit; the test should be reported as a 'high-level negative exercise test' or 'low-level', whatever the case is. Effort intolerance by itself is associated with a worse outcome and should lower the threshold for invasive evaluation.

Third, check the haemodynamic response to exercise (heart rate and blood pressure changes). Are these normal? Symptoms occurring at a low 'rate–pressure' product are of more concern than those found at higher rate–pressure product.

Fourth, look at the resting ECG, particularly for Q wave MIs and for any pre-existing ST changes. If there are pre-existing ST changes on the resting ECG this may negate the diagnostic usefulness of any exercise-induced ST depression.

Fifth, look for any exercise-induced ST depression.

Sixth, check for any postexercise ST changes.

The exercise test may then lead to a clear diagnosis and plan of action. Thus one might be confident that CAD has been excluded (high-level negative test), or conversely that severe CAD is likely and angiography required.

Not infrequently the exercise test may not lead to a clear diagnosis or plan of action. What should then be done? This really depends on the clinical situation. In some patients, especially if they have intrusive symptoms and at least some risk factors for CAD, coronary angiography may be appropriate. However, if symptoms have completely or largely settled then noninvasive imaging may well be more appropriate, and will expose the patients to fewer risks than coronary angiography. This may be an exercise or pharmacological stress myoview or cardiac ultrasound (see below)

Additional roles of the exercise ECG

The exercise test is not just used to diagnose and prognosticate in CAD. Other important roles for the exercise test include:

Evaluating other effort-induced symptoms, of which the commonest are effort-induced palpitations (in those without heart disease often due to an SVT, and in those with heart disease, especially previous MI, often due to VT). On occasions the exercise test is used to evaluate effort-induced syncope; it is vital in this situation to definitively exclude LVOT obstruction by cardiac ultrasound prior to the exercise test, as exercise in the presence of LV outflow obstruction can be dangerous. LVOT obstruction is most commonly due to valvular aortic stenosis, although it can be due to a subvalvular obstruction, eg hypertrophic cardio-myopathy.

Documenting exercise capacity. This may be undertaken to monitor a patient over time, to determine whether certain treatments should be undertaken (eg cardiac transplantation), or occasionally to clarify whether a patient's complaints of effort intolerance are genuine.

Other types of exercise stress test

Nuclear isotope exercise testing

Exercise myocardial perfusion scans involve injecting intravenously a radioisotope (usually thallium or technetium) that is taken up by healthy myocytes. These isotopes decay, emitting radioactivity which can be imaged by appropriately placed detectors ('γ-cameras'). These detectors, along with processing computers, are relatively sensitive in determining which part of the heart has given out the γ-signal; in other words, which part of the heart contains large populations of myocytes sufficiently healthy to take up the radioisotopes. Dead cells do not take up any isotope, nor do cells that are ischaemic. Thus it is possible to determine which parts of the heart become ischaemic with exercise and which parts are infarcted and dead.

Although techniques vary, the commonest approach is to inject an isotope at the peak of exercise, then image the heart. If exercise cannot be undertaken then an infusion of dobutamine, which increases the heart rate and inotropic state, can be given to mimic the effects of exercise. Alternatively, adenosine – a potent coronary vasodilator – can be given. An hour or two after exercise/stress a further injection of the radioisotope is given (if cardiac redistribution of the isotope is slow), and the resting heart imaged. Thus this technique can determine if ischaemia develops during exercise, and if it does, how large an area is affected. This can be used to estimate prognosis, as patients who develop large areas of ischaemia have a worse outlook.

It is important to realize that there are some limitations to this test. Occasionally severe CAD (eg a blocked right coronary artery with significant left main coronary disease) can be 'missed' by nuclear myocardial perfusion imaging. Furthermore, distal epicardial vessel disease or side branch disease can be missed by myocardial perfusion scans.

In other words, although this is a useful technique, it can still miss significant areas of ischaemia. One should therefore always be alert to the clinical situation, and if the test gives a completely unexpected result, be prepared to 'ignore' it, always erring on the side of caution.

Stress cardiac ultrasound imaging

In stress echo the heart is imaged by cardiac ultrasound at rest, then during pharmacological stress from agents that increase the heart rate and inotropic state – typically dobutamine and atropine. This increases myocardial oxygen demand. If a narrowed artery supplies part of the heart then this territory becomes ischaemic and contractile performance declines. The greater the decline in contractile function, and the more territories that are affected, the greater the chance of severe multivessel CAD being present

In expert hands the stress echo is a reasonably sensitive and specific means to investigate for significant CAD. However, there are a number of problems:

First, the assessment of LV function is, despite what is commonly written, one of the most difficult aspects of the cardiac ultrasound. In stress echo one must look at several different regions and compare them with each other over time. This requires a great deal of operator skill and experience. It is quite easy for the inexperienced operator to over- or underdiagnose the stress echo. This limits its use to experienced, high-volume centres.

Second, the technique is time-consuming – a full study takes at least one hour.

Third, the heart must be substantially stressed to obtain meaningful data – given that these are often patients with CAD, some post MI, the incidence of ventricular arrhythmias is higher than generally appreciated, and certainly higher than reported. Studies must always be carried out with a defibrillator close at hand and a crash team in the facility.

Chapter 12
ECG devices for remote recording of arrhythmias

There are a number of devices that allow for the recording of an ECG distant to a hospital:

- 24-hour ECG – the Holter monitor (see below)
- event recorders
- external 'loop' recorders, eg cardiomemo recorders
- implantable 'loop' recorders, eg Cardiac Reveal™ devices.

24-hour ECG recorders

A 24-hour Holter ECG monitor consists of a number of electrodes (Figure 12.1) fed into a recording device, either solid state or a tape recorder. After a period of recording (conventionally 24 hours, although up to 48 hours is often possible) the information gathered is relayed to a computer for further analysis. Although the whole 24-hour period is analysed, the patient keeps a diary so particular attention can be paid to the ECG at those times when symptoms occur.

Information on a number of cardiac functions can be obtained from this analysis:

The rhythm at the time patients experience symptoms. This is often the most helpful function of the 24-hour ECG. If one can obtain an ECG at the time of symptoms then it is possible to say conclusively whether or not symptoms relate to an arrhythmia and if so, to which one (Figure 12.2). The converse is also true, ie if a patient does not experience symptoms during the recording, one has no data on which to conclude whether or not an arrhythmia underlies symptoms. The data obtained from such asymptomatic recordings should be used with great care.

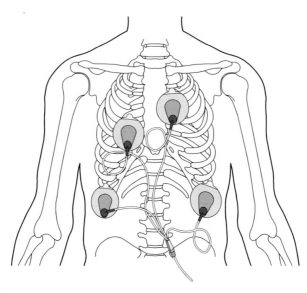

Figure 12.1
ECG setup for recording a Holter tape. In this setup the data are used to obtain (modified) lead V1 and V5 traces, ie a two-channel recording is obtained.

Presence of asymptomatic arrhythmias. Usually one is most concerned about the presence of symptomatic arrhythmias (as above). The significance of asymptomatic arrhythmias can be quite uncertain. Asymptomatic arrhythmias may bear some or no relationship to the presence of symptomatic arrhythmias. It is therefore wise to be very careful in extrapolating from asymptomatic arrhythmias to the cause of symptoms. For example, ventricular premature contractions (VPCs) are very commonly found on a 24-hour recording: symptoms may relate to them, to the ventricular tachycardia (VT) that may be associated with them in those with structural heart disease, to the atrial fibrillation (AF) that is equally associated with structural heart disease, or to a heightened appreciation of sinus tachycardia. One can only definitively say whether a rhythm disturbance is relevant if patients have definitely experienced typical symptoms when the ECG-documented rhythm disturbance occurred.

Heart rate. The 24-hour heart rate (usually divided into 2–3 minute averages) is plotted out against time (Figure 12.3). This can be quite useful in determining how fit the patient is (from the heart rate response to day-to-day levels of exercise – the less fit a patient is, the more the heart speeds up with

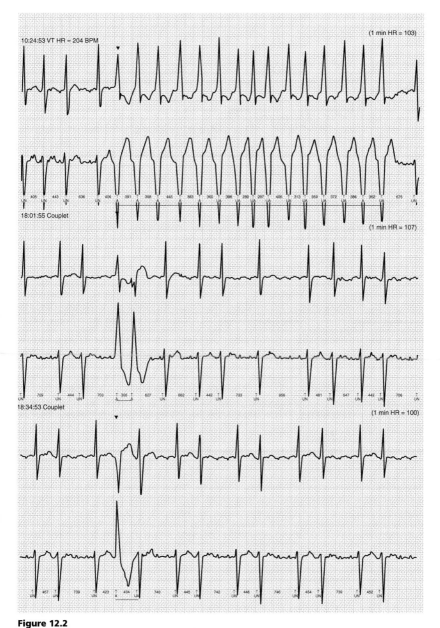

Figure 12.2

ECG printout at the time when palpitations were experienced. A 15-beat episode of ventricular tachycardia is shown in the top trace; the middle trace shows a couplet, with the underlying rhythm being an atrial tachycardia; there is an isolated ventricular premature contraction in the lower trace.

271

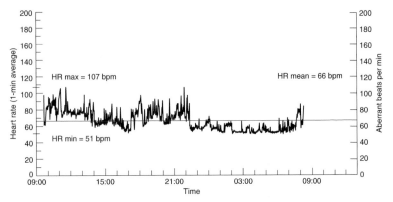

Figure 12.3
A 24-hour heart rate (HR) record from the 24-hour ECG. The heart rate (1-minute averages) is plotted out against the time of day. It can be seen when the patient is active and when they are asleep. The line plotted out at a heart rate of (about) 65 bpm is the average heart rate for this patient over the 24 hours of monitoring. max, maximum; min, minimum.

any given level of exercise) and whether there is any sinus node disease (inappropriate tachy- or bradycardias). Sudden 'step' increases in heart rate often indicate the sudden onset of a tachyarrhythmia (Figure 12.4) and this can be confirmed by analysing the printout of the ECG trace at this time. In patients with AF, the 24-hour monitor can produce good data as to whether the patient needs more or less atrioventricular node-blocking drugs.

ST segment variability. This function of the 24-hour ECG has some use in those with known coronary artery disease (CAD). Here, there is some evidence that the more ST segment depression during the 24-hours, the worse the outlook, and this should probably be factored into the decision as to whether or not coronary angiography should be undertaken. However, it has little use in those who do not have unambiguous CAD. For example, patients with left ventricular hypertrophy (LVH) free from CAD can have substantial and variable ST segment depression, as can middle-aged men and women with entirely normal hearts. It is therefore best to ignore ST segment data from 24-hour Holter monitors unless CAD is unambiguously known to be present.

Measurement of heart rate variability. This is a commonly measured variable in research practice but, perhaps surprisingly in view of its prognostic importance, a rather infrequently measured function in clinical practice (see p. 283).

A normal 24-hour ECG

One of the key questions in looking at a 24-hour ECG is to decide whether or not deviations from sinus rhythm are relevant. Indeed, the range of what is considered normal on a 24-hour recording is quite substantial.

Atrial extrasystoles can be found quite frequently in completely normal subjects, up to 1–200 in 24 hours. There is some evidence to suggest that the greater the atrial extrasystolic activity, the more likely are sustained atrial arrhythmias, eg AF. Thus frequent atrial ectopy may indicate that sustained irregular palpitations in a patient are due to a sustained atrial arrhythmia, such as atrial tachycardia or fibrillation (although as mentioned above it need not necessarily indicate the presence of such an arrhythmia).

Atrial tachycardia: short episodes (ie ≤10–15 beats) of asymptomatic atrial tachycardia likewise often have no great significance as they occur frequently in completely normal asymptomatic individuals. On occasions, however, they indicate that symptoms relate to an atrial arrhythmia.

Ventricular extrasystoles likewise can be quite frequent (up to 1–200 in 24 hours) in entirely normal subjects. However, although subjects with structurally entirely normal hearts can occasionally have many thousands of ventricular extrasystoles in a 24-hour period, as a generalization the more frequent the VPCs, the more likely there is to be heart disease present. Furthermore, in the presence of known cardiac disease it is important to note that the more frequent the VPCs, the greater the risk of sudden cardiac death. Thus if VPCs are very frequent (say ≥200 beats in 24 hours), it is worth undertaking a cardiac ultrasound to be certain that the ventricular extrasystolic activity does not reflect LV dysfunction, as if it does, intensive investigations to determine the best treatment may be appropriate.

Nonsustained VT (NSVT) can be normal, with normal subjects infrequently showing occasional episodes of up to 8–10 beats. The heart rate during nonsustained VT occurring in normal subjects is usually quite slow, often ≤ 120–130 bpm. If NSVT is seen, it is wise to be absolutely certain that the heart is structurally normal, especially if the heart rate is ≥ 140 bpm (normal cardiac ultrasound and normal exercise test) and equally to be certain that any symptoms are not due to higher-grade ventricular arrhythmias, via appropriate prolonged ECG recordings. NSVT in those with structurally damaged hearts is moderately strongly associated with sudden cardiac death due to ventricular arrhythmias, which in turn can be prevented or treated effectively with an implantable cardioverter defibrillator. Finding NSVT in those with cardiac disease should therefore substantially lower the threshold at which angiography and VT stimulation studies are undertaken.

Nocturnal atrioventricular (AV) block is not infrequently seen in the fit young adults in whom vagal tone is high. The clue that nocturnal AV block relates to high vagal tone is that the heart rate decelerates quite significantly in the 30–60 seconds before the 'dropped' beat, indicative of 'vagal switch-on'. AV block occurring without vagal switch-on raises the possibility of intrinsic AV conducting tissue disease. Daytime AV block is almost always pathological.

Indication for 24-hour ECG recording

The chance that a 24-hour tape will be diagnostically useful varies in proportion to the frequency of symptoms. If symptoms occur ≥ once a week then a 24-hour tape is moderately useful. If attacks occur less frequently then, even though it is still reasonable to carry out a 24-hour ECG, other techniques (such as an event or loop recorder) are more likely to be productive.

The 24-hour ECG may be diagnostically useful in:

- *Evaluation of palpitations*: common findings include diagnosis of 'appreciation of sinus tachycardia', extrasystoles (especially ventricular), AF and atrioventricular node reentrant tachycardia (AVNRT). It is important to appreciate that one can only be confident that one has excluded or diagnosed an arrhythmia if symptoms coincide with the ECG abnormality.
- *Evaluation of syncope*: although 24-hour ECGs are frequently and appropriately undertaken in the evaluation of unexplained syncope, the diagnostic yield is very low. Indeed, many patients have entirely or virtually normal post-syncope 24-hour ECG recordings, even if they have serious arrhythmias underlying their syncope. One can only be certain that one has excluded (or proven) the diagnosis if an ECG recording is made during a syncopal attack. Some clues as to the cause of syncope can sometimes be made from the presence of asymptomatic arrhythmias. These diagnostic clues include finding daytime AV block (see above), sinus node disease (especially inappropriate bradycardias) or NSVT (as above).
- *Evaluation of the heart rate response in atrial fibrillation.*

How to read a 24-hour ECG

The following should be specifically checked:

Patient's name and date of birth on the report, as 24-hour ECGs frequently find their way into the wrong set of notes!

Patient's diary. Did the patient have any symptoms during the recording, and if so were they typical of the symptoms that had brought them to medical attention?

ECG at the time symptoms occurred, and a few minutes either side. Typical symptoms during the recording allow for a definitive ECG diagnosis as to whether or not an arrhythmia is present.

Heart rhythm over the entire 24 hours, from the technician's report, ie whether or not the rhythm was sustained sinus rhythm, whether any arrhythmias were present, and if so what they were. If arrhythmias have been reported, confirm the accuracy of the report by looking at the ECG during a reported arrhythmia yourself. A key feature is to determine whether or not the patient experienced any symptoms whenever an arrhythmia occurred, as many arrhythmias can be asymptomatic epiphenomenona, unrelated to patients' symptoms.

Heart rate over the entire 24-hour time period. This can be found on a chart at the front of the document (Figure 12.3). Much data can be usefully determined from an analysis of the heart rate over 24 hours, particularly data on:

- how fit or unfit the patient is: unfit patients have dramatic increases in heart rate on minimal effort (Figure 12.4)
- whether or not sustained tachyarrhythmias were present during the recording. Sustained tachyarrhythmias lead to a sudden ('jump') increase in heart rate to a new and fixed (ie no variation) high heart rate (see Figure 12.4), except for AF, which gives rise to a sudden but varying increase in heart rate
- if AF is present, how good or poor heart rate control is, and whether there is a need for more (or less) AV nodal blockade.

Number of atrial and ventricular ectopics present over the 24-hour time period (from the histograms and charts usually found at the start of the report; Figure 12.5). A large number of ventricular ectopics raises the possibility of underlying myocardial disease (consider ordering a cardiac ultrasound), particularly if 'higher' grade ventricular arrhythmias are present, such as ventricular couplets or triplets.

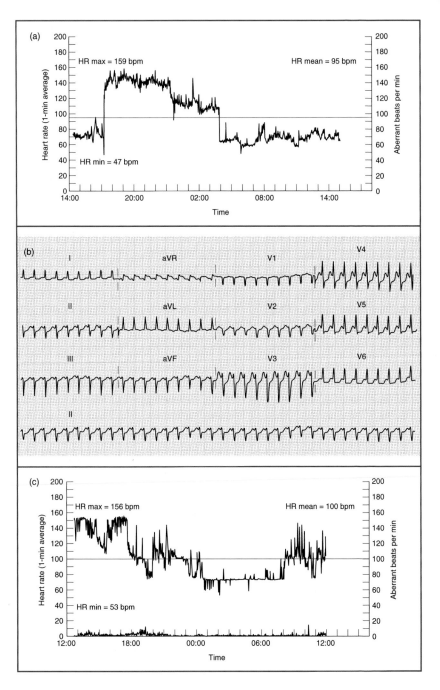

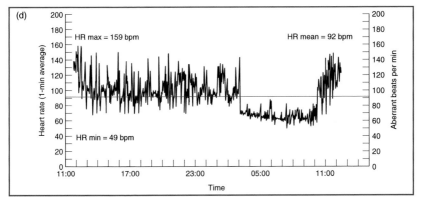

Figure 12.4
(a) Step-change in heart rate (HR) on 24-hour ECG recording, indicating the onset and offset of tachyarrhythmia. Interestingly, in this recording the arrhythmia results in two quite distinct heart rates, one of about 140–150 bpm from 17.00 to 23.00 and the second around 120 bpm until 04.00 when the arrhythmia 'breaks' (ie terminates). (b) The relevant arrhythmia is shown to be an atrial tachycardia. This patient shows considerable anterior lead ST depression during the tachycardia. (c) This tachogram shows a 'fixed' heart rate of around 75 bpm during the night, with some evidence that the heart rate during the day is 'capped' at 150 bpm. The night time fixed heart rate could be due to a pacemaker; alternatively, and as is the case here, it could be due to an atrial arrhythmia, such as atrial flutter, with four-to-one block during the night. This latter diagnosis is also supported by the daytime 'capping' of the heart rate at 150 bpm (two-to-one block). (d) Heart rate chart from 24-hour ECG showing episodes of marked sinus tachycardia, corresponding to rather minor exercise, and due to physical deconditioning. It can be seen that the heart rate during sleep, at night, shows an unremarkable resting heart rate of 60–70 bpm. This is normal, and makes thyrotoxicosis as a cause of the daytime tachycardias rather unlikely. max, maximum; min, minimum.

Heart rate variability and QT interval duration/variability, if these analytical packages have been used.

Other devices for recording arrhythmias

There are several other devices that allow the remote recording of an arrhythmia.

An 'event' recorder

This is a device that contains its own electrodes: when symptoms occur, the device is applied to the chest, allowing for the recording of a single-channel ECG (Figure 12.6). The device is lent to patients for a two- to three-week period. The ECG made when symptoms occur can sometimes be transmitted

(a)

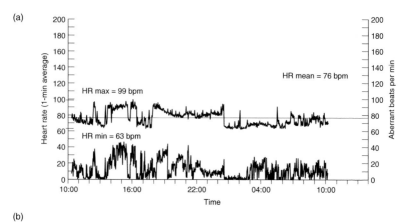

(b)

Time since recording began (hours)	QRS	Normal	Premature normal	SVT	Isolated aberrant	Premature aberrant	Couplet	Triplet	Salvo	VT
1	3195	3133	0	0	1	5	0	0	0	0
2	8984	8819	0	0	0	115	0	0	0	0
3	8188	8013	0	0	0	150	0	0	0	0
4	7320	7223	0	0	0	70	0	0	0	0
5	8706	8604	0	0	0	54	0	0	0	0
6	8135	7986	0	0	0	111	0	0	0	0
7	6267	6009	0	0	0	231	2	0	0	0
8	5433	5246	0	0	0	178	2	0	0	0
9	6524	6369	0	0	0	134	0	0	0	0
10	6566	6482	0	0	0	69	0	0	0	0
11	6054	6033	0	0	0	20	0	0	0	0
12	5132	5111	0	0	0	20	0	0	0	0
13	5039	4980	0	0	0	55	0	0	0	0
14	4377	4339	0	0	0	34	2	0	0	0
15	4355	4298	0	0	0	53	2	0	0	0
16	4440	4390	0	0	0	46	2	0	0	0
17	4480	4425	0	0	0	47	2	0	0	0
18	4499	4437	0	0	0	53	4	0	0	0
19	4572	4523	0	0	0	40	1	0	0	0
20	4556	4508	0	0	0	46	1	0	0	0
21	6069	6021	0	0	0	68	0	0	0	0
22	6633	6575	0	0	0	45	0	0	0	0
23	5557	5517	0	0	0	20	0	0	0	1
24	5922	5783	0	0	0	128	0	0	0	0
	141030	138824	0	0	0	1792	18	0	0	1

Patient name: / Patient no: / Recording date:

Figure 12.5
(a) Graph and (b) chart of ectopic frequency over the 24-hour time period of the recording.

trans-telephonically back to the physician. These devices have the advantage that patients are not connected all the time to them, and so they are not as intrusive. They have the disadvantage that they miss the start of an event, which in some situations (eg syncope) is a serious problem, although missing the onset may not be relevant for many other problems, such as the diagnosis of sustained palpitations.

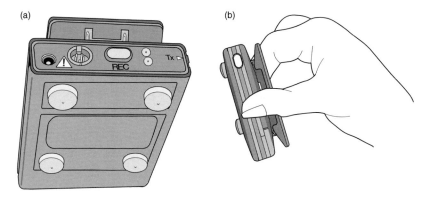

Figure 12.6
ECG event recorder. (a) Diagram of the basic device: a small electronic box with several external electrodes. A button is depressed during recording allowing the data to be stored in the box's memory. (b) Application of the device to the chest wall during a recording.

External 'loop' recorders

These allow continual recording of an ECG over a prolonged time period, typically over seven to 14 days. Patients wear electrodes connected to the loop recorder (Figure 12.7). The data is continually recorded, but only the immediately preceding 10–30 minutes is stored. If an event occurs, the patient can 'alert' the device, which 'freezes' the immediately preceding data in a memory store, ready for downloading. External loop recorders can be highly effective at diagnosing modestly frequent palpitations (ie those occurring every two to three weeks). They have little or no role in the diagnosis of syncope, and here an implantable loop recorder is the preferred diagnostic equipment.

Implantable 'loop' recorders

Advances in solid-state technology have allowed recorders to be miniaturized such that they can be implanted in the prepectoral pouch (Figure 12.8). They act as a very small ECG machine and record a one-channel signal. They can be set to automatically record all arrhythmias faster or slower than certain prespecified limits (eg ≤140 bpm and ≥120 bpm), and can also be externally activated to record an ECG when a patient has symptoms. Typically the recorder stores the 10–40 minutes of an ECG prior to activation, then 5–10 minutes following activation. This allows ECG

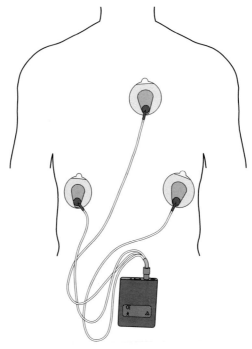

Figure 12.7
External loop recorder. The device is attached by three electrodes to the chest wall.

storage by those who have syncopal events followed by some postevent confusion (obviously provided this confusion lasts less than 10–40 minutes).

Indications

Although implantable 'loop' recorders have some use in palpitations that are intrusive and have defied diagnosis despite intensive conventional external ECG recordings, their greatest utility is in the investigation of unexplained syncope (see Chapter 8).

Common findings

Common findings recorded by implantable loop recorders activated at the time of symptoms are either sinus rhythm or a diagnostic arrhythmia, often high-grade AV block (found in about 50% of cases of unexplained

(a)

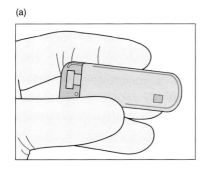

Figure 12.8

(a) Implantable loop recorder. From Medtronic.com. (b) Recording from an internal loop recorder. The patient has symptoms compatible with a vasomotor form of syncope, probably neurocardiogenic syncope. The tilt-table test, however, was negative, so further definition of the mechanism of syncope was sought from internal loop recording. This is a recording made during a typical episode; progressive sinus node slowing gives way to a prolonged period of sinus arrest, during which occasional junctional 'escape beats' occur. This patient elected to have a pacemaker, which 'cured' him from further syncopal spells.

(b) 12.5 mm/s, 25.0 mm/mV

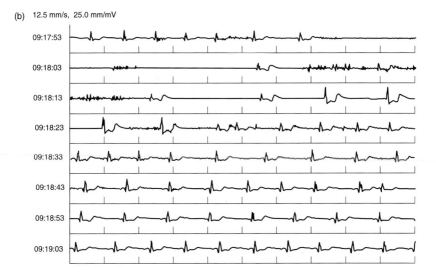

syncope in whom a loop recorder has been implanted). Occasionally VT is found in those with syncope and structural heart disease.

In those with vasomotor syncope, startlingly long periods of sinus arrest can be seen (a consequence of very high vagal tone), with asystole lasting 10, 20 or even 30 or 40 seconds. The temptation here is to immediately rush and implant a pacemaker. However, provided that the diagnosis is genuinely vasomotor syncope, one can sit back and discuss at length with the patient the advantages and disadvantages of such a choice.

First, the pacemaker will not prolong life (as the prognosis in vasomotor syncope is for a normal life expectancy). Second, a pacemaker may not relieve symptoms. Patients differ as to how great a vasodilator response they have in addition to the bradycardic response. The more marked the vasodilator response, the less likely that a pacemaker will remove symptoms. Thus in patients with no vasodilator response and a 'pure' bradycardic response, a pacemaker may remove attacks. Such patients are rather rare. More common are patients with a mixed bradycardic–vasodilator response. Here a pacemaker may modify attacks, but will not remove them. A few patients have a very marked vasodilator response and will have almost no symptom relief from pacemaker implantation. There is a 'down' side to pacemaker implantation, in that it is an invasive procedure (with attendant risks) and patients will need generator replacements every 8–12 years and new electrodes every 20 or so years. Thus if patients are young, pacemaker implantation, in theory an easy decision to make, may expose the patient to substantial further surgical intervention with its own attendant risks.

What if 'observational' ECG studies are nondiagnostic?

If observational ECG studies from 24-hour ECGs and loop/event recorders fail to lead to an unambiguous diagnosis, what should be done? This depends on the clinical circumstances. In many situations it is appropriate to operate according to the clinical diagnosis: for syncope this often means assuming that syncope is vasomotor in origin (which is a benign diagnosis). For palpitations this means assuming that symptoms relate either to 'an appreciation of the normal heartbeat' or to a benign rhythm disturbance such as AVNRT. These are benign diagnoses and as such in most cases a 'cast-iron' diagnosis should not be pursued aggressively.

However, in some situations it is important to be absolutely clear about the diagnosis. These include palpitations with syncope, if the diagnosis is not clearly 'vasomotor', and palpitations or syncope post MI (which often indicate syncopal ventricular arrhythmias, which can readily proceed to sudden cardiac death).

Syncope with injury, indicating a sudden loss of cardiac output, should also be rigorously investigated. In 'vasomotor' syncope cardiac output is often (but not always) lost gradually, so the body's various homeostatic reflexes have time to come into play, often preventing serious injury. Thus the presence of serious injury suggests a sudden and total loss of postural reflexes, and so may indicate a serious primary bradyarrhythmia, eg episodic complete heart block, or syncopal tachyarrhythmia, eg syncopal VT, rather than vasomotor syncope.

Provocative ECG studies

In some situations 'provocative' ECG studies may be appropriate. The aim of such studies is to provoke symptoms and at the same time obtain diagnostic ECGs. Such 'provocative' studies include:

- exercise ECG tests
- carotid sinus massage
- tilt-table testing, the 'circulatory stress test'
- electrophysiological studies (both supraventricular and ventricular stimulation studies as well as invasive measurement of the efficacy of the conducting system).

Other strategies

Sometimes observational and invasive studies are either inappropriate or nondiagnostic. It may then be best to proceed according to a 'best guess' strategy. If episodic complete heart block is under serious consideration then sometimes it is reasonable to empirically implant a pacemaker, especially if the patient is elderly. Likewise, aggressive anti-VT pharmacology can be appropriate in those in whom syncopal VT is strongly felt to be the diagnosis but in whom it has not been proved. This usually means amiodarone and β-blocker therapy, and sometimes ICD therapy.

Assessing 24-hour heart rate variability

Heart rate variability (HRV) is a much-underused function of the 24-hour ECG. The heart rate at rest is not 'fixed', rather it varies continuously (Figure 12.9a). The degree of variability (ie the HRV) can be determined (see below). This, in the absence of sinus node disease, relates to the state of the autonomic nervous system. The 'fitter' the person is, the greater the vagal outflow, and the higher the HRV. A high HRV post MI is associated with a lower risk of ventricular arrhythmias and so of sudden cardiac death (SCD). Conversely, low HRV post MI is associated with a higher risk of ventricular

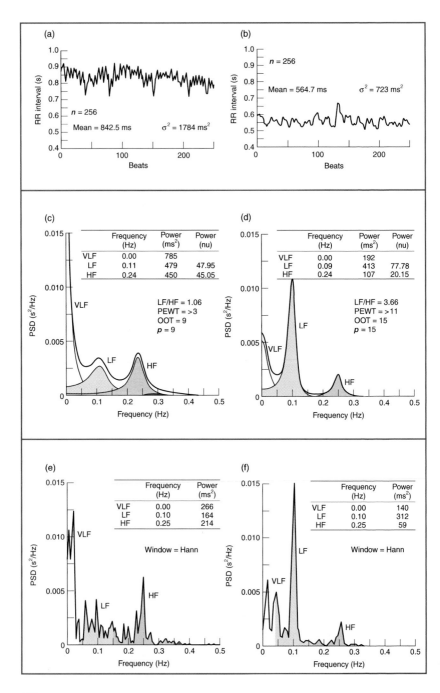

arrhythmias and thus of SCD. Drugs that increase or decrease HRV post MI usually also decrease or increase the risk of VT and SCD.

Pattern of heart rate variability

Analysis of the pattern of variability shows that there are (at least) two components of heart rate variability: a high-frequency component (the same frequency as respiration) of about 0.4 Hz (this has been interpreted as relating to vagal outflow – partly as respiration is known to enhance vagal outflow, and the high-frequency component to heart rate variability is altered by respiratory frequency) and a low-frequency component of about 0.1 Hz (this has been interpreted as relating to sympathetic outflow).

The relative strength of the sympathetic versus the parasympathetic outflow is perhaps more important physiologically than the absolute value of either, from which arises the concept of 'sympathovagal balance'.

'Routine' measures of heart rate variability

There are numerous methods of measuring HRV. However, in clinical practice the so-called time domain methods are the simplest and the most reliable. There are a few that should perhaps be used routinely:

Figure 12.9
Heart rate variability analysis. Tachograms (instantaneous RR interval plotted out against beat number) from an individual (a) resting and (b) with head-up tilt (which activates the sympathetic nervous system). The increase in heart rate (decreases RR interval) can be seen, as can the loss of high-frequency variation. Total heart rate variability can also be seen to decrease. Graphs (c) and (d) show the power spectral analysis of this heart rate variability at rest and with head-up tilt respectively. The frequency of the variation in heart rate is plotted out against the absolute amount of variability (the power spectral density, PSD). It can be seen that in this short-term recording there are two prominent peaks of variation, one around 0.1 Hz, the low-frequency peak (believed to relate to sympathetic outflow), and another around 0.25 Hz, the high-frequency peak (believed to relate to vagal outflow). Tilting the subject increases the low-power peak relative to the high-power peak, although the absolute amount of heart rate variability (shown in the size of the shaded area in the charts) is reduced. Sympathovagal balance, measured by the low:high-power ratio, is increased. Fast Fourier transform (FFT) nonparametric analysis [(e) at rest and (f) with head-up tilt] shows rather similar results. VLF, very low-frequency; LF, low-frequency; HF, high-frequency; nu, normalized units; PEWT, prediction error whiteness test (which provides information about the 'goodness' of the fitting model); OOT, optimal order test (checks the suitability of the order of the model used). Reprinted with permission from Task Force of the ESC and the North American Society of Pacing and Electrophysiology. Heart rate variability: standards of measurement, physiological interpretation, and clinical use. *Eur Heart J* 1996; **17**: 354–81.

24-hour day and night average heart rate. Much data can be obtained from knowledge of the heart rate alone, provided that patients are not on any drugs that alter heart rate (the majority unfortunately are!) and that there is no sinus node disease. However, with these provisos, the lower the heart rate during the night, the fitter the patient and the better the outlook.

Standard deviation of all the RR intervals during the full 24 hours. This is an estimate of the total variability of the heart rate over the full 24 hours.

Measures of high-frequency variability (which loosely correlates with vagal activity). A number of different measures can be used, of which the easiest to understand is the NN50 measure, which is the number of normal sinus beats that are more than 50 ms shorter or longer than the immediately preceding beat. A measure of the same index, which has greater statistical reliability, is the RMSSD, the square root of the mean squared differences in successive RR intervals (ie the average modulus of the difference between successive beats).

Other measures of heart rate variability

There are a plethora of means of measuring the variability of the heart rate, in addition to the ones mentioned above. They fall into two broad categories.

Time domain methods. Here the normal-to-normal (NN) sinus beat intervals are measured and then differences between succeeding beats analysed. Common analyses include looking at the absolute interval between beats for variation. The modulus of the difference is one common measure, as is the standard deviation of the NN intervals, or the standard deviation of the 5-minute average NN interval. Alternatively, the NN intervals can be plotted out as a histogram and analyses made of the shape found, often a triangle (the so-called 'triangularity index').

Frequency domain methods. These fit RR intervals into a number of spectral patterns using complex mathematical processing algorithms. Nonparametric analysis (eg fast Fourier transform) is the most reliable of the geometric methods, it has a quick processing speed and (as it uses few assumptions) is less prone to error than the 'autoregressive' method (Figure 12.9c). Autoregressive power spectral analysis is an extraordinarily complex mathematical parametric technique, which, although it can produce highly accurate results in very controlled situations (such as in the research laboratory), is very prone to generating artefactual and thus meaningless data. It has the advantage over nonparametric methods that meaningful data can be obtained from shorter recordings. Furthermore, it produces visually more appealing results (Figure 12.9b)!

All frequency domain analyses identify various frequencies of spectral components, varying according to whether the recording is made over a short or long time period.

In recordings made over 2–5 minutes, three components are identified: very low-frequency (VLF; 0.003–0.04 Hz), low-frequency (LF; 0.04–0.15 Hz) and high-frequency (HF; 0.15–0.4 Hz). LF and HF spectral components vary according to changes in autonomic tone. The HF component is interpreted as relating to vagal outflow and the LF component is interpreted as relating to sympathetic outflow. The meaning of the VLF component is much less clear and is therefore usually removed from subsequent analysis. The units of these spectral components are ms^2, although the LF and HF components may be normalized to the total HF and LF spectral power. If spectral analysis is carried out over 24 hours then, in addition to VLF, LF and HF components, an additional ultralow-frequency component can be identified, the meaning of which, like that of the VLF component, is unclear.

Causes of low heart rate variability

For reasons that are not entirely clear, decreases in vagal outflow and increases in sympathetic outflow (seen as a low HRV) commonly occur with:

- aging
- physical deconditioning (conversely physical reconditioning is a very powerful means of reversing an adverse sympathovagal balance, whether or not cardiac disease is present)
- post MI: the stronger the vagal outflow is prior to an MI, the lower is the chance of a dangerous/lethal ventricular arrhythmia complicating the infarct
- heart failure
- other factors can also have a substantial influence on sympathovagal balance, eg (unknown) genetic factors.

Consequences of low heart rate variability

The above conditions result in adverse changes in sympathovagal balance, that is, increased sympathetic and decreased vagal outflow both to the heart and to the peripheral arterioles. These changes are fairly strongly associated with an increased cardiovascular risk, mainly due to an increased risk of dangerous ventricular arrhythmias. Not only does a low vagal tone/high sympathetic tone (an adverse sympathovagal balance) promote ventricular arrhythmias, but manoeuvres that enhance vagal outflow and lessen sympathetic tone (a beneficial sympathovagal balance) also protect against such ventricular arrhythmias. The reasons for this are not entirely clear. However, whatever the reasons, a high vagal/low sympathetic tone is regarded as a good sympathovagal balance, whereas the reverse is regarded as bad.

Methods to increase heart rate variability

What improves sympathovagal balance? Certain drugs beneficially alter sympathovagal balance, predictably from their actions. Drugs that lessen sympathetic outflow improve sympathovagal balance; angiotensin-converting enzyme inhibitors, angiotensin receptor blockers (ARBs), β-blockers and low-dose scopolamine (perhaps paradoxically, as it is a muscarinic antagonist) all enhance vagal outflow. Physical fitness has a very strong influence on sympathovagal balance, and increasing physical fitness, regardless of whether or not there is any underlying heart disease, improves sympathovagal balance.

Chapter 13
Provocative electrophysiological studies

Although it is often possible to diagnose and treat (suspected) arrhythmias from 'observational' ECGs obtained noninvasively, this is not always the case. Often in this situation it is reasonable to make a presumptive diagnosis of the cause of the arrhythmia on the basis of symptoms and demographics and then proceed 'empirically' by adopting a 'wait-and-see' strategy. However, sometimes the clinical situation suggests that a 'dangerous' arrhythmia (either a high-grade ventricular arrhythmia or episodic high-grade heart block) may be responsible, and a correct diagnosis may be life-saving. In such a situation it is reasonable to go to considerable lengths to establish the correct diagnosis.

'Alarm' features suggestive of dangerous arrhythmias

The presence of structural heart disease [eg following myocardial infarction (MI), heart failure or hypertensive heart disease], especially if associated with excess ventricular ectopy on a 24-hour ECG, particularly (although not exclusively) if complex ventricular arrhythmias are seen [eg couplets, triplets or nonsustained ventricular tachycardia (VT)] suggests that VT may underlie symptoms, such as new-onset palpitations or pre-syncope. In this situation provocative and/or invasive studies may be used to establish the diagnosis, or at least, if negative, may provide greater reassurance than noninvasive studies.

Stokes–Adams attacks in the elderly (see p. 162); along with evidence of conducting tissue disease on the ECG, suggest that episodic heart block may be responsible. Many clinicians, faced with such a strong possibility that intermittent high-grade atrioventricular (AV) block (eg complete heart block) underlies symptoms, will empirically implant a pacemaker rather than undertaking complex and possibly only poorly predictive investigations. Occasionally, however, it is reasonable to measure the efficacy of the conducting tissue directly and exclude VT, using invasive studies. This is particularly true if symptoms occur following an MI.

Another 'alarm' signal would be an ECG showing Wolff–Parkinson–White (WPW) syndrome or a genetically determined pro-arrhythmic condition.

Types of provocative studies

Provocative studies vary greatly in their complexity:

Exercise testing is appropriate if symptoms are effort-dependent (see Chapter 11). If syncopal ventricular arrhythmias are being considered then an advanced cardiac life support (ACLS)-trained physician should supervise the test. Consideration should be given to inserting an intravenous cannula prior to exercise, in case antiarrhythmic medication needs to be given quickly.

Tilt-table testing, a 'circulatory stress test', has its main role in evaluating patients who are felt to be syncopal or near-syncopal due to a disorder in the control of the circulation. There are a large number of such disorders, the nomenclature of which is confusing. However, traditionally they are felt to include any condition in which the blood pressure falls unacceptably and reflexly from a low heart rate and/or from peripheral vasodilatation (see p. 153).

Carotid sinus massage involves determining the strength of the carotid sinus reflex noninvasively (see below). Carotid sinus hypersensitivity syndrome underlies some cases of 'collapse', especially syncope in the elderly. It responds moderately well (certainly better than neurocardiogenic syncope) to pacing.

Invasive electrophysiologic studies may be appropriate if there is a high probability of a ventricular arrhythmia, eg if patients experience symptoms post MI for the first time, or if noninvasive studies suggest that an accessory pathway is responsible for symptoms.

Tilt-table testing

Tilt-table testing is used in the investigation of vasomotor syncope and is best regarded as a form of 'circulatory stress test'. In vasomotor syncope the control of the circulation is periodically inappropriate. The aim with the tilt-table test is therefore to stress the circulation to determine how well the circulatory control systems respond. Patients are placed in a quiet darkened room, and 'strapped' to a table initially in the horizontal position, which then moves progressively towards the vertical using an electric motor. Heart rate and blood pressure are measured continuously on a beat-to-beat basis (see Figure 8.3).

There are several possible responses to tilt-table testing:

- Normal: the patient is asymptomatic, and heart rate and blood pressure both increase a little with head-upright tilting.
- Cardioinhibitory: the heart rate slows down, and ≥3 second asystole occurs during which the patient develops (pre-) syncope. After the heart rate slows down, the blood pressure falls away.
- Vasodepressor: the blood pressure falls away dramatically (≥50 mmHg fall), although the heart rate remains fairly constant or only drops marginally. As the blood pressure falls, the patient develops typical symptoms.
- Mixed cardioinhibitory and vasodepressor: blood pressure and heart rate fall away simultaneously as symptoms occur.
- 'Cerebral' neurocardiogenic syncope: a very rare finding, in which patients have typical symptoms, but no abnormality of heart rate or blood pressure. This has been interpreted as being due to cerebral hypoxia, a consequence of problems in the regulation of cerebral blood flow due to abnormalities intrinsic to the cerebral circulation.

If a 'standard' tilt-table test as described above is negative then some authorities recommend that drugs be given to increase the level of circulatory stress, eg intravenous glyceryl trinitrate or isoprenaline. This approach increases the number of both true and false positives.

There are some advantages to tilt-table testing; first, to prove the diagnosis. Thus a typical history, with symptoms replicated along with a blood pressure fall during tilt-table testing, is diagnostic in many, and highly suggestive in others, of 'vasomotor' or 'neurocardiogenic' syncope. However, one should be aware that (for the reasons listed below) a 'false-positive' tilt-table test can coexist with more serious causes of syncope. Accordingly, do not be guided by the tilt-table test alone – consider the results along with the clinical situation.

Tilt-table testing can also be used to guide therapy, and in particular to determine if patients might respond to a pacemaker ('pure' bradycardic neurocardiogenic syncope responds to pacing, there is no response at all in the 'pure' vasodilator form of neurocardiogenic syncope, and a partial response occurs in the mixed cardioinhibitory/vasodilator form of the syndrome).

There are a number of problems with tilt-table testing. It is very difficult to produce 'standardized' results, so the 'hit' rate (ie genuine positive rate) varies greatly between different cardiology units. There are high false-negative and false-positive rates. In other words, the tilt-table test can be completely normal in those with 'clear-cut' neurocardiogenic syncope, and abnormal in those 'clearly' without neurocardiogenic syncope. The reproducibility is low: patients with a positive test one day may have, in the absence of any treatment or resolution of symptoms, a negative test the next day. Positive testing is a poor predictor of benefit from any particular treatment.

These problems with tilt-table testing mean that many clinicians reach a diagnosis of vasomotor syncope on the clinical features alone and either prescribe no treatment or 'empirical' therapy (ie not tilt-table testing-guided), for example β-blockers or selective serotonin reuptake inhibitors.

Carotid sinus massage

Carotid sinus massage assesses the power of the carotid sinus reflex. In some patients, especially the elderly, the brain misinterprets day-to-day pressures on the carotid artery baroreceptors as being due to arterial hypertension. 'Overtight' neck collars, turning the head, etc, may generate such neck pressures. Messages are then sent out (often via the vagal nerve) to lower the blood pressure, by either slowing the heart rate, vasodilating the circulation, or both. The blood pressure falls to such an extent that faintness or actual syncope occurs.

Prior to the test, high-grade carotid narrowings are excluded using the clinical history (no strokes or transient ischaemic attacks) and by auscultating the carotid arteries (a bruit is present in about 50% of patients with high-grade stenosis). Patients are 'wired-up' to an ECG machine that has a paper printout (hard copy recording of the data is vital). Blood pressure is measured, preferably continuously using a beat-to-beat device (eg Finapress or similar). The carotid arteries are then firmly massaged, one at a time, at the level of the cricoid cartilage (Figure 13.1). A diagnostic test is held to be one that leads to symptoms of presyncope, or frank syncope, along with a fall in systolic BP >50 mmHg or asystole >3 seconds. Symptoms with lesser changes than these may be accepted as evidence of some degree of carotid reflex hypersensitivity. The treatment for bradycardic/asystolic carotid hypersensitivity syndrome is a pacemaker.

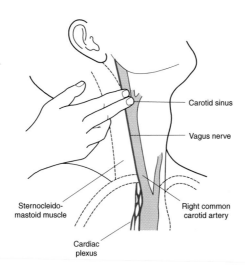

Figure 13.1
Carotid sinus massage. The carotid artery is massaged for 3–5 seconds at the level of the cricoid cartilage, after excluding carotid disease. Reprinted with permission from Sandøe E, Sigurd B. *Arrhythmia Diagnosis and Management: A Clinical Electrocardiographic Guide*. St Gallen: Fachmed.

Electrophysiological studies

Electrophysiological studies (EPSs) involve passing electrodes into the heart and stimulating it to provoke an arrhythmia. In addition, conduction times can be measured, which if prolonged may predispose to bradyarrhythmias.

The most common forms of EPS are described below.

Ventricular stimulation studies

The patient is sedated and an arterial line inserted. A single electrode is inserted transvenously into the apex of the right ventricle, and then first one, then two, and finally three sequential extrasystoles are introduced (the Wellens protocol; Table 13.1), close to the refractory period of the preceding beat, at varying heart rates (normal sinus rhythm, and pacing at a heart rate of 100, 120 and 140 bpm). The earlier sustained monomorphic VT occurs, the more likely it is to be clinically relevant. The less well tolerated the arrhythmia is haemodynamically, the greater danger the patient is in of experiencing sudden cardiac death in the community, and thus the lower is the threshold for implanting an implantable cardioversion defibrillator. Perhaps paradoxically, ventricular fibrillation, particularly if it occurs at a high level of the Wellens protocol, may be a 'nonspecific' response of the heart to electrical stimulation and not of great predictive value.

Table 13.1 The Wellens protocol

Stage	Rhythm	Heart rate	Number of VPCs
1	Sinus	Spontaneous	1
2	Sinus	Spontaneous	2
3	V paced	100	1
4	V paced	100	2
5	V paced	120	1
6	V paced	120	2
7	V paced	140	1
8	V paced	140	2
9	Sinus	Spontaneous	3
10	V paced	100	1
11	V paced	120	2
12	V paced	140	3

VPC, ventricular premature contraction; V, ventricular.
Reprinted with permission from Wellens HJJ, Brugada P, Stevenson WG. Programmed electrical stimulation of the heart in patients with life-threatening ventricular arrhythmias. What is the significance of induced arrhythmias, and what is the correct stimulation protocol? *Circulation* 1985; **72**: 1–7

Invasive measurement of conducting tissue efficacy

To perform this investigation an electrode is inserted into the venous system, to lie along the atrioventricular node and the bundle of His. The AH and HV conduction times are measured, and evidence of conducting tissue disease sought (see Figure 9.4b). Prolonged intra-Hissian conduction times are associated with episodic symptomatic AV block.

Full electrophysiological study

To perform a full EPS multiple electrodes are inserted, via the venous system, into the right side of the heart. One electrode is placed in the right atrium, another along the bundle of His, a third in the coronary sinus and a fourth in the right ventricle. Conduction times can be measured (AH and HV intervals). During a full supraventricular study atrial extrasystoles are introduced using the atrial electrode and conduction times lower down are measured. Dual AV nodal pathways (capable of sustaining AV nodal reentrant tachycardia) can be detected in this fashion, as can more remote AV accessory pathways.

Ablation

Energy, in the form of radiofrequency current, can be passed down the electrode to 'coagulate' the immediately adjacent tissue and so kill it. In due course, the dead tissue will be replaced by scar tissue. The common reasons for wishing to 'kill' parts of the heart are to:

'Ablate' an accessory pathway in WPW syndrome. This can be either when the WPW syndrome is causing frequent symptomatic supraventricular tachycardias or if the side-effects of the drugs needed to suppress such arrhythmias are considered unacceptable by the patient. An additional reason to ablate the pathway is when invasive studies have demonstrated that the pathway is capable of transmitting atrial impulses down to the ventricle at a very fast rate (ie the WPW pathway is very 'slick'). If the patient were to go into AF (and the WPW syndrome itself is associated with an increased chance of AF of about 25%) then the heart rate could exceed 250 bpm. Such high heart rates in AF are dangerous as they compromise cardiac filling and so can reduce cardiac output and provoke sudden cardiac death (SCD). All those with WPW should have the conducting potential of their accessory pathway determined, and if a 'slick' pathway is found, unless there is other comorbid disease, the pathway should be ablated to prevent SCD.

'Ablate' the pathway underlying atrial flutter. Most forms of atrial flutter are due to a continuous circuit movement within the right atrium. Most atrial flutter can be adequately treated pharmacologically – and in particular the heart rate at rest and during exercise can be controlled. However, this is not true for all patients, and furthermore some suffer unacceptable side-effects with the drugs. These patients can benefit from ablation of the atrial flutter circuit, a relatively minor procedure given advances in catheter technology.

Modify conduction through the AV node. AV nodal reentrant tachycardia is a common, benign disorder, usually controlled by vagotonic manoeuvres or drugs. Sometimes drugs are only partially effective or cause unacceptable side-effects. In this situation one may wish to consider removing the substrate for the arrhythmia. Usually the substrate is a second pathway contained within the AV node – this pathway can be removed, so-called 'slow pathway modification'. This is quite an effective procedure, with low risks, the major one being that in modifying the slow pathway the normal AV node is totally ablated, resulting in iatrogenic complete heart block and the need for a permanent pacemaker.

AV nodal ablation. There are two indications for completely ablating the AV node. First, when AF occurs – either with an unacceptably high heart rate despite drugs or if (despite adequate heart rate control) the patient is symptomatic from the irregular nature of the heartbeat. In either of these situations the AV node can be permanently ablated; a permanent pacemaker is then implanted (VVI-R for established AF, 'mode-switching' for paroxysmal AF). Second, other unacceptable atrial tachyarrhythmias (eg atrial tachycardia, especially if associated with a 'rate-related' cardiomyopathy, or atrial flutter with inadequate heart rate control) are rare but standard indications for AV node ablation with pacemaker implantation.

Interventional therapies to prevent AF. There are two approaches. First, some AF is related to an 'automatic' focus near the pulmonary veins. This can be ablated, removing the drive to AF. Unfortunately in many patients, despite ablation of one focus, all the atrial tissue near the pulmonary veins appear to have the potential to become 'irritable' and so underlie further episodes of AF. What tends to happen is that following pulmonary vein focus ablation patients are symptom-free for a while, possibly 12–18 months, until a new focus develops. This treatment is therefore still regarded as experimental. A second experimental approach to AF involves trying to remove the atrial reentry substrate for AF. The 'old' approach to this involved open-heart surgery and cutting the atria into seven or more pieces, each one not large enough to sustain reentry. In effect, this created a 'maze' of passages within the atria (Figure 13.2). Some investigators feel that they can do this percutaneously, by 'burning' multiple areas within the left and right atria, the so-called 'percutaneous maze' procedure. Unfortunately this is still not a dramatically effective procedure, and AF recurrence rates remain high.

Ablation of a VT focus. This is an unusual, although increasingly frequent, form of interventional EP therapy. Some patients who have VT are found to have a 'focus', usually somewhere within the septum of the left ventricle.

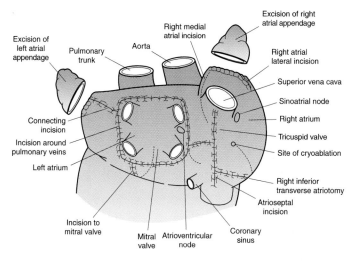

Figure 13.2

'Maze' procedure. The multiple reentrant waves found in atrial fibrillation need a large atrium to be self-sustaining. If the atria are too small, the reentrant wave will return to the start of the circuit to find the atria still refractory, and the wave will extinguish. This explains why atrial fibrillation is an uncommon arrhythmia in small mammals (eg mice) and is also rare in children. One way to reduce the substrate for reentrant circuits in adult humans is to make multiple incisions in the atria, which heal by forming electrically inert scar tissue, as in the 'open' surgical approach illustrated here. Another is the still experimental percutaneous approach. Reprinted with permission from Crawford MH, DiMarco JP. *Cardiology*. London: Mosby, 2001.

This can be identified, often by 'pace-mapping', ie moving the electrode around in the ventricle. When the paced complexes look the same as those found during an episode of spontaneous VT, the focus has been identified and can then be destroyed ('ablated').

Chapter 14

The ECG in hypertension

In those with hypertension ECGs are useful to guide prognosis, estimate LV mass and follow response to treatment.

Hypertensive patients with a normal ECG have the best prognosis; those with ECG evidence of left ventricular hypertrophy (LVH) have an intermediate outlook; and those with LVH and 'strain' (lateral lead ST changes) have the worst outlook.

Prolonged and/or severe hypertension increases LV mass. Electro-cardiographic LVH (see p. 34) bears some relation to actual LV mass but the relationship is not as good as is popularly believed. If the ECG is normal, many patients can still have significant increases in echocardiographic LV mass. If patients have ECG evidence of LVH (especially if this is associated with 'lateral lead ST changes') then they almost certainly have substantial echocardiographic LVH. Thus an abnormal ECG is very likely to reflect substantial LVH, whereas a normal ECG does not exclude significant LVH.

If LVH is present then an important objective of treatment is to ensure that this regresses. The ECG has some use in following LVH regression; diminution of LV voltages and normalization of ST changes are associated with an improved prognosis. However, the ECG is not as sensitive to regression of LVH as the cardiac ultrasound, and neither is as sensitive as cardiac magnetic resonance imaging.

Problems with the exercise ECG in hypertension

Hypertension can lead to a number of traps for the unwary when it comes to interpreting the exercise ECG, as effort can lead, in the presence of LVH and in the absence of coronary artery disease (CAD), to substantial ST segment changes, particularly ST segment depression. Thus when patients with hypertension are being evaluated for possible ischaemic heart disease (IHD) it can often be very difficult to know if exercise-induced ST segment changes relate to the LVH by itself or to CAD. There is no easy way past this issue, as the ST segment changes can be morphologically identical. This problem can be resolved by performing a cardiac ultrasound. If no LVH is present then the ECG changes are more likely to be due to CAD. If LVH is present then the situation is still unclear, and may require either:

- nuclear isotope imaging of the myocardium during an exercise test
- coronary angiography.

Which approach is best depends on the clinical situation and on the patient's preferences. However, if symptoms are atypical then exercise isotope imaging is often best, whereas if symptoms are typical for angina then coronary angiography is often best. Factor into this decision what the exercise capacity is like: a good effort capacity usually equates to a good prognosis, whereas a poor effort capacity usually implies a worse outlook and identifies patients who would probably benefit from a more invasive approach.

The ECG in hypercholesterolaemia

Hypercholesterolaemia is a powerful risk factor for the development of atheromatous CAD. However, before overt angiographically visible atheroma develops, endothelial dysfunction occurs. The normal endothelium reacts to increased blood flow by releasing a variety of vasodilators, particularly nitric oxide. This mechanism allows exercise to vasodilate the coronary arteries, which increases coronary blood flow, allowing for the increased metabolic needs of the exercising heart. If the mechanisms underlying exercise-induced coronary vasodilatation are damaged then exercise can result in an inadequate blood supply to meet the metabolic needs of the heart, with resultant myocardial ischaemia and ST segment depression during the exercise ECG. Thus a patient with hypercholesterolaemia can demonstrate ST depression on an exercise test in the absence of conventional angiographically 'fixed' flow-limiting atheromatous CAD. A corollary of this is that when the hypercholesterolaemia is vigorously treated endothelial function can improve and exercise-induced ST depression can disappear.

Thus endothelial dysfunction in hypercholesterolaemia can lead to diagnostic problems if the exercise ECG is being undertaken to determine whether or not flow-limiting atheromatous CAD is present. The key question then arises: how can one determine the meaning of ST segment depression found during an exercise test in a hypercholestrolaemic individual? The standard rules apply: the higher the pretest likelihood of CAD, the more likely it is that any ST segment depression found relates to CAD. Thus the more CAD risk factors present, and the more profound they are, the greater the chance of CAD. The presence of typical angina substantially increases the chance of finding epicardial CAD (Figure 14.1). If doubt remains this can be clarified in the standard manner. If the chance of coronary disease being present is low (atypical symptoms with few CAD risk factors) then a myocardial perfusion scan may well be appropriate, whereas if the chance of major CAD being present is high (limiting symptoms of typical angina, with multiple CAD risk factors) then angiography may be the best approach.

The ECG in electrolyte disturbance

Hypokalaemia

This is a common clinical finding, and can have a number of ECG manifestations (Figure 14.2), including:

Asymptomatic flattening of the ST segment and T wave. This is the most common finding. The differential diagnosis of flat ST/T segments is given on p. 71, and includes anxiety, hyperventilation, any myocardial disease process (especially that due to IHD), and any old pericardial disease process.

Increase in arrhythmia incidence. The K^+ level influences the frequency of many different arrhythmias, especially ventricular premature contractions (VPCs) and ventricular tachycardia (VT)/ventricular fibrillation (VF). This is true in the chronic phase of many diseases, especially IHD but is particularly the case during acute coronary syndromes, where the incidence of acute myocardial infarct (MI)-related VF relates rather strongly to the level of K^+.

Long QT intervals in those with heart failure. Low levels of K^+ promote QT interval lengthening and, conversely, K^+ supplementation leads to QT interval shortening.

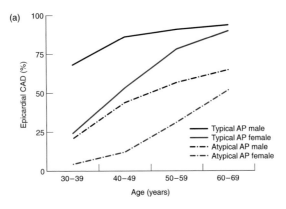

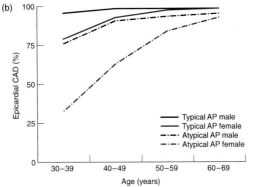

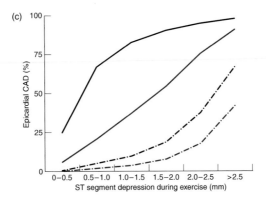

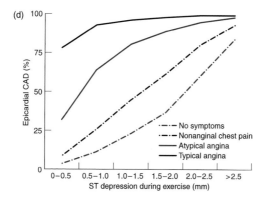

Figure 14.1

Relationship between nature of chest pain and presence of epicardial coronary artery disease (CAD). (a) Patients with 0.5–1 mm ST segment depression during exercise. (b) Patients with 2–2.5 mm ST segment depression during exercise. Probability of CAD depends on age and the typicality or otherwise of the symptoms for angina. Graphs (c), men aged 30–39 years, and (d), men aged 60–69 years, show that the extent of ST depression, in addition to age, determines the probability of CAD. Reprinted with permission from Diamond GA, Forrester JS. Analysis of probability as an aid in the clinical diagnosis of coronary artery disease. *N Engl J Med* 1979; **300**: 1350–8.

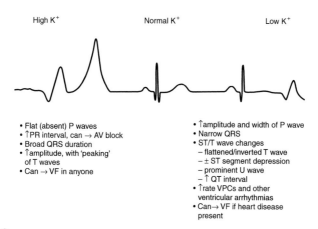

Figure 14.2

The influence of K^+ on the ECG. VF, ventricular fibrillation; VPC, ventricular premature contraction.

Hyperkalaemia

This is a rather rare electrolyte abnormality. Progressive increases in K^+ level lead to:

- decrease in the P wave amplitude, and eventually the disappearance of the P wave
- progressive broadening of the QRS complex
- increase in the height of the T wave.

The latter two lead to the QRS/T complex taking on a 'saw tooth' appearance. This is an ominous sign because VF/asystole is likely to follow soon after. The patient who experiences a hyperkalaemia-related ventricular arrhythmia usually cannot be resuscitated until the potassium level has been brought down – something that is almost impossible to do once cardiac arrest has occurred. In other words, unless the cardiac arrest occurs when the patient with hyperkalaemia is connected to a haemodialysis machine, the patient will almost invariably die. Thus if a 'saw tooth' ECG is seen, dialysis (and medical treatment for hyperkalaemia, for example insulin/glucose infusion or calcium resonium) should be commenced immediately.

Hyponatraemia and hypernatraemia

Surprisingly, these two conditions have no particular ECG features in the vast majority of affected individuals.

Hypocalcaemia and hypercalcaemia

Hypocalcaemia has the same ECG appearances as hyperventilation, with flat ST/T waves together with QT interval lengthening. If extreme, hypocalcaemia can lead to cardiac arrest. Unsurprisingly, QT interval shortening is found in hypercalcaemia.

The ECG in endocrine disease

Hyperthyroidism

Hyperthyroidism can have many ECG manifestations:

Sinus tachycardia. This is the commonest and most reliable sign of thyrotoxicosis. It not only gives a good clue to the diagnosis but also allows the effectiveness of treatment to be easily determined. Thyrotoxicosis causes a sinus tachycardia not only during the day, but also during sleep; this fact can help differentiate it from the daytime-only sinus tachycardia caused by an 'appreciation of sinus tachycardia'.

Atrial fibrillation (AF) is a particularly common complication of thyrotoxicosis, especially in older women who smoke (Figure 14.3). Interestingly, patients with apparent 'lone' AF have increased free thyroxine levels and lower thyroid-stimulating hormone levels (although both are still within the normal range). In other words, unsurprisingly, increased physiological levels of thyroxine increase the tendency towards AF.

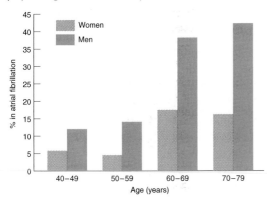

Figure 14.3
Risk factors for atrial fibrillation in thyrotoxicosis. This figure shows the proportion of people with thyrotoxicosis who have atrial fibrillation. Age and sex are powerful factors influencing whether or not an individual with thyrotoxicosis develops atrial fibrillation. Reprinted with permission from Kumar PJ, Clark ML. *Clinical Medicine.* Philadelphia: WB Saunders.

Diffuse and widespread ST/T wave flattening. Although these findings can occur in the absence of a thyroid–heart disease, their presence increases the chance of finding a dilated heart with impaired LV systolic contractile function, so-called thyrotoxic cardiomyopathy.

Increased QRS amplitude, which may reflect a thinner chest wall, but which may also be due to a direct effect of thyroxine on myocyte cell function.

QT interval shortening in those with hypercontractile hearts; QT interval lengthening develops once thyrotoxicosis-induced LV dysfunction has occurred.

Hypothyroidism

This condition has several effects on the ECG (Figure 14.4), including:

- *sinus bradycardia,* in part proportional to the severity of the thyroxine deficit

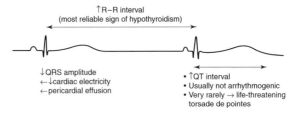

↑R−R interval
(most reliable sign of hypothyroidism)

↓QRS amplitude
← ↓cardiac electricity
← pericardial effusion

• ↑QT interval
• Usually not arrhythmogenic
• Very rarely → life-threatening
  torsade de pointes

Figure 14.4
Effects of hypothyroidism on the ECG; a sinus bradycardia is the most consistent finding.

- *decreased QRS amplitude,* partly due to thyroid hormone deficit decreasing intrinsically the amount of electricity the myocytes produce – partly as thyroxine deficit leads to a laying down of mucinous tissue within the heart (myxoedema), which interferes with current propagation, and partly as hypothyroidism leads to pericardial effusions, which also interfere with the transmission of current from the heart to the detecting electrodes
- *prolongation of the QT interval.* Unlike many other causes of QT interval prolongation, the QT interval prolongation due to hypothyroidism is not (with very few exceptions) arrhythmogenic. Very occasionally a patient does develop profound recurrent ventricular arrhythmias related to the hypothyroidism-induced long QT interval. The only long-term successful treatment for this is thyroxine replacement therapy.

Diabetes mellitus

The ECG has the same usefulness in diabetics as in nondiabetics. However, the situation is different for the exercise ECG in the diagnosis and risk-stratification of diabetic patients. This is because in diabetics who have had an MI the death rate is so frighteningly high (overall death rate is approximately 50% at three years) that, rather than using the exercise test as a filter for who should or should not have an angiogram, coronary angiography is probably mandated for all post-MI diabetic patients as the best means of risk-stratification. However, as knowledge of exercise capacity and effort-induced symptoms is useful in deciding what to do with the results of the angiogram, an exercise test should probably still be carried out.

Furthermore, the risk of coronary disease is so high in type 2 (non-insulin-dependent) diabetics from the time of diagnosis, and in type 1 (obligate insulin requirement) diabetics after 15–20 years of treatment that the false-negative rate for an exercise ECG is quite high, rendering the test less useful.

However, on the contrary, diabetics have substantial endothelial dysfunction. This means that even in the absence of flow-limiting coronary lesions, many diabetics will have a 'depressed coronary flow reserve' and so ST segment depression during exercise. Thus in diabetic patients with suspected CAD the exercise ECG will generate a significant number of false-positive tests (certainly false-positive in the sense that these patients do not have flow-limiting CAD, although perhaps not in the sense that those with substantial endothelial dysfunction are those most likely to experience adverse complications over the subsequent months and years).

These facts render the exercise ECG in those with diabetes of less value than in most patients, although the exercise test itself remains a useful means by which to quantify exercise capacity. Accordingly clinical features should usually guide investigation and treatment; there should be an extraordinarily low threshold for performing angiography. If angiography is not acceptable then other forms of risk stratification should be used, such as stress cardiac ultrasound, or exercise or stress nuclear isotope imaging.

Adrenal disease

Hyperadrenalism, if associated with hypertension (for example, Cushing or Conn syndrome) will over time result in LVH. Chronic hypoadrenalism (ie Addison's disease) can lead to small QRS complexes. In an Addisonian crisis, sinus tachycardia also occurs.

The ECG in stroke

There are several reasons to look at the ECG in someone with a stroke: First, the ECG may give some clues to the stroke aetiology (Figure 14.5). Second, a cerebrovascular accident (CVA) can be a marker for more extensive vascular disease, and the ECG may give some clues as to whether or not this is indeed the case. Most patients who survive their index admission with a CVA eventually die of another vascular event, often an MI. Third, the CVA itself can affect the ECG.

ECG clues to cause of stroke

Acute or recent MI: MI is complicated by stroke in about 1% of cases due to the embolization of a ventricular mural thrombus. Thrombolytic treatment

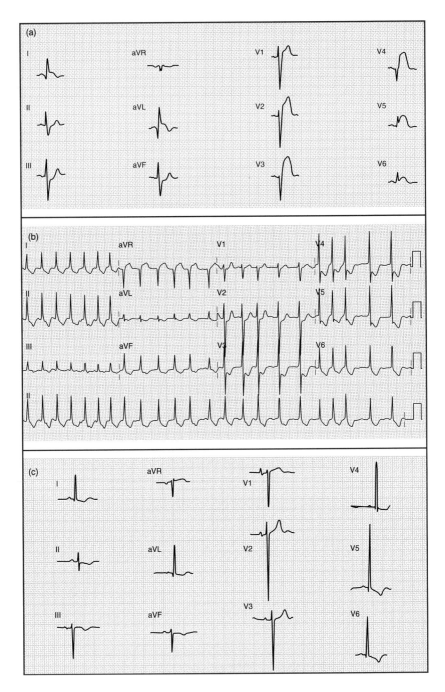

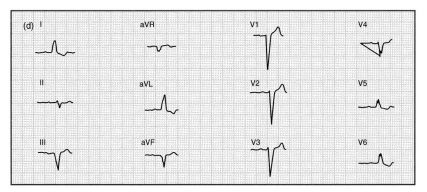

Figure 14.5
Causes of stroke that may be apparent on an ECG. (a) Acute anterior wall myocardial infarction. MI can be complicated by stroke in about 1% of cases, either from embolization from mural thrombus, or intracranial haemorrhage, a consequence of thrombolytic therapy. (b) Atrial fibrillation with a modestly slow ventricular response. There are widespread but nonspecific ST segment changes. This man had a dilated cardiomyopathy. (c) Gross left ventricular hypertrophy. This could relate to aortic valve disease, to cardiomyopathy, or, as in this case, to severe hypertension, a potent risk factor for stroke. (d) Left bundle branch block (LBBB), which can be caused by a large variety of disease processes, including heart muscle disease, ischaemic heart disease, end-stage hypertension and aortic valve disease. In addition, sarcoidosis may be responsible. Many of these can have neurological consequences. In this case a dilated cardiomyopathy resulted in LBBB and a cerebrovascular accident.

decreases the incidence of embolic strokes (which cause the vast majority of MI-related strokes) but increases the chance of haemorrhagic stroke.

LVH may be present in long-standing hypertension, which itself is a potent risk factor for both embolic and haemorrhagic stroke.

Q waves or a *diffusely abnormal ECG* may be a clue to an ischaemic or dilated cardiomyopathy, both of which predispose to stroke.

AF is a potent factor underlying some strokes, particularly in patients over 65 years and/or in those with structural heart disease.

ECG consequences of a stroke

Although stroke is widely reported as causing ECG abnormalities, it is important to realize that most reports relate to subarachnoid haemorrhage. Blood in the subarachnoid space is extremely irritant and provokes a large catecholamine surge, which results in vasoconstriction to

309

the subendocardial coronary arteries and so subendocardial myocardial ischaemia. This is seen as abnormalities in the ST/T wave. How great an abnormality occurs is directly related to how great the catecholamine surge is: T wave flattening occurs with mild 'surges', and frank pan-anterior deep symmetrical T wave inversion (of a pattern suggestive of a 'proximal LAD lesion') occurs with more substantial catecholamine release. Coincident with this latter ECG abnormality, LV function can be depressed, usually transiently. Thus, in the setting of a significant sub-arachnoid bleed, even major ST segment changes can be accepted as being the consequence of the bleed. Those with more profound ECG changes have a worse outlook due to adverse neurological events rather than adverse cardiac complications.

The situation is, however, quite different for the much more common ischaemic parenchymal stroke. Here the catecholamine surge is much less, or indeed nonexistent. No (or few) ECG changes should therefore be expected. Thus, if significant ECG changes are seen (Q waves, significant ST segment or T wave changes), it raises the possibility that the stroke is a consequence of a (recent) MI, which may have been silent. This of course has therapeutic implications, as the usual mechanism is that LV mural thrombus has complicated the infarct, some of which has broken away to cause an embolic CVA. The patient is at quite significant risk of having further thrombi break away and therefore further embolic CVAs. The patient should consequently be anticoagulated the moment it is safe to do so (ie the moment it is felt that the risk of bleeding into the brain infarct is sufficiently low).

The ECG in pneumonia

The more severe the pneumonia the more catecholamines are released and the more likely the ECG is to change. However, even in the most severe pneumonia it is still unusual to find major ECG abnormalities – if they are present they are likely to be a clue that there is also underlying heart disease. Despite this, there are two important ECG consequences of pneumonia:

Atrial fibrillation

The catecholamine surge with pneumonia makes AF more likely – indeed this is a marker of severity in pneumonia. Hence those with AF complicating their pneumonia have more severe infection and are more likely to die.

Myocardial infarction

Pneumonia results in an increase in acute phase reactants, including prothrombotic proteins, for several weeks. These are probably the cause of the threefold increase in the incidence of acute MI in the first few weeks following pneumonia.

The ECG in the elderly

Although, as discussed elsewhere in this book, the ECG can have great use in diagnosis, this is particularly true for those ≤80 years of age. The diagnostic usefulness of the ECG in the elderly (particularly those ≥80 years) is less than in the young, because many elderly patients have coincidental cardiac disease, not relevant to their presenting symptoms but sufficient to change the ECG (Figure 14.6). Furthermore, the ECG in the elderly may also not change in the typical fashion with various disease processes, especially in LVH and MI (see below).

In elderly patients it is particularly important to ensure that all the data (see below) corroborates the prime diagnosis. Inconsistencies should always be carefully explored, and, as a generalization, if the history and ECG do not correlate with each other then the ECG diagnosis should be rejected, or at the very least seriously questioned.

When taking the clinical history bear in mind that many elderly patients can have very vague symptoms. Likewise, the clinical signs can be very subtle and other investigations may have greater limitations in the elderly. For example, diastolic heart failure is especially prevalent in the elderly, where it may account for 20–40% of all heart failure. The cardiac ultrasound, at least in routine clinical practice, is really very poor at reliably detecting diastolic failure. Thus in the setting of a breathless elderly patient, a near-normal ultrasound can be quite falsely reassuring in excluding heart failure.

Presence of ECG changes in the elderly

Changes in the ECG that may not be of great relevance in this age group include:

- minor ST segment changes, especially flattening
- conducting tissue disease (eg right or left bundle branch block), especially if the PR interval is normal in the absence of any symptoms suggestive of

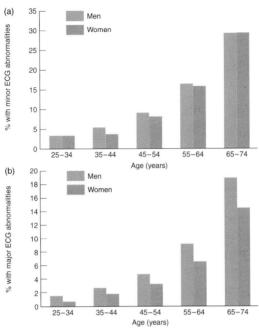

Figure 14.6
Incidence of (a) minor and (b) major ECG changes relates to age. Major ECG abnormalities are classified as (1) ST segment depression, (2) T wave inversion, (3) 2nd- or 3rd-degree heart block, (4) complete left or right bundle branch block, (5) frequent VPCs and (6) atrial fibrillation or flutter. Minor ECG abnormalities are (1) borderline Q waves, (2) left or right axis deviation, (3) QRS high voltage, (4) borderline ST segment depression, (5) T wave flattening and (6) QRS low voltage. Over the whole age spectrum, major ECG changes are associated with an 80% increase in total mortality whereas minor ECG changes have no impact on mortality. Reproduced with permission from De Bacquer D, De Backer G, Kornitzer M. *Heart* 2000; **84**: 625–33.

high-grade atrioventricular (AV) block. Furthermore, conducting tissue disease is less likely to be associated with clinically significant myocardial pathology than in a younger age group. Clearly in the presence of presyncope or Stokes–Adams attacks the finding of conducting tissue disease can be highly relevant

- many 'low-grade' arrhythmias in the absence of symptoms, eg atrial or ventricular extrasystoles.

Changes that are likely to be as relevant in the elderly as in the young include:

- Q waves

- LVH – if ECG evidence of LVH is found then it is very likely to be present; the converse, however, does not apply
- sustained arrhythmias, eg AF.

Absence of ECG changes in the elderly

The absence of ECG changes is also a less reliable guide to the absence of cardiac disease than in the young.

Left ventricular hypertrophy

Substantial LVH can be present in the elderly with no or minor ECG changes. This has significant implications for the management of many conditions, but especially of aortic stenosis. This valve lesion is very common in the elderly, where it may not infrequently underlie heart failure. One clue to the presence of symptomatic aortic stenosis in a younger population is the finding of an aortic systolic murmur with electrocardiographic LVH. Systolic aortic murmurs without ECG evidence of LVH are rarely associated with significant aortic stenosis in the young: this is not true in the elderly population, where for unknown reasons substantial LVH can occur while the ECG remains normal or near-normal. Thus if significant aortic stenosis is a possible diagnosis, and if the clinical signs have been unreliable, then the only way to rule this out is by performing a cardiac ultrasound examination.

Myocardial infarction

Here the changes can be very mild, even if the infarct is large. Furthermore, as ECG changes are very common in this population, these background changes can mask any changes due to new pathology. Finally, and most unfortunately, symptoms can also be quite atypical or even absent. Indeed up to one-third of MIs in this age range are silent, ie patients experience no chest pain (or certainly none severe enough to report to a physician or a hospital). There is no reliable way past this problem, other than to always have a high level of clinical suspicion for IHD and its complications in the elderly.

The ECG in confusion

An acute confusional state is an extraordinarily common cause for emergency hospital admission. There is a vast array of potential diagnoses, but the commonest are:

Acute septic illness and mild (+) pre-existing cognitive impairment (ie dementia) – typically a urinary tract infection, although chest infections are also common. The ECG in cognitive impairment is described below.

Severe sepsis (including pneumonia, meningitis) – this usually causes a sinus tachycardia, and often rather nonspecific ST segment changes.

Biochemical derangement – most commonly hyponatraemia, also deranged diabetes (eg diabetic ketoacidosis or hyperosmolar nonketotic coma). These often cause no specific ECG changes.

MI occasionally presents as an 'acute confusional state'. This can be a difficult diagnosis to make as chest pain may often not be commented on by the patient and the ECG changes may be minor and easily confused with the 'background' changes found in the elderly. Troponin assays have to some extent helped establish this diagnosis.

The ECG in falls

Falls are common. Often they are caused by simple trips or musculoskeletal problems, but they can relate to syncopal episodes. Interestingly, older patients recall only about 50% of witnessed syncopal episodes – thus it is always important to have a high index of suspicion that falls relate to unremembered syncope. The resting ECG may give a clue that the patient is prone to bradyarrhythmias (extensive conducting tissue disease, evidence of sinus node disease) or tachyarrhythmias (old Q wave MI, very frequent VPCs or nonsustained VT on a 24-hour ECG). One should have a low threshold for undertaking a 24-hour ECG, although this is remarkably unproductive in diagnosing many causes. If falls are frequent and do not clearly relate to some alternative pathology (dementia, postural instability or hypotension, musculoskeletal problems, etc) then one should go to some lengths to document an ECG during an attack, by external or internal loop recording.

The ECG in neurological disease

Many neurological conditions are associated with cardiac disease:

Duchenne muscular dystrophy

This condition is strongly associated with cardiomyopathy, and indeed many if not most patients with Duchenne muscular dystrophy die from such cardiac involvement. The commonest ECG manifestations are a dominant R wave in leads V1 and V2 (this probably reflects the fact that Duchenne muscular dystrophy does not affect the heart globally; rather there is a regional basis to the fibrosis, and it is particularly severe in the posterior wall) and a 'pseudo-infarction' pattern, with Q waves, especially in the anterior or lateral leads.

Freidrich's ataxia

This is another disorder commonly associated with a dominant R wave in V1 as well as the pseudoinfarction pattern described above. In addition, up to one-third of patients have a form of hypertrophic cardiomyopathy.

Myotonic dystrophy

Myotonic dystrophy is the commonest inherited neuromuscular disease in adults. It is due to CTG trinucleotide repeats on chromosome 19q13.3. It often affects the conducting tissue, so various forms of heart block are common, including both PR interval prolongation and right or left bundle branch block. Sudden cardiac death, in part relating to high-grade AV block, is not infrequent in myotonic dystrophy, and may be more common in those with a PR interval ≥240 ms. Pacemakers are useful to prevent such bradyarrhythmias. Unfortunately, it is increasingly recognized that ventricular tachyarrhythmias may also underlie sudden cardiac death in some affected individuals but their accurate prediction is difficult. Once found, they should probably be treated with an implantable cardioverter defibrillator.

Neurodegenerative conditions

Parkinson's disease and multiple sclerosis are the most common neuro-degenerative conditions. They do not have specific cardiac manifestations, and thus the ECG will only reflect coincidental comorbid disease. Some Parkinson's disease is vascular in origin, and has rather little in the way of tremor but marked bradykinisia, especially of the lower limbs. These patients often have rather extensive vascular disease and this can be reflected in the ECG: loss of R wave height, Q waves and T wave changes are all common.

Dementia

There are many causes of dementia: Alzheimer's disease, Pick's disease, prion disease, etc. However, one of the most common causes is 'multi-infarct' dementia, wherein the brain experiences multiple small infarcts, which add up to produce cognitive loss. In this condition the ECG may show evidence of a predisposing cardiac pathology:

- atrial fibrillation
- Q wave or loss of R wave height, reflecting an old MI
- LVH, reflecting long-standing and severe hypertension, and so generally rather extensive vascular disease
- ST/T wave changes, reflecting a cardiomyopathy, which in turn has been the source of central nervous system emboli.

The ECG in vasculitis

There are several different sorts of ECG changes (Table 14.1) that can occur in vasculitis.

Acute MI is a rare but dangerous complication of systemic lupus erythematosus (SLE) and polyarteritis nodosum (PAN).

Table 14.1 ECG findings in vasculitis

ECG finding	Interpretation	Disease
Normal	Does not exclude cardiac involvement in many vasculitides	Any
'Concave-up' anterolateral ST segment elevation	Pericarditis	SLE, RA
'Concave-down' ST segment elevation	Myocardial infarction	SLE Kawasaki disease (from coronary artery aneurysms)
Prominent LV voltages, ± lateral ST segment changes	LV hypertrophy	SLE (with renal disease), scleroderma (with renal failure-related hypertension) Polyarteritis nodosum (renal hypertension)
Dominant R wave in lead V1	RV hypertrophy	Scleroderma lung disease
Low QRS voltages	Myocardial fibrosis	Scleroderma
PR interval prolongation, second mothers or third degree heart block pregnancy	Conducting tissue disease	Common in children from with active SLE during Rheumatic fever Polymyositis, dermatomyositis, ankylosing spondylitis
Arrhythmias	Atrial or myocardial involvement	Found in many vasculitis illnesses, though not common.

SLE, Systemic lupus erythematosus; RA, rheumatoid arthritis.

ECG changes of pericarditis are common in SLE as well as in rheumatoid arthritis (in the latter it is usually asymptomatic).

Congenital complete heart block occurs in about 20% of children born to women who have active SLE during the pregnancy.

Heart block, especially PR interval prolongation (but also right or left bundle branch block), is a common manifestation of acute rheumatic fever. Other manifestations include nonspecific ST segment changes and arrhythmias, especially atrial arrhythmias.

LVH is common in any vasculitis complicated by renal disease, especially scleroderma, but also SLE and PAN.

The ECG in preoperative assessment

Operative risk depends on many factors, including the presence of:

- severe aortic stenosis (peak gradient ≥50 mmHg, or valve area ≤ 1 cm²)
- a rhythm other than sinus. AF and excess VPCs both significantly increase operative risk. Untreated AV block has a major adverse impact on outcome
- severe angina (Canadian class III or IV)
- recent MI (within six months). The presence of Q waves on the ECG substantially increases risk
- heart failure, especially if there has been recent pulmonary oedema (within one week) or some other form of decompensation
- comorbid disease, especially respiratory or renal failure. Diabetes has a lesser adverse impact
- coronary artery disease: severity should be assessed
- a poor functional state, (but the presence of cardiac and comorbid disease is perhaps more important)
- a need for emergency surgery: this increases the risk, especially in the elderly (≥70 years)
- a high-risk procedure: aortic and peripheral vascular surgery, and any operation involving major blood loss. Intermediate-risk surgery includes carotid, head and neck, intraabdominal or thoracic, orthopaedic, or prostate surgery. Low-risk surgery includes endoscopic procedures, superficial operations, and cataract and breast surgery.

Some US studies have suggested that the most important preoperative risk factors are Q waves on the ECG, history of angina, history of VPCs requiring treatment, diabetes mellitus, other than diet-controlled, and age ≥70 years. It has been suggested that:

- those with three or more of these risk factors are at very high risk of an adverse cardiac complication, and should have coronary angiography performed preoperatively
- those with one or two risk factors should have preoperative stress tests, which if positive should lead to coronary angiography
- those with no risk factors (suggesting low risk) have no need for preoperative coronary studies.

(It should be noted that treating VPCs was common in the 1980s when this study was undertaken. Symptomatic VPCs were probably a marker for symptomatic LV dysfunction. This aspect of the data is probably not relevant nowadays.)

From the above list it can be seen that much preoperative risk stratification depends on the history, the physical examination, and the resting ECG.

Drugs and the ECG

Drugs can have multiple effects on the ECG, and it is always wise when interpreting the ECG to question whether or not an abnormality could relate to a drug.

Drugs and arrhythmia

Sinus bradycardia can relate to β-blockers, some Ca^{2+} channel blockers and amiodarone. Clearly, if sinus bradycardia relates to β-blockers or Ca^{2+} channel blocker usage, it will reverse rapidly once the drug is discontinued. Amiodarone can lead to a profound and long-lasting bradycardia, due to its long half-life of around 20–30 days.

Sinus tachycardia can relate to drugs that enhance sympathetic outflow, such as tricyclic antidepressants when taken in overdose. The withdrawal of β-blockers can lead to a reflex sinus tachycardia (cardiac β-receptors are upregulated by long-term β-blocker therapy and sudden withdrawal leads to unopposed β-adrenergic stimulation of these upregulated receptors). Sinus tachycardia in patients on amiodarone can relate to amiodarone-induced thyrotoxicosis (a not infrequent side-effect of amiodarone therapy).

Atrial extrasystoles and ventricular extrasystoles can relate to many drugs, including any that deplete the body of potassium, including diuretics, and especially to psychoactive agents taken in overdose.

There are several drugs that may cause atrial fibrillation. The best described are those that cause AF in overdose. These include tricyclic antidepressants, antipsychotic drugs, and some of the drugs with so-called antiarrhythmic action (especially class I agents). Thyroxine if taken in high dosage can lead to AF. Digoxin in overdose can provoke many different atrial arrhythmias, but especially atrial tachycardia.

Ventricular tachycardia (VT) can relate to an adverse drug reaction. There are several classes of drugs that are particularly powerful provokers of VT. These include the antiarrhythmic drugs (all classes, but especially class I, which are particularly good in provoking VT in those with structural heart disease) and those drugs that prolong the QT interval (see below), which can provoke ventricular arrhythmias in those without any structural heart disease. An example of the latter is the macrolide antibiotics, especially erythromycin, which can lead to QT interval prolongation and torsade de pointes-type polymorphic VT

Drug and conducting tissue abnormalities

Long PR interval can relate to drugs that interfere with the autonomic supply to the heart. β-blockers can clearly slow AV conduction, as can vagotonic drugs.

Bundle branch block may relate to amiodarone.

High-grade AV block, such as type II heart block or complete heart block, can be provoked by drugs that slow AV conduction time (eg β-blockers, Ca^{2+} channel blockers, amiodarone), but usually only in those with pre-existing and severe conducting tissue disease. Clearly, stopping the drugs provoking the episode of AV block is helpful, but although this may well lead to apparently 'normal' AV conduction on the surface 12-lead ECG, it is usually held that the disease already affecting the AV conduction system is so severe as to justify a permanent pacemaker. The combination of verapamil and a β-blocker, especially if given intravenously, can by itself lead to heart block, which can proceed to fatal asystole.

Drugs and QRST abnormalities

Q waves are almost always pathological and are unlikely to relate to an adverse reaction to a drug. Occasionally, however, drugs do provoke MI and so can produce Q waves (see below).

Mild ST segment and T wave changes may relate to many drugs, including the tricyclic antidepressants, antipsychotics and drugs with class I antiarrhythmic action. Drugs that deplete the body of potassium, such as the loop diuretics, can lead to ST segment flattening via hypokalaemia. Digoxin has an interesting and dose-dependent effect on the ST segment and T wave – mainly it leads to ST segment flattening, and 'reverse tick' T wave inversion.

ST segment elevation can occur if a drug has provoked:

- MI – possible with cocaine and amphetamine-type drugs
- pericarditis – a number of drugs can provoke 'serositis' as a side-effect. These include minocycline, and drugs that can induce SLE such as hydralazine and procainamide. Thus drugs must be included in the differential diagnosis of chest pain, especially if central and pleuritic in nature.

QT interval prolongation not infrequently relates to drugs, again particularly the antipsychotic drugs, macrolide antibiotics such as erythromycin, as well as both amiodarone and the β-blocker sotalol. This is important, as arrhythmogenic QT interval prolongation is an under-diagnosed condition; in many cases it relates to a combination of cardiac disease and drug adverse reaction. Drug reactions must therefore always be considered in the differential diagnosis of syncope, particularly in the elderly, who are commonly prescribed multiple different drugs.

Drugs that commonly affect the ECG

Digoxin has multiple effects on the ECG. It can lead to ST segment flattening and frequently to T wave inversion of the so-called 'reverse-tick' form. The reasons for this are obscure. In those with heart failure digoxin leads to shortening of the prolonged QT interval. It can interfere with the interpretation of the exercise test, in that even if ST segment depression or T wave inversion have not occurred on the resting ECG, digoxin may cause them to appear on the exercise ECG even in the absence of coronary disease. Thus exercise-induced ST/T wave changes in patients taking digoxin should be interpreted with great caution. Digoxin in overdose leads to malaise, nausea, vomiting, confusion and xanthopsia (lights appear yellow). Any atrial or ventricular arrhythmia can occur, especially atrial tachycardia (often with two- or three-to-one block) and ventricular arrhythmias. The diagnosis is confirmed by measuring blood levels; toxicity is more likely when hypokalaemia is also present.

Class I antiarrhythmics can lead to QRS broadening (often not detectable clinically) and QT interval lengthening.

Tricyclic antidepressants can have profound effects on the manner in which the heart generates and transmits electrical impulses. These effects are particularly marked in overdose, where they lead to a sinus tachycardia, hypotension, any supra- or indeed ventricular arrhythmia (so the patient should be monitored until the overdose wears off), QT interval lengthening, and nonspecific ST/T flattening or frank depression. The diagnosis is confirmed from the history and clinical signs.

Antipsychotic drugs can lead to QT interval prolongation (which may underlie ventricular arrhythmias) as well as ST/T wave changes. The QT prolonging effect and ventricular pro-arrhythmogenesis is probably at least in part responsible for the excess in sudden cardiac death seen with these drugs.

Amiodarone, particularly in those on long-term chronic therapy, can lead to sinus bradycardia, including frank and rather profound sinus node disease, AV block and, almost universally, prolongation of the QT interval. Amiodarone is held not to affect the ST/T wave, and not to alter the normal response of this segment of the ECG to exercise. In other words, the exercise ECG retains its utility. Sotalol, another class III antiarrhythmic, also leads to QT interval lengthening.

β-blockers, obviously, result in a sinus bradycardia, which largely determines their therapeutic efficacy. They also tend to lengthen the QT interval at low heart rates, and shorten it at high heart rates.

Some Ca^{2+} *channel blockers* also lead to a sinus bradycardia, especially verapamil and diltiazem, although they have no marked effect on the QT interval.

Macrolide antibiotics, particularly erythromycin, can lead to prolongation of the QT interval, and this can underlie life-threatening episodes of VT, both in those with underlying heart disease and, perhaps much more worryingly, in those without. For this reason, anyone taking a macrolide antibiotic (or any other drug known to prolong the QT interval) who has a syncopal episode should be treated as having a life-threatening illness and immediately admitted to a monitored bed in hospital.

Non-sedating antihistamines, particularly terfenadine, can lead to QT interval prolongation and, in a similar fashion to erythromycin, to life-threatening ventricular arrhythmias of the torsade de pointes variety.

Chapter 15
Pacemakers and the ECG

Pacemakers are designed to prevent and/or treat brady- and tachycardias.

Bradycardias – these are the indication for ≥98% of UK pacemaker implants. In essence, the pacemaker counts the number of P/R waves and if they are insufficient, stimulates the heart to beat. The technology required is easy, widely disseminated and cheap.

Tachycardias – these are an increasingly common reason for pacemaker implantation. The pacemaker counts the number of P/R waves, and if there are too many, the pacemaker terminates the arrhythmia, either by pacing fast or by internally defibrillating the heart. The technology required for this is complex, not widely available and expensive. Despite this, antitachycardic pacemakers are set to become increasingly common.

Key functions of pacemakers

Given the above roles, all pacemakers must be able to recognize cardiac activity and respond to it appropriately. Pacemakers do this by detecting atrial or ventricular electrical activity (ie either P or R waves), counting their frequency and reacting appropriately. Thus the key functions of a pacemaker are:

- sensing of electrical activity
- determination of the correct response – the generator circuitry does this
- pacing of the heart.

Components of a pacemaker system

A permanent pacemaker comprises a generator and one or two electrodes.

The generator usually occupies a small pocket in the left pectoral fossa, just above the pectoral muscle (Figure 15.1). The generator consists of a long-lasting battery (usually lithium-based and with a lifespan of about 10 years) and electronic circuitry that allows incoming electrical activity to be counted and an appropriate response to be determined, and, by passing electrical charge down the electrode, paces the heart.

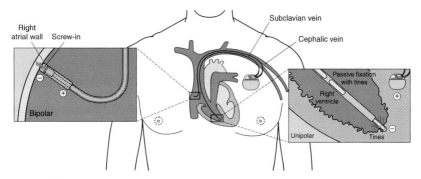

Figure 15.1
The key components of a permanent pacing system. A permanent pacemaker is shown with attached electrodes. Electrodes can either be implanted into the heart passively and held in position by plastic hooks (by far the commonest approach) or be actively 'screwed' into the heart (as here). Screwing, or 'active fixation', is useful for some atrial electrodes (which have a relatively high rate of displacement), especially if the atrial appendage has been removed (most commonly following cardiopulmonary bypass). 'Active' fixation is also useful for right ventricular electrodes in those who have substantial tricuspid regurgitation, as this tends to 'spit' the electrode out of the right ventricle.

The electrodes are used both to detect cardiac electrical activity and to pace the heart. There are two forms of electrodes (Figure 15.2): unipolar and bipolar. Unipolar electrodes are cheap, reliable and effective. They have the disadvantage that their current circuit uses the pectoral muscle, so failure to pace can occur if pectoral muscle activity is misinterpreted as heart activity. Bipolar electrodes are expensive and much more prone to failure (especially atrial ones). However, they reliably sense the heart (not the pectoral muscle), so inappropriate failure to pace does not occur. The pacing artefacts (the spike of current made by the generator) is much larger with unipolar than bipolar electrodes – so much so that occasionally the bipolar pacing artefact may not be seen.

Nomenclature of pacemakers

There is an international standard for classifying pacemakers (Table 15.1):

- The first letter refers to the chamber paced.
- The second letter refers to the chamber sensed.
- The third letter refers to the response of the pacemaker to the detection of a signal.

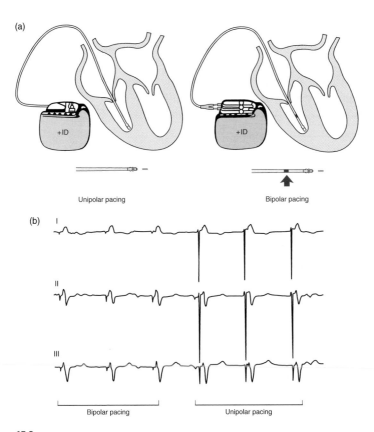

Figure 15.2
(a) Different forms of electrodes. In a unipolar electrode the current passes out of the generator, along the electrode and out into the heart. The circuit is completed with the current passing through the heart into the extracardiac tissue, and so back into the generator through the indifferent electrode in the generator casing. In a bipolar electrode the current passes out of the generator, along the electrode, out of the distal tip, along the cardiac tissues and back into the indifferent electrode situated a few centimetres back from the tip. Reprinted with permission from Sandøe E, Sigurd B. *Arrhythmia Diagnosis and Management: A Clinical Electrocardiographic Guide.* St Gallen: Fachmed. (b) Uni- versus bipolar pacing. The pacing artefact is much larger with uni- than with bipolar pacing.

- The fourth letter refers to special attributes of the pacemaker, particularly whether or not there is a 'sensor' of some description that detects activity and increases the pacing rate.
- The fifth letter (not widely used) refers to the antitachycardic functions of the pacemaker.

Table 15.1 International classification for pacemakers

Letter	Refers to	Code	Meaning
1st	Chamber paced	A	Atrium
		V	Ventricle
		D	Dual (both chambers)
2nd	Chamber sensed	A	Atrium
		V	Ventricle
		D	Dual
		O	None
3rd	Response to sensing	I	Inhibited
		T	Triggered
		D	Dual (inhibited or triggered)
		O	None
4th	Programmability, rate modulation	P	Simple program
		M	Multiprogram
		C	Communicating
		R	Rate-responsive pacemaker
5th	Antitachycardic functions	P	Pacing of tachycardias
		S	Shock delivered
		D	Dual (pacing and shock)
		O	None

There are special pacemakers that 'defy' this classification system: atrial defibrillators, ventricular defibrillators [usually termed 'implantable cardioverter defibrillators' (ICDs)], and anti-heart failure pacemakers – so-called resynchronization therapy, or multi-site pacing that uses multiple electrodes, one in the right atrium, one in the right ventricle and one (via the great cardiac vein) in the left ventricle.

Common pacing modalities

AOO or VOO

No modern pacemaker has this as a permanent function, although pacemakers manufactured in the 1950s and 60s did. The disadvantage of VOO pacing is that electricity can be delivered to the heart during its 'vulnerable' period (ie around and just after repolarization), when it may trigger ventricular fibrillation. For this reason it is not a desirable modality for long-term pacing. However, this pacing mode is still widely used when checking whether a pacemaker is working correctly. To activate the AOO, VOO or DOO function, a magnet is placed over the generator, which temporarily turns off all the sensing functions of the pacemaker (for as long as the magnet remains over the generator). With the magnet applied, the pacemaker obligatorily paces the heart at a set rate, usually around 70 bpm, regardless of whether or not there is any spontaneous electrical cardiac activity. This allows one to check whether the pacing function of the pacemaker is working, and also often to check the threshold (Figure 15.3). The way threshold-checking works is that (when the AOO or VOO mode is triggered) some pacemakers automatically decrease their output by a set amount with each successive paced beat – by knowing the output of the pacemaker with each beat, and from seeing when the pacemaker fails to capture the heart, the threshold can be deduced. Knowledge of the threshold is used to set the pacemaker output to the right level (see below).

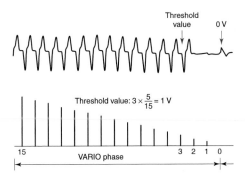

Figure 15.3
Scheme of VOO pacing used to check the threshold. The pacemaker is activated to start pacing at full output, and then to decrease this in 15 equal steps to an output of 0 V. The threshold can be determined from knowledge of the pacing output when the ventricle fails to capture. Reprinted with permission from Lindgren A, Jansson S. *Heart Physiology and Stimulation: An Introduction.* Sweden: Siemens-Elema ab Solna, 1992.

VVI-R

This is probably the commonest form of pacing system; a single electrode is sited in the right ventricle so only ventricular electrical activity is detected and only the ventricle is paced – all atrial activity is ignored (Figure 15.4). When right ventricular activity occurs, the pacemaker remains silent (ie is inhibited); when no activity is detected, the ventricle is paced.

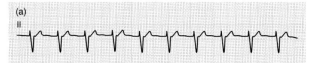

(a)

II

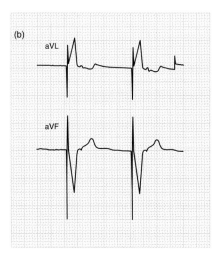

(b)

aVL

aVF

Figure 15.4
(a) VVI pacing: the pacing spike is followed by a broad QRS beat. Interestingly the P wave occurs just after every QRS complex. This is due to retrograde activation of the atria from the ventricles. This is further shown in (b). This is an unusual finding: most patients with intact atrioventricular tracts do not need ventricular pacing – atrial pacing is often sufficient. Retrograde P wave activation can lead to hypotension (partly due to excess atrial natriuretic peptide release – so-called 'pacemaker syndrome').

AAI-R

A single electrode is sited in the right atrium, allowing detection and pacing of the atrium only (Figure 15.5). This pacemaker is indicated for sinus node disease and some atrial arrhythmias – it is contraindicated if there is any evidence of coexisting atrioventricular (AV) block, when a DDD system is required.

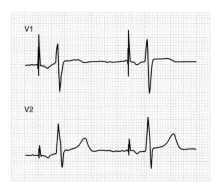

Figure 15.5
AAI pacing; the pacing artefact is seen, followed by a low-voltage P wave. Then, after the PR interval, a narrow QRS complex is seen.

DDD-R

Here there are two electrodes within the heart; one in the right atrium and one in the right ventricle (Figure 15.6). If electrical activity is detected in both chambers then the pacemaker is inhibited. If activity is only detected in the atrium then the P wave triggers (after an appropriate delay) pacing of the ventricle. If the atrium is silent then it is paced, as is the ventricle if an R wave does not spontaneously follow the P wave after an appropriate interval. As the pacemaker can be both triggered and inhibited, in the pacemaker classification system the third letter is D, standing for dual response.

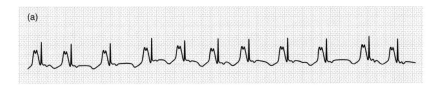

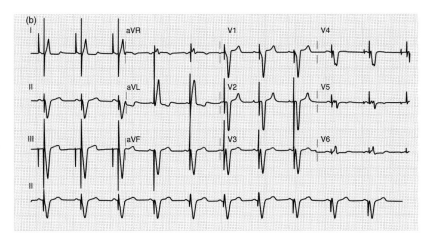

Figure 15.6
DDD pacing. (a) Atrial tracking: the P wave is normal but is following by a paced ventricular beat. The pacing 'spike' is clearly seen. (b) In this ECG both the atrium and the ventricle are paced – this is the case as both the P wave and the QRS complex are preceded by a pacing 'spike' in many of the beats.

Implantable cardiac defibrillators

These devices are increasingly commonly used. They detect sustained ventricular arrhythmias (eg ventricular tachycardia and ventricular fibrillation) and then treat them either by overdrive pacing – the preferable modality as it is does not drain the battery of power – or by internally defibrillating the heart (energy-expensive; most ICDs contain only 50–200 DC shocks). The indications are increasing all the time – currently ICDs are used for prevention of dangerous recurrences of symptomatic ventricular arrhythmias that are not preventable with more standard cardiological treatments and for prophylaxis in those who are at high risk of dangerous ventricular arrhythmias. The system consists of a sophisticated electrode, which is implanted into the apex of the right ventricle (RV). The 'shocking' poles are usually between the electrode at the RV apex, and a 'plate' contained within the electrode and sited in the superior vena cava (SVC). Often the system also has an atrial electrode so that antibradycardic DDD pacing can also occur. The most sophisticated pacemakers include antitachycardic functions (overdrive pacing and shocking therapy), antibradycardic functions and resynchronization therapy (multisite pacing).

Rate-responsive pacemakers

Although the cardiac output of the normal heart is surprisingly constant over a wide range of heart rates at rest, due to the Frank–Starling 'law of the heart', many patients with heart disease do benefit from pacing the heart faster during exercise. To do this, a pacemaker must be able to recognize exercise and then increase the pacing rate, and equally, recognize rest so that the pacing rate can be lowered. The common ways by which pacemakers detect physical activity include:

Motion detectors

If motion is detected (often using piezoelectric crystals) then the pacemaker interprets this as physical activity, and increases the pacing rate.

QT interval measurement

The QT interval shortens on physical activity regardless of whether or not the heart rate increases (Figure 15.7). This is because sympathetic activation and vagal withdrawal, which both occur on exercise, both shorten the duration of the action potential and hence shorten the QT interval. Thus a shortening of the QT interval can be used as an indirect measure of whether or not physical activity is taking place. The QT interval is measured from the electrogram obtained from the RV electrode.

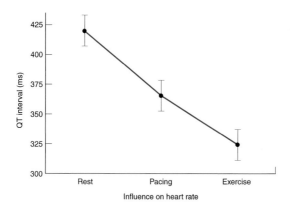

Figure 15.7

QT interval shortening during exercise. The data presented here show subjects who had dual chamber pacemakers. In 'pacing' the heart rate was increased to 110 bpm by turning up the pacing rate. In 'exercise', subjects exercised to obtain a heart rate of 110 bpm. The pacing-induced changes in QT interval are due to the effects of changing heart rate alone, whereas the exercise changes in QT interval relate not only to the change in heart rate, but also to the autonomic changes induced by exercise (vagal withdrawal and sympathetic stimulation, both of which shorten the QT interval). These data therefore show that about two-thirds of the QT interval shortening of exercise is due to heart rate, and about one-third is due to the effects of exercise. Reprinted with permission from Davey P, Bateman J. *Clin Cardiol* 1999; **22**: 513–18.

Temperature measurement

Exercise increases the body core temperature. Thus if a rise in temperature is detected from a temperature probe sited within the electrode, the generator increases the pacing rate.

Lung electrical impedance

During exercise people breathe more deeply and frequently. This alters the electrical impedance between the inside of the heart and the outside of the thorax, ie between the electrode tip and the generator. This can be used to detect activity and so to increase the pacing rate.

There is no entirely ideal way of detecting exercise. Probably the 'best' method is that using motion detectors.

Recognition by the pacemaker of cardiac electrical activity

Both antibradycardic and antitachycardic pacemakers make use of the same basic mechanism to detect the electrical activity of the heart. An electrode is situated in the cardiac chamber of interest (usually the right atrium and/or ventricle). When the atria or ventricle depolarize, a wave of electricity passes through the chamber, up through the electrode and into the generator, where it is detected. The size of the voltage detected by an intracardiac electrode varies between the different chambers: the normal atrium develops about 2–5 mV of electricity; the normal ventricle develops about 8–16 mV.

Pacemaker output

The generator circuit counts the number of P/R waves in a prespecified time period, and reacts according to how it has been programmed. For antibradycardic pacemakers this means that if the electrical activity falls below a programmed level, the heart is paced at a rate of 40–90 bpm.

For antitachycardic pacing the generator is programmed to either 'overdrive' or defibrillate the heart.

Overdrive pacing

The generator will 'overdrive'-pace the heart if the arrhythmia is felt to be a relatively haemodynamically stable form of ventricular tachycardia (VT). This is usually done by determining that VT in that patient is at least moderately haemodynamically stable, ie either spontaneous or electrophysiological study (EPS)-induced VT has been shown to be reasonably well tolerated.

Internal defibrillation

The generator will 'defibrillate' the heart if either overdrive pacing fails or the rhythm is felt to be haemodynamically unstable. This usually means that either the arrhythmia has been shown to be unstable previously (by observing the patient during spontaneous or EPS-induced VT) or it is very fast. The generator battery is used to charge the generator capacitor, and then discharges this charge through the electrode 'shocking' plates. Usually the defibrillation charge is rather small, 4–20 J.

Programming the generator to detect cardiac, not other, electrical activity

When it comes to the generator detecting electrical activity, only current that exceeds a prespecified voltage (the sensitivity of the pacemaker; Figure 15.8) is counted as constituting cardiac electrical activity. Thus if the R wave is, say, 10 mV, and the sensitivity of the pacemaker is set at, say, 8 mV, all those beats in which the R wave exceeds 8 mV will be counted. If a heartbeat generates an R wave of 7 mV then it will not be counted. As there will be a variability in the size of the R waves, particularly in those from ventricular premature contractions (which are smaller than average), setting the

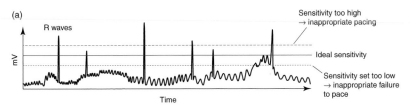

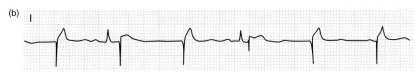

Figure 15.8
(a) Pacing sensitivity. 1–4 mV. The sensitivity can be programmed into the generator system. The level at which it is set is determined mainly by the size of the R wave at implantation – the larger the R wave, the higher the sensitivity can be set, to avoid inappropriately detecting nonrelevant electrical activity. Conversely, the lower the R wave, the lower the sensitivity needs to be set, with the risk that nonrelevant noncardiac electrical activity will be detected. (b) Failure to sense. In this rhythm strip the second paced beat falls on the T wave of a naturally occurring beat, which has not been sensed by the pacemaker. Failure to sense may relate to setting the sensitivity too high, or to electrode failure, or to scar tissue occurring around the electrode tip, interfering with flow of electricity into the electrode.

sensitivity far below the R wave found at the time of implantation allows all the heartbeats to be detected and so counted. Thus one wishes to set the sensitivity as low as possible, so that all cardiac electrical activity is appropriately detected, but not so low that nonrelevant activity is picked up (see below).

Conversely, if the sensitivity of the pacemaker is set too low then the pacemaker may inadvertently pick up nonrelevant electrical activity. The most important nonrelevant electrical signal that a pacemaker might pick up (particularly a unipolar system – see electrode types above) comes from the pectoral muscle. Typically, the electrical activity of this muscle is around 1–4 mV. Thus if the sensitivity of the pacemaker is set below this then the pacemaker can misinterpret pectoral muscle activity as cardiac activity (eg when an arm is being used). The pacemaker will believe that there is cardiac electrical activity and will not pace the heart. If, in fact, there is no cardiac activity then this failure to pace is inappropriate and the patient may blackout. To prevent this problem, one wishes to set the sensitivity of the pacemaker at a level as high as possible above nonrelevant electrical activity, but below that of the P or R wave.

To set the sensitivity appropriately, one wishes to detect the largest possible P/R wave. For this it is vital that the electrode is positioned, at the time of implantation, where the largest P or R waves are to be found. Acceptable implant values are:

- P waves ≥1.5 mV. Anything over 3 mV is excellent. The P wave sensitivity is usually set to about two-thirds of the implant P wave value.
- R waves ≥5 mV. Any value over 10 mV is excellent. As pectoral muscle activity is ≤4 mV, the R wave sensitivity should preferably be set to ≥4 mV.

Another source of nonrelevant electrical activity is the discharge of a remote cardiac chamber, occurring either spontaneously or as a consequence of pacing a distant chamber. For example, if the R wave is very large or if the current passed down the ventricular electrode is large then current flow from this can sometimes be detected in the atrium. This might prevent the atrial electrode firing, as the pacemaker thinks the atrial chamber is working when in fact it is not. To prevent this particular problem, the pacemaker is programmed to ignore electrical activity in certain parts of the cardiac cycle – these times are known as 'blanking periods'. These periods not only prevent the pacemaker not working when it should not but also help prevent pacemaker-mediated tachycardia (see over).

Cardiac pacing

During pacing a small electric charge is passed from the generator down the electrode and through the electrode tip to the immediately adjacent cardiac tissue. This results in the depolarization of the nearest cells, which triggers the firing of an action potential within these cells. The depolarized cells adjacent to the electrode tip then have an electrotonic depolarizing effect on cells further from the electrode tip, which in turn will trigger action potentials within them. This results in further, more distant electrotonic depolarization, more action potentials and even more distant electrotonic depolarization.

Thus the triggering of action potentials in the area of the heart immediately adjacent to the electrode results in a wave of electricity passing throughout that chamber. If the chamber is the atrium, and AV conduction is intact, then atrial activity spreads down the AV node to activate the whole heart. The cardiac electrical activity triggered in this fashion leads to cardiac mechanical activity.

Threshold

The amount of electricity that the pacemaker passes down the electrode and into the heart can be adjusted. In particular both the duration of the electrical impulse and the voltage can be altered, usually between 0.2 and 2 ms and 2 and 10 V. The output is set so that the charge is large enough for the heart to be reliably activated but small enough for the life of the generator to be prolonged.

These are conflicting aims! How does one estimate what charge is needed? The amount of electricity needed to just stimulate the heart can be found by turning the output of the pacemaker down until the heart only just does not pace, and then back up again so that the heart paces (but only just). This voltage is known as the threshold. Usually, in chronic use, the pacemaker electrical output is set to 50% above the threshold as this has been empirically found to reliably pace the heart during day-to-day usage.

Indications for pacemaker implantation

Bradyarrhythmias

- High-grade AV block, such as type II, or complete heart block are straightforward indications for immediate pacing.

- Sick sinus syndrome if symptoms are present.
- A high suspicion that bradyarrhythmias underlie symptoms is, in the elderly, a reasonable basis for implanting a pacemaker – one will 'be right' in about 50% of cases, which is acceptable, provided that patients have been informed that they have about a 50% chance of losing their symptoms.
- Vasomotor syncope with a predominant bradycardic mechanism.

Tachyarrhythmias

- VT, if the substrate cannot be dealt with using a more conventional approach. There are two pacemaker-based approaches to VT. Some (rather rare) forms of VT are entirely bradycardia-dependent (often long QT interval-dependent torsade-de-pointe type VT); thus if one can remove bradycardias with 100% reliability (which antibradycardic pacing does do) then these forms of VT can be suppressed entirely reliably. The more usual approach is to put in an ICD, which does not suppress VT, but when VT is detected tries to terminate it, either by overdrive pacing or by internal cardioversion.
- Ventricular fibrillation. Again, if the substrate cannot be treated conventionally (eg by revascularization) then ICD implantation is appropriate.
- Atrial fibrillation (AF) is an increasingly common reason for implanting a pacemaker. This may be employed when sick sinus syndrome underlies the AF – then AAI pacing is appropriate suppressive therapy; when pause-dependent atrial ectopics underlie the AF – preventing the atrial ectopics by pacing at a sufficiently high heart rate helps to suppress the AF; or sometimes when AF can be terminated by a 'burst' of atrial pacing. Even more complex algorithms are being developed.

Novel indications

There is now increasing recognition that in many cases of heart failure depolarization is prolonged – seen on the ECG as QRS interval prolongation. The degree of QRS prolongation relates inversely to prognosis. Although QRS prolongation may well reflect the fact that cell-to-cell communication is damaged, and may thus reflect the overall level of cardiac damage, it also allows for 'dyscoordinate' LV contraction. That is, one part of the heart starts contracting well before another, and by the time the latter part of the heart starts to contract, the first part is relaxing. This dyscoordinate contraction removes effective mechanical force from the heart and lowers cardiac output. If all the different areas of the heart can be activated simultaneously then cardiac output can be improved. To do this, electrodes are implanted not only in the right ventricle, but also in one of the branches of the great cardiac vein, allowing simultaneous left ventricular activation. This is 'resynchronization' therapy and has been shown to reduce symptoms, and increase life-expectancy in those with broad QRS complexes and heart failure. There are now some pacemakers available that can resynchronize the heart and can also incorporate an internal defibrillator. These are likely to be used more and more frequently.

Problems with pacemakers

Infection

Pacemaker infection is more common than usually realized (Table 15.2). It can occur early on, within the first month or so, when it relates to microorganism implantation at the time of surgery. To reduce this risk, prophylactic antibiotics are given at the time of surgery. The common infecting pathogens are staphylococci. Unfortunately the only effective treatment is to completely remove the infected system, disinfect the body with systemic antibiotics, then reimplant a totally new system. Usually the infection is rather florid, with systemic signs of sepsis, fever and redness over the generator, and/or a gaping wound. Occasionally the symptoms and signs can be rather subtle.

Table 15.2 Pacemaker infections

	Acute infection	Chronic infection
Time of presentation post-implantation	4 days (range 1–12 days)	25 months (range 1–>120 months)
Impaired immunity (diabetes, renal failure, cancer, etc)	25%	25%
Fever	90%	85%
Pain over generator site	40%	55%
↑ESR/CRP	90%	95%
↑White cell count	50%	65%
TTE abnormalities	5%	30%
TOE abnormalities	90%	95%
Culture-positive	70%	95%
Staphylococcus aureus	50%	15%
Staphylococcus epidermidis	30%	75%
Gram-negative infection	10%	*10%*

ESR, erythrocyte sedimentation rate; CRP, C-reactive protein; TTE, transthoracic echocardiography; TOE, transoesophageal echocardiography.

Later on, infection often relates to a blood-borne pathogen. Any persisting fever in a patient with a permanent pacemaker should be considered as being a pacemaker infection until proved otherwise. The diagnosis is best made from blood culture (and finding a raised erythrocyte sedimentation rate, C-reactive peptide and/or low haemoglobin level). Occasionally the cardiac ultrasound is useful, and shows vegetations on the electrode, usually around the SVC or tricuspid valve. There are many possible pathogens, but again staphylococci are the commonest implicated organisms. Again, the only treatment is to completely remove all the hardware of the old system, decontaminate the body, then reimplant a new system.

Generator failure

Very rarely, generator failure can occur. Perhaps the commonest way for a generator to fail is for the battery to run out. Although patients are seen frequently to determine exactly when this will happen, so that the generator can be replaced prophylactically, the odd patient fails to keep their appointments or moves away without arranging follow-up. Generator failure is recognized by the pacemaker failing completely – it is not possible to pace the heart at all, and on attempted interrogation of the device no meaningful data can be obtained.

Electrode failure

This can occur in a number of ways.

Electrode breakage

The electrode can 'snap', that is, it can break. This usually happens just as the electrode passes under the clavicle. The break in the electrode can cause either permanent failure to pace and sense, or, perhaps more usually, intermittent failure – this can be rather difficult to diagnose. These result in two patterns of abnormality. With a complete breakage the electrode neither detects any cardiac activity nor can pace the heart. Interrogation of the generator reveals that the generator itself is still working. The impedance of the lead, measured noninvasively, is either very or immeasurably high. An incomplete breakage usually causes intermittent failure to capture the ventricle – this can be very hard to diagnose, as when the system is checked all may be working satisfactorily. Sometimes a clue is that the lead impedance is high. The best clue is symptoms of syncope recurring in a pacing-dependent patient known not to have any other cause for syncope. A chest X-ray may show that the lead passes under the clavicle very medially, in the gap between the clavicle and the first rib, where it is often crushed. The treatment is to replace the electrode.

'Exit' block

Scar tissue can form around the electrode just after it makes contact with the heart – this can occur early on, within the first few weeks, when it is known as acute exit block, or it can occur later, usually after the first few months, often not until a year or two has passed, when it is known as chronic exit block. The consequences of exit block are first that more electricity is needed to pace the heart and second that less electricity flows from the heart up the electrode into the generator, so that it is possible for the generator to fail to detect that a heart beat has actually occurred, so that it may pace inappropriately.

Pacemaker-mediated tachycardia

These are nowadays quite rare, but they do still occur. Dual chamber pacemakers, in effect, introduce a bypass tract to the heart. If a ventricular ectopic beat occurs and passes retrogradely up the AV node, it can trigger a P wave and so an atrial beat. This atrial beat will be sensed by the atrial electrode and will lead to a paced ventricular beat after the programmed AV delay. This can again pass retrogradely up the AV node, initiating another atrial beat that will be sensed and therefore trigger yet another ventricular beat: a re-entrant arrhythmia can therefore occur, using the AV path as the retrograde limb and the pacing electrodes as the anterograde limb. Pacemakers are designed to prevent these arrhythmias occurring by having periods when they are unable to sense – so-called 'blanking periods'. In addition, pacemakers can occasionally 'drop' a paced beat if they suspect a pacemaker-mediated tachycardia (PMT) occurred. If a patient presents with a PMT, the application of a magnet (which results in DOO pacing) will break the arrhythmia, as will intravenous adenosine.

Further reading

Bayes De Luna, A. *Clinical Electrocardiography: A Textbook*. Oxford: Blackwell Science, 1993.

Braunwald E, Zipes DB, Libby P. *Heart Disease: A Textbook of Cardiovascular Medicine*. Philadelphia: WB Saunders, 2001.

Crawford MH, DiMarco JP. *Cardiology*. London: Mosby, 2001.

Hampton JR. *100 ECG Problems*. London: Churchill Livingstone, 1997.

Hampton JR. *The ECG Made Easy*. London: Churchill Livingstone, 2003.

Houghton AR, Gray D. *Making sense of the ECG*. London: Hodder Arnold, 2003.

Kaddoura S. *Echo Made Easy*. London: Churchill Livingstone, 2001.

Malik M, Camm AJ. *Dynamic Electrocardiography*. Oxford: Blackwell Publishing, 2004.

Morris F, Edhouse J, Brady W, Camm AJ. *ABC of Clinical Electrocardiography*. London: BMJ Books, 2003.

Sandøe E, Sigurd B. *Arrhythmia Diagnosis and Management: A Clinical Electrocardiographic Guide*. St Gallen: Fachmed, 1984.

Schamroth L, Schamroth C. *An Introduction to Electrocardiography. 7th Edition*. Oxford: Blackwell Science, 1990.

Surawicz B. Knilans TK. *Chou's Electrocardiography in Clinical Practice. 5th edition*. London: WB Saunders, 1996.

Timmis AD, Nathan AW, Sullivan ID. *Essential Cardiology. 3rd Edition*. Oxford: Blackwell Science, 1997.

Wagner GS. *Marriot's Practical Electrocardiology, 10th edn*. Philadelphia: Lippincott, Williams and Wilkins, 2001.

Ward D. *Clinical Electrophysiology of the Heart (Current Topics in Cardiovascular Medicine, Vol 1)*. London: Edward Arnold, 1987.

Zaza A, Rosen MR. *Introduction to Cardiac Electrophysiology*. London: Martin Dunitz, 2000.

Zipes DP, Jali J. *Cardiac Electrophysiology*. London: WB Saunders, 2004.

Index

Page numbers in *italics* refer to information that is shown only in a figure or table.

3